Update in Sepsis

Guest Editor

MITCHELL M. LEVY, MD

CLINICS IN CHEST MEDICINE

www.chestmed.theclinics.com

December 2008 • Volume 29 • Number 4

SAUNDERS an imprint of ELSEVIER, Inc.

W.B. SAUNDERS COMPANY
A Division of Elsevier Inc.

1600 John F. Kennedy Boulevard • Suite 1800 • Philadelphia, Pennsylvania 19103

http://www.theclinics.com

CLINICS IN CHEST MEDICINE Volume 29, Number 4
December 2008 ISSN 0272-5231, ISBN-13: 978-1-4160-6280-6, ISBN-10: 1-4160-6280-7
Editor: Sarah E. Barth

Developmental Editor: Jamie Babbitt

© **2008 Elsevier ■ All rights reserved.**

This journal and the individual contributions contained in it are protected under copyright by Elsevier, and the following terms and conditions apply to their use:

Photocopying
Single photocopies of single articles may be made for personal use as allowed by national copyright laws. Permission of the Publisher and payment of a fee is required for all other photocopying, including multiple or systematic copying, copying for advertising or promotional purposes, resale, and all forms of document delivery. Special rates are available for educational institutions that wish to make photocopies for non-profit educational classroom use. For information on how to seek permission visit www.elsevier.com/permissions or call: (+44) 1865 843830 (UK)/(+1) 215 239 3804 (USA).

Derivative Works
Subscribers may reproduce tables of contents or prepare lists of articles including abstracts for internal circulation within their institutions. Permission of the Publisher is required for resale or distribution outside the institution. Permission of the Publisher is required for all other derivative works, including compilations and translations (please consult www.elsevier.com/permissions).

Electronic Storage or Usage
Permission of the Publisher is required to store or use electronically any material contained in this journal, including any article or part of an article (please consult www.elsevier.com/permissions). Except as outlined above, no part of this publication may be reproduced, stored in a retrieval system or transmitted in any form or by any means, electronic, mechanical, photocopying, recording or otherwise, without prior written permission of the Publisher.

Notice
No responsibility is assumed by the Publisher for any injury and/or damage to persons or property as a matter of products liability, negligence or otherwise, or from any use or operation of any methods, products, instructions or ideas contained in the material herein. Because of rapid advances in the medical sciences, in particular, independent verification of diagnoses and drug dosages should be made.

Although all advertising material is expected to conform to ethical (medical) standards, inclusion in this publication does not constitute a guarantee or endorsement of the quality or value of such product or of the claims made of it by its manufacturer.

Clinics in Chest Medicine (ISSN 0272-5231) is published quarterly by Elsevier Inc., 360 Park Avenue South, New York, NY 10010-1710. Months of issue are March, June, September, and December. Business and Editorial Offices: 1600 John F. Kennedy Blvd., Suite 1800, Philadelphia, PA 19103-2899. Customer Service Office: 11830 Westline Industrial Drive, St. Louis, MO 63146. Periodicals postage paid at New York, NY and additional mailing offices. Subscription prices are $251.00 per year (domestic individuals), $400.00 per year (domestic institutions), $122.00 per year (domestic students/residents), $275.00 per year (Canadian individuals), $491.00 per year (Canadian institutions), $342.00 per year (international individuals) $491.00 per year (international institutions), and $171.00 per year (international and Canadian students/residents). International air speed delivery is included in all Clinics subscription prices. All prices are subject to change without notice. **POSTMASTER:** Send address changes to *Clinics in Chest Medicine,* 11830 Westline Industrial Drive, St. Louis, MO 63146. Customer Service (orders, claims, online, change of address): Elsevier Periodicals Customer Service, 11830 Westline Industrial Drive, St. Louis, MO 63146. Tel: 1-800-654-2452 (U.S. and Canada). Fax: 314-523-5170. E-mail: journalscustomerservice-usa@elsevier.com (for print support); journalsonlinesupport-usa@elsevier.com (for online support).

Reprints. For copies of 100 or more of articles in this publication, please contact the Commercial Reprints Department, Elsevier Inc., 360 Park Avenue South, New York, NY 10010-1710. Tel.: 212-633-3812; Fax: 212-462-1935; E-mail: reprints@elsevier.com.

Clinics in Chest Medicine is covered in *MEDLINE/PubMed (Index Medicus), Current Contents/Clinical Medicine, EMBASE/ Excerpta Medica, Science Citation Index,* and *ISI/BIOMED.*

Printed in the United States of America.

Contributors

GUEST EDITOR

MITCHELL M. LEVY, MD
Professor of Medicine, Division of Pulmonary and Critical Care Medicine, Brown University; Director, Medical Intensive Care Unit, Rhode Island Hospital, Providence, Rhode Island

AUTHORS

DAVID AMPONSAH, MD
Department of Emergency Medicine, Henry Ford Health Systems, Detroit, Michigan

DJILLALI ANNANE, MD, PhD
Director and Professor in Medicine, Assistance Publique Hôpitaux de Paris, General Intensive Care Unit, Hôpital Raymond Poincaré, Université de Versailles SQY (UniverSud Paris), Garches, France

ALFRED AYALA, PhD
Division of Surgical Research, Department of Surgery, The Warren Alpert Medical School of Brown University, Providence, Rhode Island

JAN BAKKER, MD, PhD
Department of Intensive Care, Erasmus MC University Medical Center, Rotterdam, The Netherlands

BRIAN CASSERLY, MD
Critical Care Fellow, Division of Pulmonary, Critical Care, and Sleep Medicine, The Warren Alpert Medical School of Brown University, Providence, Rhode Island

CHEE M. CHAN, MD
Division of Pulmonary and Critical Care Medicine, Washington Hospital Center, Washington, District of Columbia

EMMANUEL CHARBONNEY, MD
Research Fellow, Interdepartmental Division of Critical Care; and Department of Surgery, Li Ka Shing Knowledge Institute, St. Michael's Hospital, University of Toronto, Toronto, Ontario, Canada

VICTOR COBA, MD
Department of Surgery, Henry Ford Health Systems, Detroit, Michigan

GWENHAËL COLIN, MD
Senior Registrar, Assistance Publique Hôpitaux de Paris, General Intensive Care Unit, Hôpital Raymond Poincaré, Université de Versailles SQY (UniverSud Paris), Garches, France

R. PHILLIP DELLINGER, MD
Division of Critical Care Medicine, Cooper University Hospital, Robert Wood Johnson Medical School at Camden, University of Medicine and Dentistry of New Jersey, Camden, New Jersey

PATRICIA DUQUE GONZALEZ, MD
Clinical Fellow, Interdepartmental Division of Critical Care; and Department of Surgery, Li Ka Shing Knowledge Institute, St. Michael's Hospital, University of Toronto, Toronto, Ontario, Canada

CAN INCE, PhD
Department of Intensive Care, Erasmus MC
University Medical Center, Rotterdam, The
Netherlands

EVA KLIJN, MD
Department of Intensive Care, Erasmus MC
University Medical Center, Rotterdam, The
Netherlands

JAMES R. KLINGER MD
Division of Pulmonary Critical Care Medicine,
Rhode Island Hospital, Brown University,
Providence, Rhode Island

HAKAN ATALAN KORKUT, MD
Intensivist, Department of Intensive Care,
Erasme Hospital, Université Libre de Bruxelles,
Brussels, Belgium

ANAND KUMAR, MD, FCCM
Associate Professor, Sections of Pulmonary
and Critical Care Medicine and Infectious
Diseases, Department of Medicine, University
of Manitoba, Winnipeg, Manitoba, Canada;
Department of Medicine, University of
Medicine and Dentistry of New Jersey,
Camden, New Jersey

STEVEN P. LAROSA, MD
Assistant Professor of Medicine, Warren Alpert
School of Medicine, Brown University; Division
of Infectious Diseases, Rhode Island Hospital,
Providence, Rhode Island

MARCEL LEVI, MD, PhD
Department of Medicine, Academic Medical
Center, University of Amsterdam, Amsterdam,
The Netherlands

MITCHELL M. LEVY, MD
Professor of Medicine, Division of Pulmonary
and Critical Care Medicine, Brown University;
Director, Medical Intensive Care Unit, Rhode
Island Hospital, Providence, Rhode Island

JOHN C. MARSHALL, MD, FRCSC
Professor of Surgery, Interdepartmental
Division of Critical Care; and Department of
Surgery, Li Ka Shing Knowledge Institute,
St. Michael's Hospital, University of Toronto,
Toronto, Ontario, Canada

STEVEN M. OPAL, MD
Professor of Medicine, Warren Alpert School
of Medicine, Brown University, Providence;
Division of Infectious Diseases, Memorial
Hospital, Pawtucket, Rhode Island

EMANUEL P. RIVERS, MD, MPH
Department of Emergency Medicine; and
Department of Surgery, Henry Ford Health
Systems, Detroit, Michigan

CHRISTA SCHORR, RN
Division of Critical Care Medicine, Cooper
University Hospital, Robert Wood Johnson
Medical School at Camden, University of
Medicine and Dentistry of New Jersey,
Camden, New Jersey

SAT SHARMA, MD, FRCPC, FCCP
Professor, Sections of Pulmonary and Critical
Care Medicine, Department of Internal
Medicine, University of Manitoba, Winnipeg,
Manitoba, Canada

MERVYN SINGER, MBBS, MD, FRCP
Professor of Intensive Care Medicine,
University College London, London, United
Kingdom

B. TAYLOR THOMPSON, MD
Director and Associate Professor, Department
of Medicine, Pulmonary and Critical Care Unit,
Medical Intensive Care Unit, Massachusetts
General Hospital, Harvard Medical School,
Boston, Massachusetts

SEAN R. TOWNSEND, MD
Division of Pulmonary and Critical Care
Medicine, Rhode Island Hospital, Brown
University, Providence, Rhode Island

C.A. DEN UIL, MD
Department of Cardiology, Erasmus MC
University Medical Center, Rotterdam,
The Netherlands

COREY E. VENTETUOLO, MD
Division of Pulmonary, Allergy, and Critical
Care Medicine, Department of Medicine,
College of Physicians and Surgeons, Columbia
University, New York City, New York

JEAN-LOUIS VINCENT, MD, PhD
Head, Department of Intensive Care, Erasme
Hospital, Université Libre de Bruxelles,
Brussels, Belgium

ALVARO VISBAL, MD
Department of Pulmonary and Critical Care
Medicine, Henry Ford Health Systems, Detroit,
Michigan

MELISSA WHITMILL, MD
Department of Surgery, Henry Ford Health
Systems, Detroit, Michigan

NICHOLAS S. WARD, MD
Associate Professor of Medicine, Division of
Pulmonary, Critical Care, and Sleep Medicine,
The Warren Alpert Medical School of Brown
University, Providence, Rhode Island

Contents

Definitions have been considered important in all fields of medicine, both at a patient level to facilitate accurate diagnosis and treatment, and at a research level to clarify patient inclusion criteria and interpretation of study results. Although there is agreement that sepsis refers to the host response to infection, the complexity of this response and of the patient groups affected, however, has meant that establishing accepted definitions of sepsis has been difficult. Recent consensus has provided global definitions of sepsis and infection, but further work is necessary to provide a means of more completely characterizing the sepsis response in individual patients, such that new interventions can be targeted better as physicians strive to decrease the still high mortality rates associated with this condition.

Prompt diagnosis, intervention, and risk assessment are critical in caring for septic patient but remain difficult with currently available methods. Biomarkers may become useful adjuncts to clinicians and ultimately serve as targets for future therapeutic trials in sepsis. The most relevant markers are reviewed in this article, including interleukin-6, C-reactive protein, procalcitonin, triggering receptor expressed on myeloid cells-1, and biomarker panels.

The mammalian immune system comprises a complex network of physical and molecular elements that protect the individual from danger in the environment. An evolutionarily ancient innate immune system recognizes danger through pattern-recognition receptors that are encoded in the genome and mobilizes a rapid and potent but nonspecific response. This response is responsible for the clinical syndromes of sepsis and the multiple organ dysfunction syndrome. The adaptive immune system is highly selective in its targets and is endowed with memory but is slow in initial activation. Critical illness results in derangements of all components of the immune response, but the very complexity of the process has frustrated attempts to correct these derangements and to affect significantly the clinical course of sepsis.

Like the systemic inflammatory response syndrome (SIRS), the compensatory anti-inflammatory response syndrome (CARS) is a complex pattern of immunologic responses to severe infection or injury. The difference is that while SIRS is a proinflammatory response tasked with killing infectious organisms through activation of the immune system, CARS is a global deactivation of the immune system tasked with restoring homeostasis. Much research now suggests that the timing and relative magnitude of this response have a profound impact on patient outcomes.

Sepsis is often associated with systemic intravascular activation of coagulation, potentially leading to widespread microvascular deposits of fibrin, and thereby contributing to multiple organ dysfunction. A complex interaction exists between activation of inflammatory systems and the initiating and regulating pathways of coagulation. A diagnosis of sepsis-associated disseminated intravascular coagulation can be made by a combination of routinely available laboratory tests, for which simple diagnostic algorithms have become available. Strategies to inhibit coagulation activation may theoretically be justified and are being evaluated in clinical studies.

Microcirculation, a complex and specialized facet of organ architecture, has characteristics that vary according to the function of the tissue it supplies. Bedside technology that can directly observe microcirculation in patients, such as orthogonal polarization spectral imaging and sidestream dark field imaging, has opened the way to investigating this network and its components, especially in critical illness and surgery. These investigations have underscored the central role of microcirculation in perioperative disease states. They have also highlighted variations in the nature of microcirculation, both among organ systems and within specific organs. Supported by experimental studies, current investigations are better defining the nature of microcirculatory alterations in critical illness and how these alterations respond to therapy. This review focuses on studies conducted to date on the microcirculatory beds of critically ill patients. The functional anatomy of microcirculation networks and the role of these networks in the pathogenesis of critical illness are discussed. The morphology of microvascular beds that have been visualized during surgery and intensive care at the bedside are also described, including those of the brain, sublingual region, skin, intestine, and eyes.

Cellular dysfunction is a commonplace sequelum of sepsis and other systemic inflammatory conditions. Impaired energy production (related to mitochondrial inhibition, damage, and reduced protein turnover) appears to be a core mechanism underlying the development of organ dysfunction. The reduction in energy availability appears to trigger a metabolic shutdown that impairs normal functioning of the cell. This may well represent an adaptive mechanism analogous to hibernation that prevents a massive degree of cell death and thus enables eventual recovery in survivors.

Right ventricular dysfunction is common in sepsis and septic shock because of decreased myocardial contractility and elevated pulmonary vascular resistance despite a concomitant decrease in systemic vascular resistance. The mainstay of treatment for acute right heart failure includes treating the underlying cause of sepsis and reversing circulatory shock to maintain tissue perfusion and oxygen delivery. Decreasing pulmonary vascular resistance with selective pulmonary vasodilators is a reasonable approach to improving cardiac output in septic patients with right ventricular dysfunction. Treatment for right ventricular dysfunction in the setting of sepsis should concentrate on fluid repletion, monitoring for signs of RV overload, and correction of reversible causes of elevated pulmonary vascular resistance, such as hypoxia, acidosis, and lung hyperinflation.

Every patient who has sepsis and septic shock must be evaluated appropriately at presentation before the initiation of antibiotic therapy. However, in most situations, an abridged initial assessment focusing on critical diagnostic and management planning elements is sufficient. Intravenous antibiotics should be administered as early as possible, and always within the first hour of recognizing severe sepsis and septic shock. Broad-spectrum antibiotics must be selected with one or more agents active against likely bacterial or fungal pathogens and with good penetration into the presumed source. Antimicrobial therapy should be reevaluated daily to optimize efficacy, prevent resistance, avoid toxicity, and minimize costs. Consider combination therapy in septic shock *Pseudomonas* infections in neutropenic patients. Combination therapy should be continued for no more than 3 to 5 days and de-escalation should occur following availability of susceptibilities. The duration of antibiotic therapy typically is limited to 7 to 10 days. Longer duration is considered if response is slow, if there is inadequate surgical source control, or if immunologic deficiencies are evident. Antimicrobial therapy should be stopped if infection is not considered the etiologic factor for a shock state.

Key links in the chain of survival for the management of severe sepsis and septic shock are early identification and comprehensive resuscitation of high-risk patients. Multiple studies have shown that the first 6 hours of early sepsis management are especially important from a diagnostic, pathogenic, and therapeutic perspective, and that steps taken during this period can have a significant impact on outcome. The recognition of this critical time period and the robust outcome benefit realized in previous studies provides the rationale for adopting early resuscitation as a distinct intervention. Sepsis joins trauma, stroke, and acute myocardial infarction in having "golden hours," representing a critical opportunity early on in the course of disease for actions that offer the most benefit.

superantigens, as well endogenous proinflammatory cytokines are considered important to the pathogenesis of sepsis-induced organ failure and are being targeted with numerous molecules and removal devices. Additional therapeutic strategies are aimed at restoring the natural anticoagulant levels, blocking deleterious effects of the complement cascade, reversing cytopathic hypoxia, and inhibiting excessive lymphocyte apoptosis. Molecules with pluripotent activity, such as interalpha inhibitor proteins and estrogen-receptor ligands, are also being investigated.

Clinics in Chest Medicine

RELATED INTEREST

Sleep Medicine Clinics March 2009 (Vol. 4. No. 1)
Epidemiology of Sleep
Edward Bixler, *Guest Editor*

Critical Care Clinics January 2009 (Vol. 25, No. 1)
Hemoglobin-Based Oxygen Carriers
Lena Napolitano, *Guest Editor*

THE CLINICS ARE NOW AVAILABLE ONLINE!

Access your subscription at:
www.theclinics.com

Preface

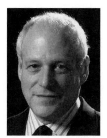

Mitchell M. Levy, MD
Guest Editor

The management of sepsis is a common challenge for anyone who works in a critical care setting. The diagnosis and management of sepsis, severe sepsis, and septic shock are a familiar process to clinicians who are in the emergency department, acting as part of a rapid response team taking care of patients who deteriorate on the wards, or are in the intensive care unit.

Over the past ten years, insights into the host response to infection have deepened. Multiple studies have identified specific genotypic variants associated with worse outcomes in patients who have sepsis. Also, many studies have evaluated the phenotypic expression of inflammatory markers in the evolution of the sepsis response. Over time, clinicians will likely be able to use this information in the diagnosis, risk assessment, and management of sepsis. More recently, new technology and bench studies have led to a greater understanding of the important role of the endothelium and microcirculation in the progression of sepsis. Although the clinical impact of these studies has to be determined yet, these studies offer promising new targets for ongoing trials. One of the most important advances in the field has been in clinical trials. Large-scale, multi-center trials, previously limited to industry-sponsored testing of new therapeutic agents, are no longer unusual. As a result, pathophysiologic insights may be tested now in large-scale clinical trials that sometimes are funded by national funding agencies and conducted on a global scale.

In this issue, an impressive line-up of scientists, clinical trialists, and experts in clinical practice have been assembled. The articles cover the gamut of sepsis, discussing the host response to infection from the molecular to the macroscopic level. In addition, although the results of sepsis trials still have yet to provide a definitive answer for the management of sepsis, there are enough data available in the articles to provide the basis for large scale quality improvement efforts that are focused on creating a minimum standard of care.

The last decade in sepsis research and clinical practice holds great promise for the future of sepsis management. As technology allows for better and more rapid identification of the molecular derangements that become prevalent in severe sepsis and septic shock, this information may be used more precisely to shape the clinical approach to caring for critically-ill patients. More careful titration of clinical interventions, supported by a deeper understanding of pathophysiology, may allow clinicians to provide better care and reduce mortality in this commonly-encountered illness in the intensive care unit.

Mitchell M. Levy, MD
Medical Intensive Care Unit
Rhode Island Hospital
593 Eddy Street
Providence, RI 02903, USA

E-mail address:
mitchell_levy@brown.edu (M.M. Levy)

Clin Chest Med 29 (2008) xiii
doi:10.1016/j.ccm.2008.08.002

Defining Sepsis

Jean-Louis Vincent, MD, PhD*, Hakan Atalan Korkut, MD

KEYWORDS

- Infection • Septic shock • Inflammatory response

The word definition has its roots in the Latin term, definire, meaning to limit or to place boundaries. It first was used in the sense of providing a meaning for words in the mid-16th century (*Online Etymology Dictionary*). A quick search in various English-language dictionaries provides the following definitions of definition:

> "A statement of the exact meaning of a word or the nature or scope of something" (*Oxford English Dictionary*)
> "A statement expressing the essential nature of something" (*Merriam-Webster*)
> "A description of a thing by its properties" (*Webster*)
> "The clear determination of the limits of anything, as of a disease process" (*Dorland's Illustrated Medical Dictionary*)

Importantly, definitions can range from the very simple to the much more detailed and complex, and this will depend not only on what is being defined, but also the purpose for which the definition is required.

Definitions in medicine help provide a relatively concise and clear description of the condition in question, enabling a diagnosis to be determined precisely and rapidly. Without a specific definition, it is difficult to make a diagnosis, choose an appropriate therapy, select homogeneous groups of patients for clinical trials, or clearly assess the effect of new interventions on a specific disease process. In recent years, attempts have been made to standardize definitions for various conditions within intensive care medicine, so that the same definition is used each time the condition in question is discussed, whether in individual patient care or for clinical trial purposes. For some conditions it has been relatively easy to develop a working and widely accepted definition; however, sepsis has proved much more difficult to define for several reasons, including the complex nature of the septic process and the huge variety of patients it can affect.

DEFINING SEPSIS

Clinicians recognize sepsis as an important cause of mortality in the intensive care setting. Increasingly, it is becoming clear that early recognition and accurate diagnosis of a patient with sepsis are imperative, as early resuscitation and antibiotic therapy are key to ensuring the best possible outcome for that patient.[1,2] To be able to achieve early diagnosis, however, one needs a good understanding of the concepts underlying sepsis and, ideally, good working definitions. And therein lies a problem. Sepsis is a complex disease state, or syndrome, that can affect many diverse groups of patients, originate from multiple sites, be triggered as a result of infection by many different microorganisms, and present with assorted symptoms and signs. There is no single sign, symptom, or test with 100% specificity and sensitivity for sepsis. Hence, while acute myocardial infarction can be defined relatively simply for most patients according to typical symptoms (eg, chest pain, breathlessness, nausea), signs (eg, ST elevation on EKG), and biomarkers (raised creatine kinase or troponin levels), the situation for patients who have sepsis is much more complex.

Over the years, there has been much discussion about how best to define sepsis, and the following section will run through the developments in this field in chronologic order to the current situation in which, perhaps, the focus is beginning to shift more to the importance of the concept of sepsis rather than to any specific definition.

Department of Intensive Care, Erasme Hospital, Université Libre de Bruxelles, 808, Route de Lennik, 1070 Brussels, Belgium
* Corresponding author.
E-mail address: jlvincent@ulb.ac.be (J-L. Vincent).

Clin Chest Med 29 (2008) 585–590
doi:10.1016/j.ccm.2008.06.001
0272-5231/08/$ – see front matter © 2008 Elsevier Inc. All rights reserved.

A Little History

The word sepsis is derived from a Greek word meaning decay or putrefaction, and the term originally was used with no knowledge of the microbial origins of the condition. Indeed, although some of the first descriptions of bacteria were made in the 1680s, it was another 200 years before the link between bacteria and infection finally began to be realized, and only in 1914 did Schottmueller[3] report that the release of pathogenic germs into the bloodstream was responsible for systemic symptoms and signs, thus changing the modern understanding of the term sepsis.[4]

Sepsis Syndrome

In 1989, Bone and colleagues[5] made a notable attempt to define severe sepsis and proposed the term sepsis syndrome. Sepsis syndrome was defined as hypothermia (temperature less than 96 °F [35.5 °C]) or hyperthermia (greater than 101 °F [38.3 °C]), tachycardia (greater than 90 beats/min), tachypnea (greater than 20 breaths/min), clinical evidence of an infection site, and at least one end-organ demonstrating inadequate perfusion or dysfunction expressed as poor or altered cerebral function, hypoxemia (PaO_2 less than 75 torr), elevated plasma lactate, or oliguria (urine output less than 30 mL/h or 0.5 mL/kg body weight/h without corrective therapy). There were several problems with this definition, including the fact that not all patients with severe sepsis will have tachycardia or tachypnea, and that altered cerebral function is difficult to quantify. This definition thus largely has been replaced by the term severe sepsis.

Systemic Inflammatory Response Syndrome

Following on from the sepsis syndrome, in 1991 the American College of Chest Physicians (ACCP) and the Society of Critical Care Medicine (SCCM)[6] convened a consensus conference of 35 experts in an attempt to create a set of standardized definitions for patients who have sepsis. It had been realized for some time that sepsis was the result of an inflammatory response to infection, but that this systemic response could occur in response to other conditions, including acute pancreatitis, trauma, ischemia/reperfusion injury, and burns. The goal of the conference, therefore, was to provide a framework to define the systemic inflammatory response and to differentiate that occurring because of infection (ie, sepsis) from that occurring as a result of other processes (systemic inflammatory response syndrome [SIRS]).

SIRS was defined as being the presence of at least two of four clinical criteria:[6]

1. Body temperature greater than 38 °C or less than 36 °C
2. Heart rate greater than 90 beats/min
3. Respiratory rate greater than 20 breaths/min or hyperventilation with a $PaCO_2$ less than 32 mm Hg
4. White blood cell count greater than 12,000/mm^3, less than 4000/mm^3, or with greater than 10% immature neutrophils

Sepsis was defined as the presence of SIRS with a confirmed infectious process. Sepsis associated with organ dysfunction, hypoperfusion abnormality, or sepsis-induced hypotension was called severe sepsis, and septic shock was defined as severe sepsis with sepsis-induced hypotension persisting despite adequate fluid resuscitation.

Worldwide, many adopted the SIRS approach rapidly, and it has been used to define populations of patients in many interventional clinical trials. A study in 2005 reported that 69% of clinical trials in sepsis published after the consensus conference used the consensus conference definitions as standard.[7] Nevertheless, in a survey of 1058 physicians conducted in 2000, only 5% (22% of the intensivists) gave the ACCP/SCCM definition when asked to define sepsis;[8] only 17% of physicians agreed on any one definition for sepsis, and six different definitions were mentioned by at least 1 in 10 physicians. Indeed, the SIRS criteria have been criticized for being too sensitive and nonspecific, limiting their clinical usefulness.[9] It is true that most ICU patients and many general ward patients meet the SIRS criteria;[10–14] for example, in the Sepsis Occurrence in Acutely ill Patients (SOAP) study, 93% of ICU admissions had at least two SIRS criteria at some point during their ICU stay.[14] Moreover, each of the SIRS criteria can be present in many varied conditions, so that a label of SIRS provides little information about the underlying disease process. For example:

Fever can be present in sepsis, after myocardial infarction or pulmonary embolism, or postoperatively
Tachycardia and tachypnea may be present in heart failure, anemia, respiratory failure, hypovolemia, and sepsis
A raised white blood cell count can be present in many other diseases encountered in ICU patients, including trauma, heart failure, pancreatitis, hemorrhage, and pulmonary edema

Indeed, presence of the SIRS criteria generally reflects an appropriate adaptive response to a physiologic insult rather than an abnormality, and SIRS in itself should not be considered as a disease entity.[15]

2001 Sepsis Definitions Conference

With advances in the understanding of the pathophysiology of sepsis, development of new biomarkers, and continuing dissatisfaction with the ACPP/SCCM definitions, particularly the clinical validity of the SIRS criteria, a consensus sepsis definitions conference of 29 international experts in the field of sepsis was held in December 2001, under the auspices of the SCCM, the European Society of Intensive Care Medicine (ESICM), the ACCP, and the Surgical Infection Societies (SIS).[16] The conference participants concluded that the definitions of sepsis, severe sepsis, and septic shock, as defined in the 1991 North American Consensus Conference,[6] remain useful both in clinical practice and for research purposes, but that the diagnostic criteria for SIRS were overly sensitive and nonspecific. The participants suggested that an expanded list of signs and symptoms of sepsis might reflect the clinical response to infection better (**Fig. 1**). By these new definitions (**Box 1**), sepsis is defined as the presence of infection plus some of the listed signs and symptoms of sepsis. Severe sepsis is defined as sepsis complicated by organ dysfunction, and septic shock as severe sepsis with acute circulatory failure characterized by persistent arterial hypotension unexplained by other causes.

Importantly, the list of signs and markers suggested by the Sepsis Definitions Conference participants should be considered as a guide to diagnosis. Not all patients with sepsis will have all the markers included on the list, and many patients without sepsis will have several. The unexplained presence of several of the listed signs in a patient, however, should be used to raise suspicion of sepsis and to encourage a repeated, or more thorough, search for an infectious focus (**Fig. 2**). As research continues, and more potential markers are identified, this list likely will need to be adapted and expanded. A detailed evaluation of the individual biomarkers is provided in the article by Levy in this issue.

Definition of Infection

Although precise definitions of sepsis still are debated, few would argue that sepsis is the host response to infection; hence, a definition of infection is integral to the definition of sepsis. For general purposes, infection is defined as a pathologic process caused by the invasion of normally sterile tissue or fluid or body cavity by pathogenic or potentially pathogenic microorganisms.[16] More precise definitions exist that have been used widely in clinical trials,[17] but there are no definitions for specific infections as related to the patient who has sepsis. Therefore, a consensus conference was organized by the International Sepsis Forum to provide definitions for specific infections, specifically for use in clinical studies of sepsis.[18] The panel of 28 international experts in the fields of intensive care medicine, infectious diseases,

SIRS
- Fever/hypothermia
- Tachycardia
- Tachypnea
- Altered white blood cell count

Signs of Sepsis
- General signs and symptoms
  Rigor – fever (sometimes hypothermia)
  Tachypnea/respiratory alkalosis
  Positive fluid balance – edema
- General inflammatory reaction
  Altered white blood cell count
  Increased CRP, IL-6, PCT concentrations
- Hemodynamic alterations
  Arterial hypotension
  Tachycardia
  Increased cardiac output/low SVR/high SvO_2
  Altered skin perfusion
  Decreased urine output
  Hyperlactatemia – increased base deficit
- Signs of organ dysfunction
  Hypoxemia
  Coagulation abnormalities
  Altered mental status
  Hyperglycemia
  Thrombocytopenia, DIC
  Altered liver function (hyperbilirubinemia)
  Intolerance to feeding (altered GI motility)

Fig. 1. The Sepsis Definitions Conference[16] suggested that the systemic inflammatory response syndrome criteria be replaced by a longer list of possible signs and symptoms of sepsis. Although none of these is specific of sepsis, the unexplained presence of several in combination should raise suspicion of sepsis.

and clinical microbiology developed definitions for the six most frequent causes of infections in septic patients:

- Pneumonia
- Bloodstream infections (including infective endocarditis)
- Intravascular catheter-related sepsis

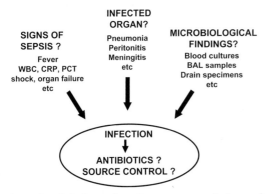

Fig. 2. In clinical practice, the presence of signs of sepsis in a patient is one factor that leads to a search for infection requiring treatment with appropriate antibiotics and effective source control; local signs of infection or positive microbiological cultures are also important clues.

- Intra-abdominal infections
- Urosepsis
- Surgical wound infections

The main aim of these definitions is to facilitate patient selection for clinical trial inclusion; by classifying patients into prospectively defined infection categories, treatments could be targeted more specifically. Such definitions, however, potentially could be used as a framework for guiding diagnostic or therapeutic decisions.

Beyond Definitions

In addition to concerns about defining sepsis, participants at the Sepsis Definitions Conference were concerned that there was no mechanism for characterizing or staging the host response to infection.[16] Sepsis can be considered as a global concept covering a large group of more specific diseases related to the type of microorganism, the degree of immunologic response, the genetic make-up of the individual, and multiple other factors.[19,20] As further advances in the understanding of the pathophysiology of sepsis are made, and potential therapeutic targets are identified, the global definition or concept of sepsis will need to be expanded by a mechanism or system that allows specific individual characteristics and profiles to be determined so that therapies can be targeted more appropriately and outcomes improved. Very few of the many randomized–controlled studies of potential new sepsis interventions that have been conducted over the last 20 years have yielded positive results. One reason for this is that the definitions of sepsis have been too broad, allowing very heterogeneous groups of patients to be included.[21] Similarly, in acute respiratory distress syndrome (ARDS), the introduction of precise definitions in 1994[22] was not associated with any increased success in clinical trials of new therapies for patients who had ARDS. As discussed already by Abraham and colleagues[23] in 2000, a key problem with the consensus conference definitions for sepsis and ARDS was that they were descriptive rather than mechanistic, based on clinical, laboratory, and radiological abnormalities, with little reference to the biochemical, immunologic, or pathophysiological changes that occur in individual patients. Whether the recent call for all studies in patients who have acute renal failure to use the risk, injury failure, loss, end-stage kidney disease criteria definition as developed by the Acute Dialysis Quality Initiative will result in more positive trial results or will prove ineffective in the search for new therapies for acute renal failure remains to be seen.

Sepsis is a process that has many different facets, and grouping all patients with sepsis together is too simplistic. A new, more specific approach to defining the sepsis patient is needed, that takes into account the numerous factors involved in an individual's response to infection. The PIRO (predisposing factors, infection, response, organ dysfunction) system has been suggested as a means of describing patients who have sepsis,[16] much as the TNM (tumor, node, metastases) staging system allows the degree of disease to be staged in patients who have cancer. Defining cancer has faced many of the same problems as defining sepsis, in that cancer can affect many different groups of patients, originate in many different organ systems, and have varied means of presentation, with no single marker or sign common to all patients who have cancer. As is likely to be the case in sepsis, treatments in cancer need to be individualized with no one cure for all cancers. Improved characterization of individual patients using a grading system could help determine which therapies are likely to be most beneficial at an individual level. The PIRO grading system is discussed in more detail in the article by Levy elsewhere in this issue.

SUMMARY

Although the notion of sepsis as a concept is important in clinical practice and for clinical trials, specific definitions of sepsis are difficult to develop and have not proved to be of great benefit for developing new therapies. New strategies need to be introduced to define the sepsis patient rather than sepsis per se. Such systems will allow specific individual characteristics and profiles to be determined, so that therapies can be targeted more appropriately and outcomes improved.

REFERENCES

1. Rivers E, Nguyen B, Havstad S, et al. Early goal-directed therapy in the treatment of severe sepsis and septic shock. N Engl J Med 2001;345: 1368–77.
2. Kumar A, Roberts D, Wood KE, et al. Duration of hypotension before initiation of effective antimicrobial therapy is the critical determinant of survival in human septic shock. Crit Care Med 2006;34: 1589–96.
3. Schottmueller H. Wesen und Behandlung der Sepsis. Inn Med 1914;31:257–80.
4. Vincent JL, Abraham E. The last 100 years of sepsis. Am J Respir Crit Care Med 2006;173:256–63.
5. Bone RC, Fisher CJ, Clemmer TP, et al. Sepsis syndrome: a valid clinical entity. Crit Care Med 1989;17: 389–93.
6. ACCP-SCCM Consensus Conference. Definitions of sepsis and multiple organ failure and guidelines for the use of innovative therapies in sepsis. Crit Care Med 1992;20:864–74.
7. Trzeciak S, Zanotti-Cavazzoni S, Parrillo JE, et al. Inclusion criteria for clinical trials in sepsis: did the American College of Chest Physicians/Society of Critical Care Medicine consensus conference definitions of sepsis have an impact? Chest 2005;127: 242–5.
8. Poeze M, Ramsay G, Gerlach H, et al. An international sepsis survey: a study of doctors' knowledge and perception about sepsis. Crit Care 2004;8: R409–13.
9. Vincent JL. Dear Sirs, I'm sorry to say that I don't like you. Crit Care Med 1997;25:372–4.
10. Pittet D, Rangel-Frausto S, Li N, et al. Systemic inflammatory response syndrome, sepsis, severe sepsis, and septic shock: incidence, morbidities, and outcomes in surgical ICU patients. Intensive Care Med 1995;21:302–9.
11. Rangel Frausto MS, Pittet D, Costigan M, et al. The natural history of the systemic inflammatory response syndrome (SIRS). A prospective study. JAMA 1995;273:117–23.
12. Salvo I, de Cian W, Musicco M, et al. The Italian SEPSIS study: preliminary results on the incidence and evolution of SIRS, sepsis, severe sepsis, and septic shock. Intensive Care Med 1995;21:S244–9.
13. Bossink AW, Groeneveld J, Hack CE, et al. Prediction of mortality in febrile medical patients: how useful are systemic inflammatory response syndrome and sepsis criteria? Chest 1998;113:1533–41.
14. Sprung CL, Sakr Y, Vincent JL, et al. An evaluation of systemic inflammatory response syndrome signs in the Sepsis Occurrence in Acutely Ill Patients (SOAP) study. Intensive Care Med 2006;32:421–7.
15. Marshall J. Both the disposition and the means of cure: Severe SIRS, sterile shock, and the ongoing challenge of description. Crit Care Med 1997;25: 1765–6.
16. Levy MM, Fink MP, Marshall JC, et al. 2001 SCCM/ESICM/ACCP/ATS/SIS International Sepsis Definitions Conference. Crit Care Med 2003;31:1250–6.
17. Garner JS, Jarvis WR, Emori TG, et al. CDC definitions for nosocomial infections. Am J Infect Control 1988;16:128–40.
18. Calandra T, Cohen J. The International Sepsis Forum Consensus Conference on definitions of infection in the intensive care unit. Crit Care Med 2005;33: 1538–48.
19. Marshall JC, Vincent JL, Fink MP, et al. Measures, markers, and mediators: toward a staging system for clinical sepsis. A report of the Fifth Toronto

Sepsis Roundtable, Toronto, Ontario, Canada, October 25–26, 2000. Crit Care Med 2003;31:1560–7.

20. Marshall JC. Sepsis research: where have we gone wrong? Crit Care Resusc 2006;8:241–3.

21. Carlet J, Cohen J, Calandra T, et al. Sepsis: time to reconsider the concept. Crit Care Med 2008;36:964–6.

22. Bernard GR, Artigas A, Brigham KL, et al. The American-European Consensus Conference on ARDS. Definitions, mechanisms, relevant outcomes, and clinical trial coordination. Am J Respir Crit Care Med 1994;149:818–24.

23. Abraham E, Matthay MA, Dinarello CA, et al. Consensus conference definitions for sepsis, septic shock, acute lung injury, and acute respiratory distress syndrome: time for a reevaluation. Crit Care Med 2000;28:232–5.

Biomarkers: Diagnosis and Risk Assessment in Sepsis

Corey E. Ventetuolo, MD[a], Mitchell M. Levy, MD[b,c],*

KEYWORDS

- Sepsis • Biomarkers • Diagnosis • Risk assessment

The challenges of diagnosing and treating sepsis only seem more daunting as incidence increases, patients become older and sicker, and pathogenic organisms evolve.[1,2] New understanding of inflammatory mediators and pathways, immunity, and genetic variability in this disease state suggests that the current definitions of systemic inflammatory response syndrome (SIRS), sepsis, severe sepsis, and septic shock are oversimplified.[3] Evidence supports early intervention[4] and diagnosis in sepsis and that the failure to intervene results in significant morbidity and mortality.[5] Early and appropriate antibiotic therapy is critical.[6] Likewise, limiting exposure when infection is absent will become exceedingly important as drug resistance increases.

These complexities have led to the search for the "troponin" of sepsis, a biomarker or set of biomarkers with compelling sensitivity and specificity for effectively identifying the disease, patients at risk for untoward outcomes, and reliably guiding treatment. Countless potential markers have been evaluated in published literature, a detailed discussion of which is beyond the scope of this article. The most relevant biomarkers are highlighted, including interleukin (IL)-6, C-reactive protein (CRP), procalcitonin (PCT), and triggering receptor expressed on myeloid cells (TREM)-1, as are composite markers or biomarker panels. A more comprehensive list of potential markers of interest is included in **Table 1**.

DEFINITIONS AND CRITERIA

Biomarkers are an appealing addition to the care of patients who have sepsis because they are non-invasive, ideally rapidly available, and may be followed over a patient's course. They may ultimately serve as potential targets for therapy and large-scale randomized control trials. Assay reliability, the establishment of cut-offs, and timely, affordable processing must be considered and addressed before the widespread adoption of a given marker.

A biomarker is defined as "a characteristic that is objectively measured and evaluated as an indicator of normal biological processes, pathogenic processes, or pharmacologic responses to a therapeutic intervention."[7] Before the widespread use of a marker of interest, it must endure *validation* (ie, have known characteristics, be well standardized, and be accurate) and *qualification* (ie, be integral to the disease process and clinical end points).[8] Depending on the intended use, the validation and qualification process may be more or less rigorous (known as the "fit-for-purpose" paradigm in drug development[9]) (**Table 2**).

A recently convened consensus panel put forth important distinctions between sepsis *measures*, *markers*, and *mediators* to address the need for a more systematic approach to clinical research in sepsis.[10] Currently, the literature is filled with countless measures and markers in various stages of preclinical, translational, and clinical

Dr. Levy receives grant support from Brahm's Diagnostics.
[a] Division of Pulmonary, Allergy, and Critical Care Medicine, Department of Medicine, College of Physicians and Surgeons, Columbia University, PH 8, Room 101, 622 W. 168th Street, New York City, NY 10032, USA
[b] Division of Pulmonary and Critical Care Medicine, Brown University, 593 Eddy Street, Main 7, Providence, RI 02903, USA
[c] Medical Intensive Care Unit, Rhode Island Hospital, 593 Eddy Street, Providence, RI 02903, USA
* Corresponding author.
E-mail address: mitchell_levy@brown.edu (M.M. Levy).

Clin Chest Med 29 (2008) 591–603
doi:10.1016/j.ccm.2008.07.001

Table 1
Potential biomarkers of interest

Cell Surface Markers	Cytokines	Apoptosis	Coagulation	Soluble Receptors	Miscellaneous	Acute Phase Proteins
CD13-HLADR[122]	TNF-α[123]	Fas/Apo-1[124]	vWF[125,126]	sIL-2R[127]	NT-proBNP[127,128]	PTX3[129]
HLA-G5[130]	IL-8[23,127]	Gas6[131]	PAI-1[132–134]	sCD163[135]	pro-ADM[136,137]	ET-1[123]
HLA-DR[138,139]	IL-12[140]	TNFRI[141]	Thrombopoietin[142]	s-TNF-R[32]	MBL[143]	—
—	IL-10[139]	Fas/FasL[141]	aPTT waveform analysis[144]	TNF-R p55[145]	HDL[146]	—
—	—	—	AT[59,147]	—	Gc-globulin[148]	—
—	—	—	—	—	Copeptin[149]	—
—	—	—	—	—	ICAM-1[150]	—

Abbreviations: aPTT waveform analysis, activated partial thromboplastin time; AT, antithrombin; CD13-HLADR, CD13-class II histocompatibility antigen; ET-1, endothelin-1; FasL, Fas ligand; Gas6, growth-arrest-specific protein 6; HDL, high-density lipoprotein; HLA-G5, human leukocyte antigen-G5; ICAM-1, intercellular adhesion molecule-1; MBL, mannan-binding lectin; NT-proBNP, N-terminal pro-brain natriuretic peptide; PAI-1, plasminogen activator inhibitor type 1; pro-ADM, pro-adrenomedullin; PTX3, pentraxin3; sIL-2R, soluble IL-2 receptor; s-TNF-R, soluble TNF-α receptor; TNF-R p55, tumor necrosis factor receptor p55; TNFRI, tumor necrosis factor type-I receptor; vWF, von Willebrand factor.

investigation. Sample sizes remain small, variable assays and cut-offs abound, and study populations vary widely, however. It is not surprising that myriad randomized control trials based on a perceived understanding of sepsis mediators have been negative.[11–17]

While we are searching for the biomarker "holy grail," clinicians at the bedside remain charged with the difficult task of diagnosing and assessing risk in sepsis. With this article, we hope to offer clinicians a summary of the current biomarker literature and identify the markers most likely to prove useful in clinical practice. Ideally, a useful biomarker should be accurate and available, enhance clinical assessment, and aid in decision making for patient care.

SELECTED BIOMARKERS
Interleukin-6

The release of inflammatory cytokines, such as tumor necrosis factor (TNF)-α, IL-1β, IL-8, and IL-6, in response to infectious pathogens and host injury leads to SIRS and multiple organ dysfunction syndrome.[18] IL-6 is induced by TNF-α and has a longer half-life, which can be measured reliably in the blood after insult to the host.[19] IL-6 is an important mediator in septic shock and has long been acknowledged to predict severity and outcome in this disease.[20–25] As a marker of infection, it is relatively nonspecific, however, and is elevated in a variety of inflammatory states.[25–31] As one of the initial cytokines released in inflammation, IL-6 may be an early predictor of more downstream effects, such as organ dysfunction. This concept has been supported by recent work in sepsis-induced acute kidney injury.[32,33] A retrospective study of the placebo arm of the Recombinant Human Activated Protein C Worldwide Evaluation in Severe Sepsis (PROWESS) trial correlated serum IL-6 levels independently with the development of acute kidney injury on multivariate analysis.[33]

As a diagnostic and prognostic tool, some evidence suggests that IL-6 performs reasonably well, although not as well as PCT.[23,34–36] Harbarth and colleagues[23] reported IL-6's moderate ability to distinguish SIRS from sepsis (area under the curve [AUC] 0.75, 95% CI 0.63-0.87). For risk assessment, they demonstrated levels of more than 1000 ng/mL to be highly predictive of sepsis-related death. A single study demonstrated IL-6 levels on day 2 of intensive care unit (ICU) admission had comparable discriminative power to day 2 PCT and Acute Physiology and Chronic Health Evaluation (APACHE II) scores in predicting hospital mortality.[24] Several studies have shown that the diagnostic and prognostic accuracy of IL-6 may

Table 2
The "fit-for-purpose" paradigm of biomarker development

Biomarker	Description	Drug Development Use
Exploration	Biomarker in research and development; in vitro and/or preclinical evidence available; no or limited data linking biomarker to outcomes in humans	Hypothesis generating
Demonstration	Biomarker with acceptable preclinical sensitivity and specificity; some data supporting association with clinical outcomes	Decision making
Characterization	Biomarker correlated to clinical outcomes; validity demonstrated by more than one prospective study	Decision making, dose finding, secondary/tertiary claims
Surrogacy	Biomarker as surrogate for clinical endpoint	Registration

Adapted from Wagner JA, Williams SA, Webster CJ. Biomarkers and surrogate end points for fit-for-purpose development and regulatory evaluation of new drugs. Clin Pharmacol Ther 2007;81:104–7; with permission.

depend on time and frequency of measurement and underlying illness severity, perhaps suggesting the importance of trending cytokine levels with clinical course and therapy.[35,36] To this end, a point-of-care assay that has been validated against the IL-6 enzyme-linked immunosorbent assay soon may be available.[37]

C-REACTIVE PROTEIN

CRP is an acute phase protein synthesized predominantly in hepatocytes but also in alveolar macrophages[38] in response to a variety of cytokines, particularly IL-6. CRP plays a role in immune modulation, with both pro- and anti-inflammatory effects. It has been shown to modulate the complement cascade and regulate bacterial opsonization and phagocytosis in the face of host infection.[39,40] Elevations in CRP have been demonstrated in a variety of noninfectious states, including in postsurgical and postmyocardial infarction settings[41,42] and in rheumatologic disease.[43] Serum CRP is appealing as a biomarker because concentrations increase rapidly in response to inflammation and half-life is short (approximately 19 hours), although its kinetics may not be as favorable as those of PCT.[44–46] Finally, the assay is inexpensive and widely available.

Numerous studies have demonstrated CRP levels to be elevated in sepsis,[47–51] but the data supporting its use as a diagnostic biomarker are less convincing.[52–54] The marker performs better than standard clinical parameters, such as white blood cell count and temperature, in predicting infection.[47,55,56] Alone and combined with five variables in a clinical prediction score, CRP had reasonable diagnostic accuracy.[56] It has been

suggested that CRP may be used to follow response to antibiotic therapy,[55,57] but CRP performs poorly in discriminating septic from nonseptic shock[52] and is less accurate than PCT in differentiating SIRS from sepsis (AUC 0.677, 95% CI 0.622-0.733, versus 0.925, 95% CI 0.899-0.952, respectively).[54] Designating an appropriate cut-off (eg, > 50 mg/mL) may help to identify infection as the cause of inflammation and improve CRP sensitivity.[50]

Just as CRP's use as a diagnostic tool in sepsis has been challenged, so has its role as a prognostic measure. In an unselected population of patients admitted to an ICU in Belgium, elevated admission CRP levels (> 10 mg/dL) were significantly associated with a higher incidence of organ failures and mortality.[58] Numerous studies, however, have shown CRP to be poorly predictive of outcome in sepsis.[24,46,52,59] It is unclear whether significant increases in CRP occur with worsening sepsis severity.[45,47,51,54] Because of the mixed results in published studies, although serial CRP monitoring may have some value in predicting infection and response to antibiotics in the ICU, its role as a singular diagnostic and prognostic biomarker in sepsis remains limited.

PROCALCITONIN

PCT is a propeptide of calcitonin that is ubiquitously expressed as part of the host's inflammatory response to a variety of insults.[60,61] Although calcitonin is a neurohormone classically produced in the thyroid and involved in calcium homeostasis, PCT is one of several calcitonin precursors involved in the immune response, acting as a so-called "hormokine"[61] in a variety of inflammatory states, including cardiogenic shock,[31] trauma,[62] necrotizing pancreatitis,[63] burns,[64] surgery,[41] and infection (**Fig. 1**). Immunologic blockade of calcitonin precursors improves organ dysfunction and outcome in animal models of sepsis.[65,66]

A growing body of literature suggests that PCT is a specific marker for severe bacterial infection[23,34,51,67–70] and, in clinical context, may distinguish patients who have sepsis from patients who have SIRS. In a population of medical and surgical ICU patients, baseline PCT was highly accurate in the diagnosis of sepsis (AUC 0.92, 95% CI 0.85-1.0) and significantly improved predictive power when added to standard clinical and laboratory parameters.[23] It has been shown to be superior to IL-6 and CRP in diagnosis[34] and in characterizing infectious from noninfectious acute respiratory distress syndrome.[53] It also may be useful in identifying septic complications in trauma[51,62] and postsurgical patients[69,71] and in predicting neonatal sepsis.[36,72,73]

Plasma PCT concentrations have been correlated to sepsis-related organ failure scores[45] and may be useful in risk assessment. Higher absolute concentrations[34] and, perhaps more important clinically, persistent elevations in PCT after ICU admission have been associated with poor outcomes, distinguishing survivors from nonsurvivors.[52,59,74,75] In a large, diverse cohort of critically ill patients followed serially with PCT, white blood cell counts, and CRP levels, only maximum PCT level and a day-to-day increase in PCT ($\geq$ 1.0 ng/mL) were associated with septic episodes and independently correlated with mortality.[70] The value of PCT in risk assessment and response to therapy also has been demonstrated in the pediatric population.[74,76] Based on the results of several encouraging studies,[23,34] the US

Food and Drug Administration has approved the use of PCT "in conjunction with other laboratory findings and clinical assessments to aid in the risk assessment of critically ill patients on their first day of ICU admission for progression to severe sepsis and septic shock."[77] In several studies, admission or baseline PCT has not proven prognostically meaningful, however, reinforcing the importance of serial measurements.[69,70]

PCT-based treatment strategies have been used successfully in the management of lower respiratory tract infections[78] and community-acquired pneumonia.[79] A single-center randomized control trial in patients with severe sepsis or septic shock examined a PCT-based protocol to limit antibiotic therapy in response to baseline and serially decreasing PCT levels.[68] The intervention group had significant reductions in antibiotic use and shorter ICU lengths of stay without increased mortality or rates of recurrent infection. It is important to realize that this study excluded patients who were immunosuppressed or had infections that warranted prolonged treatment (eg, endocarditis), which highlights the importance of using biomarkers to enhance—not replace—clinical judgment.

Although PCT remains among the most promising biomarkers in sepsis, considerable controversy surrounding its clinical utility remains.[80–82] The marker has been studied in a wide variety of clinical circumstances and different patient populations, and it is important for clinicians to consider this in the context of the patient being treated at the bedside. The most commonly used assay has been criticized as too poorly sensitive to detect subtle, day-to-day trends in PCT.[83,84] Thresholds are not well established, although based on the work of Harbarth[23] and Müller,[34] the Food

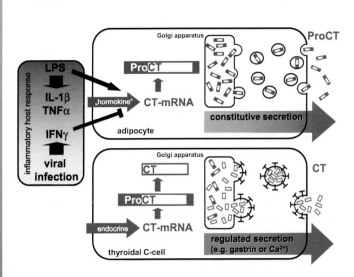

Fig. 1. Procalcitonin (ProCT) as a "hormokine." Calcitonin 1 (CALC 1) expression is restricted to neuroendocrine cells, specifically C cells of the thyroid, in the normal state. In sepsis, constitutive synthesis and release occurs in response to the host inflammatory response. (*Adapted from* Linscheid P, Seboek D, Nylen ES, et al. In vitro and in vivo calcitonin I gene expression in parenchymal cells: a novel product of human adipose tissue. Endocrinology 2003;144:5578–84; with permission.)

and Drug Administration designates < 0.5 ng/mL and > 2 ng/mL as low and high risk for illness severity, respectively.[77] PCT may be a less attractive biomarker in renal failure, because little is known about serum levels in this setting and evidence suggests that PCT is dialyzed.[85]

TRIGGERING RECEPTOR EXPRESSED ON MYELOID CELLS-1

Neutrophils and monocytes/macrophages are the primary mediators of the innate immune response to bacterial infection, promoting release of proinflammatory cytokines, such as TNF-α and IL-1β, which, when produced in excess, contribute to end-organ dysfunction and overwhelming sepsis.[18,86] TREM-1, part of the immunoglobulin superfamily, is up-regulated in response to bacteria or fungi and, when bound to ligand, stimulates release of such cytokines via signal transduction molecule DAP12.[87,88] Healthy volunteers injected with lipopolysaccharide[89] and patients with septic shock have been shown to have high levels of TREM-1 expression.[90] There is a complex and yet-to-be fully understood relationship between

TREM-1 and Toll-like receptor-4 (TLR-4)–mediated pathways, but together they act synergistically to augment the immune response (**Fig. 2**).[91–93] In contrast to infectious insults, TREM-1 is not up-regulated in noninfectious inflammatory disorders, such as inflammatory bowel disease and SIRS.[94] Moreover, its modulation has been shown to be protective in murine models of sepsis,[94–96] making TREM-1 a potentially appealing biomarker.

Several studies have investigated the use of TREM-1 as a diagnostic biomarker and shown it to be more sensitive and specific than CRP and PCT.[97,98] A soluble form of TREM-1 (sTREM-1) is shed from the membranes of activated phagocytic cells and can be quantified in human body fluids. In a prospective study of mechanically ventilated patients suspected to have pneumonia (25% of whom were admitted with shock and had mean sepsis-related organ failure scores of 7.8 ± 3.9), sTREM-1 obtained via rapid immunoblot testing from bronchoalveolar fluid was shown to be a useful marker (LR 10.38; sensitivity 98%, specificity 90% at a cut-off level of ≥ 5 pg/mL) and was the strongest independent predictor when compared with standard parameters for diagnosing

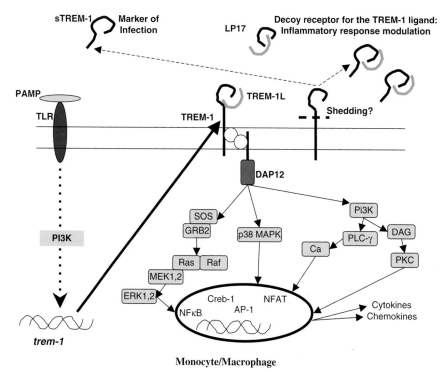

Fig. 2. TREM-1 pathway in monocytes/macrophages. DAG, diacylglycerol; ERK, extracellular signal regulated kinase; GRB, growth receptor binding protein; MAPK, mitogen-activated protein kinase; MEK, mitogen-activated protein kinase; PAMP, pathogen-associated molecular pattern; P13K, phosphatidylinositol 3-kinase; PKC, protein kinase C; PLC, phospholipase C; SOS, son of sevenless; TLR, Toll-like receptor; TREM-1L, TREM-1 ligand. (*Adapted from* Gibot S. Clinical review: role of triggering receptor expressed on myeloid cells-1 during sepsis. Critical Care 2005;9:485–9; with permission.)

pneumonia (OR 41.5).[97] The same investigators conducted a similar study of 76 patients in whom sepsis was suspected and found that plasma sTREM-1 levels were highly accurate (LR 8.6; sensitivity 96%, specificity 89% at a cut-off level of $\geq$ 60 ng/mL) in distinguishing SIRS from sepsis or septic shock.[98] sTREM-1 was a superior diagnostic marker to PCT and CRP in this study.[98] It is important to note that there were differences in illness severity between the two cohorts. Elderly (> 80 years old) and immunocompromised individuals were excluded from this study sample, and the role of TREM-1 in these groups is largely unknown.

Although TREM-1 may be a promising diagnostic marker in sepsis, less is known about its use in risk assessment and prognosis in patients with known sepsis. Gibot and colleagues[99] demonstrated elevated baseline sTREM-1 levels to be independently *protective* against death (OR 0.1, 95% CI 0.1-0.8), perhaps indicating the importance of the host's initial augmented inflammatory response, as has been suggested in murine models.[94,100] Conversely, progressive decline in sTREM-1 over the 14-day study period tracked with more favorable outcomes.[99] A second prospective study of patients with sepsis from ventilator-associated pneumonia correlated declining sTREM-1 levels with clinical resolution of ventilator-associated pneumonia and survival.[101] Finally, Tejera and colleagues[102] demonstrated sTREM-1 to be independently correlated with survival in a cohort of diverse patients who presented with community-acquired pneumonia (56% of whom were in septic shock), although these results have not been corroborated.[103]

COMPOSITE MARKERS AND BIOMARKER PANELS

No single sepsis biomarker is without limitation. The incredible complexity of the host response to overwhelming infection, host characteristics, and type and extent of the infectious pathogen involved may not, in fact, lend to the identification of a single ideal marker. As such, it may prove more useful to combine various markers. The multi-marker approach applied to risk stratification in acute coronary syndromes,[104] for example, combines individual markers to capture important pathways in acute coronary syndromes (eg, troponinI, CRP, and B-type natriuretic peptide). The unique complexity of the septic state notwithstanding, a similar approach may prove useful for diagnosis, therapeutic aim, and prognosis (eg, a panel containing valid representatives of the innate immune response, inflammatory state, and coagulation perturbation) in sepsis. The study of composite

markers may allow for considerable savings in time, cost, and amount of sample required. Data informing the use of combined markers are limited, but recent technologic advances offer promising opportunities for study.[105–107]

Sepsis-induced derangements of coagulation and fibrinolysis may precede severe sepsis and septic shock and, when present, signal end-organ failure and death.[108] Given the therapeutic benefit of recombinant human activated protein C (rhAPC),[109] the predictive accuracy of various markers of coagulation from the placebo group of the PROWESS trial was investigated retrospectively.[110] Logistic regression modeling demonstrated that baseline to day 1 changes in individual parameters of coagulation (prothrombin time, antithrombin III, D-dimer, and protein C levels) were predictive of outcome in severe sepsis. A composite coagulopathy score containing these parameters was found to be correlated with the development of multi-organ failure and death.[110] Importantly, because serum levels were obtained after enrollment criteria (ie, diagnosis of severe sepsis or septic shock) were met, no conclusions can be drawn regarding the use of these markers or the composite score in sepsis diagnosis.

Another group of investigators explored the interaction between endothelial adhesion and damage and neutrophil activation with a selection of five biomarkers in patients with and without sepsis and healthy controls.[111] Although all five biomarkers were useful in predicting severe infection, markers of endothelial activity (E-selectin, endothelial intercellular adhesion molecule-1 [ICAM-1], and von Willebrand factor antigen) were found to be more closely correlated with outcomes than markers of neutrophil activity (myeloperoxidase and lactoferrin).

Going forward, composites that contain system-specific markers may enhance the ability to identify risk for new organ failures and worsening sepsis severity. Recently, pro-atrial natriuretic peptide (pro-ANP) has been described in patients who have sepsis with myocardial depression[112] and, in a single study, admission pro-ANP performed better than PCT and CRP in predicting death from septic shock.[113] Another group of investigators examined a panel of three markers, including ANP, and their role in sepsis-induced myocardial depression.[114] A similar panel has been proposed for the identification of acute kidney injury.[115]

Multiplex bead array assays are currently available and allow for measurement of multiple markers from solution using flow cytometry. This technology has been validated and compared in several different settings, including in patients with sepsis.[107,116–118] Kofoed and colleagues[107] constructed composite diagnostic markers in a cohort of patients admitted from the community with SIRS and suspected infection. Soluble urokinase plasminogen activator receptor (su-PAR), sTREM-1, and macrophage migration inhibiting factor were evaluated using multiplex assays, along with standard measurement of CRP, PCT, and neutrophil count. Composites of the three best performing markers (CRP, PCT, and neutrophil count) and all six markers were found to be more accurate in detecting inflammatory response caused by bacterial infection than individual markers alone. Using neural network modeling, a panel of seven markers (IL-1β, -6, -8, -10, TNF-α, FasL, and chemokine [C-C motif] ligand 2) obtained using real-time reverse transcriptase-polymerase chain reaction was found to be highly accurate in predicting the development of sepsis in a recent pilot study.[119]

Ideally, multi-marker panels will add to diagnostic accuracy and risk assessment in sepsis. Several caveats, however, should be kept in mind. The discovery of each new marker, composite or individual, requires reassessment of statistical and clinical relevance with particular attention to the patient population, the outcome of interest, and the validity and appropriate weighting of individual markers. Through the science of proteomics and genomics, this will become increasingly important as new discoveries are made and as point-of-care testing becomes more widely available. Statistical modeling will become increasingly complex, and the best method for analysis has yet to be identified.[120,121] Accordingly, the validation of such marker panels requires trials of sufficient sample size and—to be clinically generalizable—varied patient populations.

SUMMARY

Scientific progress has resulted in an endless array of potential mediators in sepsis and yet-to-be-characterized interactions and pathways. Our ability to diagnose and predict severity in this disease is limited by the insensitive and nonspecific clinical and laboratory parameters that are currently available. Based on our rapidly expanding insight into the pathophysiology of the host inflammatory response to infection, biomarkers may provide a much-needed solution.

The current evidence suggests that IL-6 and CRP are likely to remain sentinel markers of inflammation and infection but are too nonspecific for further use. Based on recently published studies,

PCT likely will enhance clinicians' ability to diagnose the presence of infection in critically ill patients and perhaps guide antimicrobial therapy. TREM-1 is also a promising candidate. Clearly, the goal of devising biomarker-based treatment strategies and therapies in sepsis requires further validation and qualification. Given the incredible complexity and variability of the disease, host, and pathogen, biomarker panels or composite markers may prove most useful in examining a particular immunologic pathway, predicting organ-specific response, and, ideally, identifying at-risk individuals who require aggressive intervention and monitoring. Above all, there is a need for consensus on appropriate biomarkers for further study.

ACKNOWLEDGMENTS

The authors would like to thank Amy Palmisciano, RN, for her help in preparing the manuscript and Barbara Shott for her invaluable administrative assistance.

REFERENCES

1. Martin GS, Mannino DM, Eaton S, et al. The epidemiology of sepsis in the United States from 1979 through 2000. N Engl J Med 2003;348:1546–54.
2. Annane D, Aegerter P, Jars-Guincestre MC, et al. Current epidemiology of septic shock: the CUB-Réa Network. Am J Respir Crit Care Med 2003; 168:165–72.
3. Bone RC, Balk RA, Cerra FB, et al. Definitions for sepsis and organ failure and guidelines for the use of innovative therapies in sepsis. The ACCP/SCCM Consensus Conference Committee. American College of Chest Physicians/Society of Critical Care Medicine. Chest 1992;101:1644–55.
4. Rivers E, Nguyen B, Havstad S, et al. Early goal-directed therapy in the treatment of severe sepsis and septic shock. N Engl J Med 2001;345: 1368–77.
5. Levy MM, Macias WL, Vincent JL, et al. Early changes in organ function predict eventual survival in severe sepsis. Crit Care Med 2005;33:2194–201.
6. Kumar A, Roberts D, Wood K, et al. Duration of hypotension before initiation of effective antimicrobial therapy is the critical determinant of survival in septic shock. Crit Care Med 2006;34:1589–96.
7. The Biomarker Definitions Working Group. Biomarkers and surrogate endpoints: preferred definitions and conceptual framework. Clin Pharmacol Ther 2001;69:89–95.
8. Wagner JA, Williams SA, Webster CJ. Biomarkers and surrogate end points for fit-for-purpose

development and regulatory evaluation of new drugs. Clin Pharmacol Ther 2007;81:104–7.

9. Lee JW, Devanarayan V, Barrett YC, et al. Fit-for-purpose method development and validation for successful biomarker measurement. Pharm Res 2006;23:312–28.

10. Marshall JC, Vincent JL, Fink MP, et al. Measures, markers, and mediators: toward a staging system for clinical sepsis: a report of the Fifth Toronto Sepsis Roundtable, Toronto, Ontario, Canada, October 25-26, 2000. Crit Care Med 2003;31:1560–7.

11. Warren BL, Eid A, Singer P, et al. High-dose antithrombin III in severe sepsis. JAMA 2001;286:1869–78.

12. Abraham E, Reinhart K, Opal S, et al. Efficacy and safety of tifacogin (recombinant tissue factor pathway inhibitor) in severe sepsis: a randomized control trial. JAMA 2003;290:238–47.

13. Reinhart K, Meier-Hellmann A, Beale R, et al. Open randomized phase II trial of an extracorporeal endotoxin absorber in suspected gram-negative sepsis. Crit Care Med 2004;32:1662–8.

14. Abraham E, Wunderink R, Silverman H, et al. Efficacy and safety of monoclonal antibody to human tumor necrosis factor alpha in patients with sepsis syndrome: a randomized, controlled, double-blind, multicenter clinical trial. TNF-alpha MAb Sepsis Study Group. JAMA 1995;273:934–41.

15. Cohen J, Carlet J. INTERSEPT: an international, multicenter, placebo controlled trial of monoclonal antibody to human tumor necrosis factor-alpha in patients with sepsis. International Sepsis Trial Study Group. Crit Care Med 1996;24:1431–40.

16. Opal SM, Fisher CJ, Dhainaut JF, et al. Confirmatory interleukin-1 receptor antagonist trial in severe sepsis: a phase III, randomized, double-blind, placebo-controlled, multicenter trial. The Interleukin-1 Receptor Antagonist Sepsis Investigator Group. Crit Care Med 1997;25:1115–24.

17. Abraham E, Anzueto A, Gutierrez G, et al. Double-blind randomised controlled trial of monoclonal antibody to human tumour necrosis factor in treatment of septic shock. NORASEPT II Study Group. Lancet 1998;28:929–33.

18. Dinarello CA. Proinflammatory and anti-inflammatory cytokines as mediators in the pathogenesis of septic shock. Chest 1997;112:321S–9S.

19. Panacek EA, Kaul M. IL-6 as a marker of excessive TNF-α activity in sepsis. Sepsis 1999;3:65–73.

20. Hack CE, De Groot ER, Felt-Bersma RJ, et al. Increased plasma levels of interleukin-6 in sepsis. Blood 1989;75:1897–8.

21. Casey LC, Balk RA, Bone RC. Plasma cytokine and endotoxin levels correlate with survival in patients with the sepsis syndrome. Ann Intern Med 1993;119:771–8.

22. Pinsky MR, Vincent JL, Deviere J, et al. Serum cytokine levels in human septic shock: relation to multiple-system organ failure and mortality. Chest 1993;103:565–75.

23. Harbarth S, Holeckova K, Froidevaux C, et al. Diagnostic value of procalcitonin, interleukin-6, and interleukin-8 in critically ill patients admitted with suspected sepsis. Am J Respir Crit Care Med 2001;164:396–402.

24. Pettilä M, Hynninen M, Takkunen O, et al. Predictive value of procalcitonin and interleukin-6 in critically ill patients with suspected sepsis. Intensive Care Med 2002;28:1220–5.

25. Martin C, Boisson C, Haccoun M, et al. Patterns of cytokine evolution (tumor necrosis factor-alpha and interleukin-6) after septic shock, hemorrhagic shock, and severe trauma. Crit Care Med 1997;25:1813–9.

26. Biffl WL, Moore EE, Moore FA, et al. Interleukin-6 in the injured patient: marker of injury or mediator of inflammation? Ann Surg 1996;224:647–64.

27. Drost AC, Burleson DG, Cioffi WG, et al. Plasma cytokines following thermal injury and their relationship with patient mortality, burn size, and time postburn. J Trauma 1993;35:335–9.

28. Stimac D, Fisić E, Milić S, et al. Prognostic value of IL-6, IL-8, and IL-10 in acute pancreatitis. J Clin Gastroenterol 2006;40:209–12.

29. Berber I, Yiğit B, Işitmangil G, et al. Evaluation of pretransplant serum cytokine levels in renal transplant recipients. Transplant Proc 2008;40:92–3.

30. Chun HY, Chung JW, Kim HA, et al. Cytokine IL-6 and IL-10 as biomarkers in systemic lupus erythematosus. J Clin Immunol 2007;27:461–6.

31. de Werra I, Jaccard C, Corradin SB, et al. Cytokines, nitrite/nitrate, soluble tumor necrosis factor receptors, and procalcitonin concentrations: comparisons in patients with septic shock, cardiogenic shock, and bacterial pneumonia. Crit Care Med 1997;25:607–13.

32. Iglesias J, Marik PE, Levine JS. Elevated serum levels of the type I and type II receptors for tumor necrosis factor-alpha as predictive factors for ARF in patients with septic shock. Am J Kidney Dis 2003;41:62–5.

33. Chawla LS, Seneff MG, Nelson DR, et al. Elevated plasma concentrations of IL-6 and elevated APACHE II score predict acute kidney injury in patients with severe sepsis. Clin J Am Soc Nephrol 2007;2:22–30.

34. Müller B, Becker KL, Schächinger H, et al. Calcitonin precursors are reliable markers of sepsis in a medical intensive care unit. Crit Care Med 2000;28:977–83.

35. Oda S, Hirasawa H, Shiga H, et al. Sequential measurement of IL-6 blood levels in patients with

systemic inflammatory resposne syndrome (SIRS)/ sepsis. Cytokine 2005;29:169–75.

36. Chiesa C, Pellegrini G, Panero A, et al. C-reactive protein, interleukin-6, and procalcitonin in the immediate postnatal period: influence of illness severity, risk status, antenatal and perinatal complications, and infection. Clin Chem 2003;49:60–8.

37. Schefold JC, Hasper D, von Haehling S, et al. Interleukin-6 serum level assessment using a new qualitative point-of-care test in sepsis: a comparison with ELISA measurements. Clinical Biochemistry 2008;41:893–8.

38. Dong Q, Wright JR. Expression of C-reactive protein by alveolar macrophages. J Immunol 1996; 156:4815–20.

39. Szalai AJ, Briles DE, Volanakis JE. Role of complement in C-reactive-protein-mediated protection of mice from *Streptococcus pneumoniae*. Infect Immun 1996;64:4850–3.

40. Gershov D, Kim S, Brot N, et al. C-reactive protein binds to apoptotic cells, protects the cells from assembly of the terminal complement components, and sustains an antiinflammatory innate immune response: implications for systemic autoimmunity. J Exp Med 2001;192: 1353–64.

41. Meisner M, Tschaikowsky K, Hutzler A, et al. Postoperative plasma concentrations of procalcitonin after different types of surgery. Intensive Care Med 1998;24:680–4.

42. Nikfardjam M, Müllner M, Schreiber W, et al. The association between C-reactive protein on admission and mortality in patients with acute myocardial infarction. J Intern Med 2000;247:341–5.

43. Eberhard OK, Haubitz M, Brunkhorst FM, et al. Usefulness of procalcitonin for differentiation between activity of systemic autoimmune disease (systemic lupus erythematosus/systemic antineutrophil cytoplasmic antibody-associated vasculitis) and invasive bacterial infection. Arthritis Rheum 1997;40:1250–6.

44. Brunkhorst FM, Heinz U, Forycki ZF. Kinetics of procalcitonin in iatrogenic sepsis. Intensive Care Med 1998;24:888–9.

45. Meisner M, Tschaikowsky K, Palmaers T, et al. Comparison of procalcitonin (PCT) and C-reactive protein (CRP) plasma concentrations at different SOFA scores during the course of sepsis and MODS. Crit Care 1999;3:45–50.

46. Claeys R, Vinken S, Spapen H, et al. Plasma procalcitonin and C-reactive protein in acute septic shock: clinical and biological correlates. Crit Care Med 2002;30:757–62.

47. Póvoa P, Coelho L, Almeida E, et al. C-reactive protein as a marker of infection in critically ill patients. Clin Microbiol Infect 2004;11:101–8.

48. Yentis SM, Soni N, Sheldon J. C-reactive protein as an indicator of resolution of sepsis in the intensive care unit. Intensive Care Med 1995;21:602–5.

49. Matson A, Soni N, Sheldon J. C-reactive protein as a diagnostic test of sepsis in the critically ill. Anaesth Intensive Care 1991;19:182–6.

50. Póvoa P, Almeida E, Moreira P, et al. C-reactive protein as an indicator of sepsis. Intensive Care Med 1998;24:1052–6.

51. Castelli GP, Pognani C, Meisner M, et al. Procalcitonin and C-reactive protein during systemic inflammatory response syndrome, sepsis and organ dysfunction. Crit Care 2004;8:R234–42.

52. Clec'h C, Ferriere F, Karoubi P, et al. Diagnostic and prognostic value of procalcitonin in patients with sepsis and septic shock. Crit Care Med 2004;32: 1166–9.

53. Brunkhorst FM, Eberhard OK, Brunkhorst R. Discrimination of infectious and noninfectious causes of early acute respiratory distress syndrome by procalcitonin. Crit Care Med 1999;27:2172–6.

54. Luzzani A, Polati E, Dorizzi R, et al. Comparison of procalcitonin and C-reactive protein as markers of sepsis. Crit Care Med 2003;31:1737–41.

55. Póvoa P, Coelho L, Almeida E, et al. Early identification of intensive care unit-acquired infections with daily monitoring of C-reactive protein: a prospective observational study. Crit Care 2006;10:R63–71.

56. Bota DP, Mélot C, Ferreira FL, et al. Infection probability score (IPS): a method to help assess the probability of infection in critically ill patients. Crit Care Med 2003;31:2579–84.

57. Póvoa P, Coelho L, Almeida E, et al. C-reactive protein as a marker of ventilator-associated pneumonia resolution: a pilot study. Eur Respir J 2005;25:804–12.

58. Lobo SMA, Lobo FRM, Bota DP, et al. C-reactive protein levels correlate with mortality and organ failure in critically ill patients. Chest 2003;123:2043–9.

59. Pettilä V, Pentti J, Pettilä M, et al. Predictive value of antithrombin III and serum C-reactive protein concentration in critically ill patients with suspected sepsis. Crit Care Med 2002;30:271–5.

60. Linscheid P, Seboek D, Schaer DJ, et al. Expression and secretion of procalcitonin and calcitonin gene-related peptide by adherent monocytes and by macrophage-activated adipocytes. Crit Care Med 2004;32:1715–21.

61. Becker KL, Nylén ES, White JC, et al. Procalcitonin and the calcitonin gene family of peptides in inflammation, infection, and sepsis: a journey from calcitonin back to its precursors. J Clin Endocrinol Metab 2004;89:1512–25.

62. Wanner GA, Keel M, Steckholzer U, et al. Relationship between procalcitonin plasma levels and severity of injury, sepsis, organ failure, and mortality in injured patients. Crit Care Med 2000;28:950–7.

63. Riché FC, Cholley BP, Laisné MC, et al. Inflammatory cytokines, C reactive protein, and procalcitonin as early predictors of necrosis infection in acute necrotizing pancreatitis. Surgery 2003;133:257–62.

64. Nylen ES, Arifi AA, Becker KL, et al. Effect of classic heatstroke on serum procalcitonin. Crit Care Med 1997;25:1362–5.

65. Wagner KE, Martinez JM, Vath SD, et al. Early immunoneutralization of calcitonin precursors attenuates the adverse physiologic response to sepsis in pigs. Crit Care Med 2002;30:2313–21.

66. Nylén ES, Whang KT, Snider RH, et al. Mortality is increased by procalcitonin and decreased by an antiserum reactive to procalcitonin in experimental sepsis. Crit Care Med 1998;26:1001–6.

67. Assicot M, Gendrel D. High serum procalcitonin concentrations in patients with sepsis and infection. Lancet 1993;341:515–8.

68. Nobre V, Harbarth S, Graf JD, et al. Use of procalcitonin to shorten antibiotic treatment duration in septic patients. Am J Respir Crit Care Med 2008; 177:498–505.

69. Dahaba AA, Hagara B, Fall A, et al. Procalcitonin for early prediction of survival outcome in postoperative critically ill patients with severe sepsis. Br J Anaesth 2006;97:503–8.

70. Jensen JU, Heslet L, Jensen TH, et al. Procalcitonin increase in early identification of critically ill patients at high risk of mortality. Crit Care Med 2006;34:2596–602.

71. Mokart D, Merlin M, Sannini A, et al. Procalcitonin, interleukin 6 and systemic inflammatory response syndrome (SIRS): early markers of postoperative sepsis after major surgery. Br J Anaesth 2005;94: 767–73.

72. Turner D, Hammerman C, Rudensky B, et al. The role of procalcitonin as a predictor of nosocomial sepsis in preterm infants. Acta Paediatr 2006;95: 1571–6.

73. Vazzalwar R, Pina-Rodrigues E, Puppala BL, et al. Procalcitonin as a screening test for late-onset sepsis in preterm very low birth weight infants. J Perinatol 2005;25:397–402.

74. Hatherill M, Tibby SM, Turner C, et al. Procalcitonin and cytokine levels: relationship to organ failure and mortality in pediatric and septic shock. Crit Care Med 2000;28:2591–4.

75. Wunder C, Eichelbrönner O, Roewer N. Are IL-6, IL-10, and PCT plasma concentrations reliable for outcome prediction in severe sepsis? A comparison with APACHE III and SAPS II. Inflamm Res 2004; 53:158–63.

76. Han YY, Doughty LA, Kofos D, et al. Procalcitonin is persistently increased among children with poor outcome from bacterial sepsis. Pediatr Crit Care Med 2003;4:21–5.

77. Immunology and microbiology devices; serological reagents. 21 CFR 866 2007.

78. Christ-Crain M, Jaccard-Stolz D, Bingisser R, et al. Effect of procalcitonin-guided treatment on antibiotic use and outcome in lower respiratory tract infections: cluster-randomised, single-blinded intervention trial. Lancet 2004;363:600–7.

79. Christ-Crain M, Stolz D, Bingisser R, et al. Procalcitonin guidance of antibiotic therapy in community-acquired pneumonia: a randomized trial. Am J Respir Crit Care Med 2006;174:84–93.

80. Tang BMP, Eslick GD, Craig JC, et al. Accuracy of procalcitonin for sepsis diagnosis in critically ill patients: systematic review and meta-analysis. Lancet Infect Dis 2007;210:210–7.

81. Müller B, Christ-Crain M, Schuetz P. Meta-analysis of procalcitonin for sepsis detection. Lancet Infect Dis 2007;7:498–9.

82. Reinhart K, Brunkhorst FM. Meta-analysis of procalcitonin for sepsis detection. Lancet Infect Dis 2007; 7:500–2.

83. Becker KL, Snider RH, Nylen ES. Procalcitonin assay in systemic inflammation, infection, and sepsis: clinical utility and limitations. Crit Care Med 2008; 36:941–52.

84. Nylen E, Muller B, Becker KL, et al. The future diagnostic role of procalcitonin levels: the need for improved sensitivity. Clin Infect Dis 2003;36:823–4.

85. Dahaba AA, Rehak PH, List WF. Procalcitonin and C-reactive protein plasma concentrations in non-septic uremic patients undergoing hemodialysis. Intensive Care Med 2003;29:579–83.

86. Bone RC. The pathogenesis of sepsis. Ann Intern Med 1991;115:457–69.

87. Bouchon A, Dietrich J, Colonna M. Inflammatory responses can be triggered by TREM-1, a novel receptor expressed on neutrophils and monocytes. J Immunol 2000;164:4991–5.

88. Lanier LL, Corliss BC, Wu J, et al. Immunoreceptor DAP12 bearing a tyrosine-based activation motif is involved in activating NK cells. Nature 1998;391:703–7.

89. Knapp S, Gibot S, de Vos A, et al. Cutting edge: expression patterns of surface and soluble triggering receptor expressed on myeloid cells-1 in human endotoxemia. J Immunol 2004;173:7131–4.

90. Gibot S, Le Renard PE, Bollaert PE, et al. Surface triggering receptor expressed on myeloid cells 1 expression patterns in septic shock. Intensive Care Med 2005;31:594–7.

91. Ornatowska M, Azim AC, Wang X, et al. Functional genomics of silencing TREM-1 on TLR4 signaling in macrophages. Am J Physiol Lung Cell Mol Physiol 2007;293:L1377–84.

92. Klesney-Tait J, Colonna M. Uncovering the TREM-1-TLR connection. Am J Physiol Lung Cell Mol Physiol 2007;293:L1374–6.

93. Dower K, Ellis DK, Saraf K, et al. Innate immune responses to TREM-1 activation: overlap, divergence, and positive and negative cross-talk with bacterial lipopolysaccharide. J Immunol 2008; 180:3520–34.

94. Bouchon A, Facchetti F, Weigand MA, et al. TREM-1 amplifies inflammation and is a crucial mediator in septic shock. Nature 2001;410:1103–7.

95. Gibot S, Buonsanti C, Massin F, et al. Modulation of the triggering receptor expressed on the myeloid cell type 1 pathway in murine septic shock. Infect Immun 2006;74:2823–30.

96. Gibot S, Alauzet C, Massin F, et al. Modulation of the triggering receptor expressed on myeloid cells-1 pathway during pneumonia in rats. J Infect Dis 2006;194:975–83.

97. Gibot S, Cravoisy A, Levy B, et al. Soluble triggering receptor expressed on myeloid cells and the diagnosis of pneumonia. N Engl J Med 2004;350: 451–8.

98. Gibot S, Kolopp-Sarda MN, Béné MC, et al. Plasma level of a triggering receptor expressed on myeloid cells-1: its diagnostic accuracy in patients with suspected sepsis. Ann Intern Med 2004;141:9–15.

99. Gibot S, Cravoisy A, Kolopp-Sarda MN, et al. Time-course of sTREM (soluble triggering receptor expressed on myeloid cells)-1, procalcitonin, and C-reactive protein plasma concentrations during sepsis. Crit Care Med 2005;33:792–6.

100. Gibot S, Massin F, Marcou M, et al. TREM-1 promotes survival during septic shock in mice. Eur J Immunol 2007;37:456–66.

101. Routsi C, Giamarellos-Bourboulis EJ, Antonopoulou A, et al. Does soluble triggering receptor expressed on myeloid cells-1 play any role in the pathogenesis of septic shock. Clin Exp Immunol 2005;142:62–7.

102. Tejera A, Santolaria F, Diez ML, et al. Prognosis of community acquired pneumonia (CAP): value of triggering receptor expressed on myeloid cells-1 (TREM-1) and other mediators of the inflammatory response. Cytokine 2007;38:117–23.

103. Müller B, Mikael G, Gibot S, et al. Circulating levels of soluble triggering receptor expressed on myeloid cells (sTREM)-1 in community acquired pneumonia. Crit Care Med 2007;35:990–1.

104. Sabatine MS, Morrow DA, de Lemos JA, et al. Multimarker approach to risk stratification in non-ST elevation acute coronary syndromes: simultaneous assessment of troponin I, C-reactive protein, and B-type natriuretic peptide. Circulation 2002;105: 1760–3.

105. Jordan JA, Durso MB. Real-time polymerase chain reaction for detecting bacterial DNA directly from blood of neonates being evaluated for sepsis. J Mol Diagn 2005;7:575–81.

106. Liu Y, Han JX, Huang HY, et al. Development and evaluation of 16S rDNA microarray for detecting bacterial pathogens in cerebrospinal fluid. Exp Biol Med 2005;230:587–91.

107. Kofoed K, Schneider UV, Scheel T, et al. Development and validation of a multiplex add-on assay for sepsis biomarkers using xMAP technology. Clin Chem 2006;52:1284–93.

108. Fourrier F, Chopin C, Goudemand J, et al. Septic shock, multiple organ failure, and disseminated intravascular coagulation: compared patterns of antithrombin III, protein C, and protein S deficiencies. Chest 1992;101:816–23.

109. Bernard GR, Vincent JL, Laterre PF, et al. Efficacy and safety of recombinant human activated protein C for severe sepsis. N Engl J Med 2001;344: 699–709.

110. Dhainaut JF, Shorr AF, Macias WL, et al. Dynamic evolution of coagulopathy in the first day of severe sepsis: relationship with mortality and organ failure. Crit Care Med 2005;33:341–8.

111. Kayal S, Jaïs JP, Aguini N, et al. Elevated circulating E-selectin, intercellular adhesion molecule 1, and von Willebrand factor in patients with severe infection. Am J Respir Crit Care Med 1998;157: 776–84.

112. Mazul-Sunko B, Zarkovic N, Vrkic N, et al. Pro-atrial natriuretic peptide hormone from right atria is correlated with cardiac depression in septic patients. J Endocrinol Invest 2001;24:RC22–4.

113. Morgenthaler NG, Struck J, Christ-Crain M, et al. Pro-atrial natriuretic peptide is a prognostic marker in sepsis, similar to the APACHE II score: an observational study. Crit Care 2005;9:R37–45.

114. Hartemink KJ, Groeneveld J, de Groot MM, et al. α-Atrial natriuretic peptide, cyclic guanosine monophosphate, and endothelin in plasma markers of myocardial depression in human septic shock. Crit Care Med 2001;29:80–7.

115. Parikh CR, Devarajan P. New biomarkers of acute kidney injury. Crit Care Med 2008;36:S159–65.

116. Khan SS, Smith MS, Reda D, et al. Multiplex bead array assays for detection of soluble cytokines: comparisons of sensitivity and quantitative values among kits from multiple manufacturers. Cytometry B Clin Cytom 2004;61:35–9.

117. Liu MY, Xydakis AM, Hoogeveen RC, et al. Multiplexed analysis of biomarkers related to obesity and the metabolic syndrome in human plasma, using the Luminex-100 system. Clin Chem 2005;51: 1102–9.

118. duPont NC, Wang K, Wadhwa P, et al. Validation and comparison of luminex multiplex cytokine analysis kits with ELISA: determinations of a panel of nine cytokines in clinical sample culture supernatants. J Reprod Immunol 2005;66:175–91.

119. Lukaszewski RA, Yates AM, Jackson MC, et al. The pre-symptomatic prediction of sepsis in intensive care unit patients: a pilot study. Clin Vaccine Immunol 2008;15:CVI.0048607:1089–94.

120. Cook NR. Statistical evaluation of prognostic versus diagnostic models: beyond the ROC curve. Clin Chem 2008;54:17–23.

121. Hanley JA, McNeil BJ. The meaning and use of the area under a receiver operating characteristic (ROC) curve. Radiology 1982;143:29–36.

122. Sáenz JJ, Izura JJ, Manrique A, et al. Early prognosis in severe sepsis via analyzing the monocyte immunophenotype. Intensive Care Med 2001;27:970–7.

123. Brauner JS, Rohde LE, Clausell N. Circulating endothelin-1 and tumor necrosis factor-α: early predictors of mortality in patients with septic shock. Intensive Care Med 2000;26:305–13.

124. Torre D, Tambini R, Manfredi M, et al. Circulating levels of FAS/APO-1 in patients with the systemic inflammatory response syndrome. Diagn Microbiol Infect Dis 2003;45:233–6.

125. Ware LB, Conner ER, Matthay MD. von Willebrand factor antigen is an independent marker of poor outcome in patients with early acute lung injury. Crit Care Med 2001;29:2325–31.

126. Ware LB, Eisner MD, Thompson BT, et al. Significance of von Willebrand factor in septic and nonseptic patients with acute lung injury. Am J Respir Crit Care Med 2004;170:766–72.

127. Aalto H, Takala A, Kautiainen H, et al. Laboratory markers of systemic inflammation as predictors of bloodstream infection in acutely ill patients admitted to hospital in medical emergency. Eur J Clin Micriobiol Infect Dis 2004;23:699–704.

128. Varpula M, Pulkki K, Karlsson S, et al. Predictive value of N-terminal pro-brain natriuretic peptide in severe sepsis and septic shock. Crit Care Med 2007;35:233–6.

129. Muller B, Peri G, Doni A, et al. Circulating levels of the long pentraxin PTX3 correlate with severity of infection in critically ill patients. Crit Care Med 2001;29:1404–7.

130. Monneret G, Voirin N, Krawice-Radanne I, et al. Soluble human leukocyte antigen-G5 in septic shock: marked and persisting elevation as a predictor of survival. Crit Care Med 2007;35:1942–7.

131. Borgel D, Clauser S, Bornstain C, et al. Elevated growth-arrest-specific protein 6 plasma levels in patients with severe sepsis. Crit Care Med 2006; 34:219–22.

132. Mesters RM, Flörke N, Ostermann H, et al. Increase of plasminogen activator inhibitor levels predicts outcome of leukocytopenic patients with sepsis. Thromb Haemost 1996;75:902–7.

133. Madoiwa S, Nunomiya S, Ono T, et al. Plasminogen activator inhibitor 1 promotes a poor prognosis in sepsis-induced disseminated intravascular coagulation. Int J Hematol 2006;84:398–405.

134. Pralong G, Calandra T, Glauser MP, et al. Plasminogen activator inhibitor 1: a new prognostic marker in septic shock. Thromb Haemost 1989;61:459–62.

135. Møller HJ, Moestrup SK, Weis N, et al. Macrophage serum markers in pneumococcal bacteremia: prediction of survival by soluble CD163. Crit Care Med 2006;34:2561–6.

136. Christ-Crain M, Morgenthaler NG, Stolz D, et al. Pro-adrenomedullin to predict severity and outcome in community-acquired pneumonia [ISRCTN04176397]. Crit Care 2006;10:R96–103.

137. Christ-Crain M, Morgenthaler NG, Struck J, et al. Mid-regional pro-adrenomedullin as a prognostic marker in sepsis: an observational study. Crit Care 2005;9:R816–824.

138. Oczenski W, Krenn H, Jilch R, et al. HLA-DR as a marker for increased risk for systemic inflammation and septic complications after cardiac surgery. Intensive Care Med 2003;29:1253–7.

139. Lekkou A, Karakantza M, Mouzaki A, et al. Cytokine production and monocyte HLA-DR expression as predictors of outcome for patients with community-acquired severe infections. Clin Diagn Lab Immunol 2004;11:161–7.

140. Novotny AR, Emmanuel K, Ulm K, et al. Blood interleukin 12 as preoperative predictor of fatal postoperative sepsis after neoadjuvant radiochemotherapy. Br J Surg 2006;93:1283–9.

141. De Freitas I, Fernández-Somoza M, Essenfeld-Sekler E, et al. Serum levels of the apoptosis-associated molecules, tumor necrosis factor-α/tumor necrosis factor type-I receptor and Fas/FasL, in sepsis. Chest 2004;125:2238–46.

142. Zakynthinos S, Papanikolaou S, Theodoridis T, et al. Sepsis severity is the major determinant of circulating thrombopoietin levels in septic patients. Crit Care Med 2004;32:1004–10.

143. Siassi M, Riese J, Steffensen P, et al. Mannan-binding lectin and procalcitonin measurement for prediction of postoperative infection. Crit Care 2005; 9:R483–9.

144. Chopin N, Floccard B, Sobas F, et al. Activated partial thromboplastin time waveform analysis: a new tool to detect infection? Crit Care Med 2006;34: 1654–60.

145. Gunter P, Fraunberger P, Appel R, et al. Early prediction of outcome in score-identified, postcardiac surgical patients at high risk for sepsis, using soluble tumor necrosis factor receptor-55 concentrations. Crit Care Med 1996;24:596–600.

146. Chien JY, Jerng JS, Yu CJ, et al. Low serum level of high-density lipoprotein cholesterol is a poor prognostic factor for severe sepsis. Crit Care Med 2005; 33:1688–93.

147. Sakr Y, Reinhart K, Hagel S, et al. Antithrombin levels, morbidity, and mortality in a surgical intensive care unit. Anesth Analg 2007;105: 715–23.

148. Dahl B, Schiødt FV, Ott P, et al. Plasma concentration of Gc-globulin is associated with organ dysfunction and sepsis after injury. Crit Care Med 2003;31:152–6.

149. Müller B, Morgenthaler N, Stolz D, et al. Circulating levels of copeptin, a novel biomarker, in lower respiratory tract infections. Eur J Clin Invest 2007; 37:145–52.

150. Weigand MA, Schmidt H, Pourmahmoud M, et al. Circulating intercellular adhesion molecule-1 as an early predictor of hepatic failure in patients with septic shock. Crit Care Med 1999;27:2656–61.

The Immune System in Critical Illness

John C. Marshall, MD, FRCSC[a,b,c],*, Emmanuel Charbonney, MD[a,b,c],
Patricia Duque Gonzalez, MD[a,b,c]

KEYWORDS

- Sepsis • Innate immunity • Bacteria
- Toll-like receptors • Neutrophils
- Macrophages • Lymphocytes • Coagulation

Multicellular creatures face a daunting series of challenges if they are to survive and persist on this planet. They must feed, grow, and reproduce—processes that mandate an interaction with the surrounding world and, in particular, with other living organisms. At the same time, they must protect themselves from becoming food for others, or more generally, from the adverse consequences of this interaction with the living world. This task falls to a remarkably sophisticated network of humoral and cellular elements collectively known as the immune system.

The immune system includes physical barriers to tissue invasion, an innate response system that can be mobilized within minutes of a new threat, and an adaptive component that requires more time for its initial activation but that, once activated, is characterized by both specificity and memory. The normal function of each of these elements is altered in the critically ill patient, rendering the patient vulnerable both to infection and to the systemic consequences of a dysfunctional defense response.

THE IMMUNE SYSTEM: AN EVOLUTIONARY AND CONCEPTUAL OVERVIEW

An effective immune system has evolved over more than a billion years in response to the fundamental evolutionary imperative: living organisms that are unable to survive long enough to replicate are lost forever from the tree of life. Reproductive survival is more than simply withstanding threats arising from the microbial world. Contrary to earlier theories of the role of the adaptive immune response, the ability to discriminate self from non-self has minimal, if any, utility in promoting reproductive success (although it is the contemporary bane of the transplant surgeon). A more relevant model of immunity stemming from the work of immunologists such as Janeway and Matzinger[1] is that the primary force driving the evolution of immunity is the need to recognize and respond to danger.

Danger takes many forms. It may be invasion of tissue by bacteria, fungi, or viruses, but it also may be the invasion of tissue through traumatic injury—the bite of a predator or the prick of a thorn—or the transformation of normally growing tissues into a cancer. The immune system faces no evolutionary pressure to determine the nature of the threat, only to recognize that a threat is present. Thus the mechanisms of immunity that have evolved do not differ fundamentally in their responses to injured tissue or bacteria. The microbial world has presented humans with the most diverse group of antigenic stimuli, so responses to bacteria are the most complex and numerous in our immunologic repertoire, but they are neither exclusive nor unique. In fact, because bacteria and viruses are also living organisms, their interaction with the eukaryotic world has been particularly complex and, over time, mutually beneficial.

a Interdepartmental Division of Critical Care, St. Michael's Hospital, University of Toronto, 30 Bond Street, Toronto, Ontario, Canada M5B 1W8
b Department of Surgery, St. Michael's Hospital, University of Toronto, 30 Bond Street, Toronto, Ontario, Canada M5B 1W8
c The Li Ka Shing Knowledge Institute, St. Michael's Hospital, University of Toronto, 30 Bond Street, Toronto, Ontario, Canada M5B 1W8
* Corresponding author. Room 4-007, Bond Wing, St. Michael's Hospital, 30 Bond Street, Toronto, Ontario, Canada M5W 1B8.
E-mail address: marshallj@smh.toronto.on.ca (J.C. Marshall).

Clin Chest Med 29 (2008) 605–616
doi:10.1016/j.ccm.2008.08.001

The immune system can be thought of as comprising three elements that arose at differing times during the evolution of life (**Fig. 1**). Physical barriers—the bacterial cell wall or the epithelial barriers of the skin and mucous membranes—are the most primitive form of defense, dating back to the initial evolution of unicellular organisms. As multicellular organisms appeared about 1 billion years ago, new systems to recognize and avert danger—the coagulation and complement cascades, danger receptors, and phagocytic cells—evolved and collectively comprised the innate immune response. With the evolution of bony fishes some 600 million years ago, a third component of immunity emerged, carried out by lymphocytes and known as the "adaptive immune response." These three arms of the immune system support and interact with one other, although it is convenient to consider them separately here.

PHYSICAL BARRIERS TO MICROBIAL INVASION

The physical barriers to invasion by pathogenic micro-organisms include both cells of the host and a complex indigenous microbial flora that exists in symbiosis with the host.

The Endogenous Microbial Flora as a Component of Normal Host Defenses

A normal, healthy human being is made up of approximately 10^{13} mammalian cells and about 250 different types of cells. This same healthy individual harbors 10^{14} microbial cells on mucosal surfaces, representing at least 500 to 1000 different species of organisms and at least two to three times the number of genes expressed in a human being.[2] The normal human is seen quite appropriately as an eukaryotic scaffold for a larger, and genetically more diverse, aggregation of prokaryotic life.[3] The interaction between the micro-organism and the host has defined the evolution of the human innate response to danger. Multicellular organisms have developed complex and highly effective mechanisms to identify and respond to threats from the microbial world. The endogenous bacterial flora, however, also plays multiple key roles in the normal defenses of the mammalian host.

The mucosal surfaces of the healthy individual are carpeted with a complex, indigenous microbial flora. The presence of this flora restricts access to potential mucosal binding sites for exogenous pathogens and so plays a key role in preventing infection with organisms such as *Salmonella*;[4] conversely, when the indigenous flora is disrupted by antibiotics, the host becomes more susceptible to infection with antibiotic-resistant organisms such as *Candida*.[5] Members of the indigenous flora produce a variety of antimicrobial substances that inhibit the growth of other gut organisms and so stabilize patterns of normal flora. They also promote the development and maintenance of the normal intestinal epithelium[6] and of a normal systemic inflammatory response to injury.[7]

Symbiotic host–microbial interactions also occur at the level of the gene. For example, the baculoviral protein p35 can inhibit the programmed cell death, or apoptosis, of virally infected cells and so promotes viral persistence by blocking a key component of normal host defenses. Orthologues of the *p35* gene, however, probably reflecting the incorporation of viral DNA into the mammalian genome, are present in human and other cells as members of a family of proteins known as the inhibitor of apoptosis protein (IAP) family. IAPs inhibit apoptosis, and their expression in inflammatory neutrophils enables the neutrophil

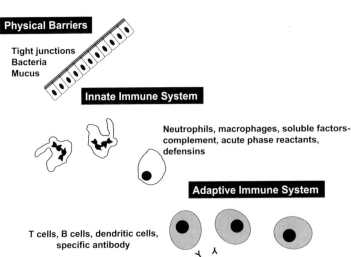

Fig. 1. The immune system can be conceptualized as comprising three main components: the mucocutaneous barriers that separate the internal organs from the external environment, an innate immune system that responds aggressively but nonspecifically to an acute threat, and an adaptive immune system that is delayed in its expression but demonstrates exquisite specificity for its targets and thus results in minimal collateral damage to the host.

Physical Barriers

Tight junctions
Bacteria
Mucus

Innate Immune System

Neutrophils, macrophages, soluble factors-complement, acute phase reactants, defensins

Adaptive Immune System

T cells, B cells, dendritic cells, specific antibody

to survive longer during an acute inflammatory response.[8] Similarly, Nampt, a bacterial protein that enables the micro-organism to synthesize nicotinamide adenine dinucleotide (NAD), has become incorporated into the eukaryotic genome both as an enzyme in a pathway of NAD synthesis and as an anti-apoptotic factor for a variety of cell types.[9]

Perhaps the most remarkable example of the complex and mutually beneficial symbiotic relationships that have arisen between eukaryotes and prokaryotes is the role played in innate immunity by bacterial lipopolysaccharide, or endotoxin. Endotoxin is an intrinsic component of the cell wall of gram-negative bacteria and so is present ubiquitously in the mammalian gut. Although elevated levels of endotoxin induce inflammatory symptoms (and, if levels are high enough, death), the capacity to respond to endotoxin confers protection against opportunistic pathogens such as Candida,[10] and endotoxin triggers the release of cardinal inflammatory mediators such as tumor necrosis factor (TNF) and interleukin (IL)-1 that amplify the host response to bacterial challenge. Indeed, mammals have evolved a dedicated carrier protein for endotoxin, along with a receptor complex that triggers a beneficial innate immune response in the cell, suggesting that endotoxin may be better considered as an exogenous hormone.[11]

Mucosal Barriers

The skin and mucous membranes are the interface between the individual and the external world and are the most important defense against danger in the environment. Microbial invasion normally is prevented by a number of mechanisms. Tight junctions between cells create a physical barrier, and a surface layer of mucous prevents microbial binding to the cell. In the airway, the hairs of the nares filter out bacteria and particulates, and the movement of the cilia serves to propel inhaled particles back to the oropharynx where they are swallowed. Normal gastric acidity kills gram-negative bacteria,[12] and bile contains factors that inhibit the growth of some gram-positive species.[13]

These physical barriers are compromised in the patient in the ICU, often by the injury that precipitated ICU admission and almost invariably by iatrogenic intrusions in the form of devices such as venous or arterial catheters, endotracheal tubes, and urinary catheters. A variety of other ICU interventions—for example, the use of broad-spectrum antimicrobial agents, narcotics, or acid-reduction therapy—further jeopardizes immunity at the mucosal surface.

An endotracheal tube bypasses the anatomic defenses of the upper airway, allowing oropharyngeal secretions to pass into the distal airway and impairing the efficacy of clearance through coughing.[14] The presence of an endotracheal tube decreases mucociliary clearance,[15] and when the intubated patient is nursed in the semirecumbent position to minimize aspiration, mucus flows preferentially toward the distal airways.[16] Moreover the tube itself supports the establishment of colonies of bacteria in biofilms on its surface and so becomes a reservoir for continuing colonization of the tracheobronchial tree.[17]

Mechanical ventilation alters the humidification of the airway and even may promote bacterial overgrowth through epithelial cell acidification induced by cyclic stretch.[18] Experimental studies have shown that injurious ventilation strategies predispose a patient to developing subsequent bacteremia, possibly through stretch-mediated activation of inflammatory pathways.[19]

Other invasive devices such as urinary or central venous catheters provide a conduit for bacteria to reach normally sterile anatomic sites. Micro-organisms that are capable of forming biofilms, including Staphylococcus aureus, coagulase-negative Staphylococci, Pseudomonas, and Candida, are common causes of nosocomial infection in the critically ill patient,[20] in part because they share this property. Microbial colonies within the biofilm serve as a source of organisms that can be shed from the surface of the device, and the biofilm protects the micro-organism from the host's normal antimicrobial defense mechanisms.

The barrier function of the gastrointestinal tract incorporates multiple elements. Digestive enzymes in the oropharynx degrade carbohydrates and proteins into smaller molecules that are less immunogenic. Gastric acid and bile salts exert antibacterial activity,[21] and normal intestinal peristalsis inhibits gut colonization by potential pathogens. Mucus produced by goblet cells found from the nasal cavity to the rectum prevents potential pathogens from accessing binding sites on the gut epithelium; the anaerobic flora of the distal small bowel and colon plays a similar role.[22]

The brush border microvilli of the intestinal epithelial cells inhibit bacterial adhesion, and tight junctions between the cells further prevent bacterial invasion. Intestinal epithelial integrity is preserved further by trefoil factors, reparative proteins secreted by goblet cells, and defensins, which are antimicrobial peptides secreted by Paneth cells.[23] The gut flora provides a continuous immune signal to the colonic epithelium through epithelial Toll-like receptors (TLRs) and acts to suppress an inflammatory reaction and to maintain local homeostasis.[24] The mucosa-associated lymphoid tissue integrates the barrier function of the gut with the activation of an adaptive immune response. For example, dendritic cells penetrate the epithelial monolayer through tight junctions and can sample bacterial antigens on the luminal side.[25]

A complex interaction between the gut epithelium, the innate and adaptive immune system within the gut wall, and the endogenous colonizing flora promotes a state of normal homeostasis; conversely, disruption of any of these three elements can result in disease.[26]

Alterations in patterns of mucosal colonization in critical illness are particularly well described. Johanson and colleagues[27] reported that the oropharynx of the critically ill ventilated patient rapidly becomes colonized with gram-negative bacteria. Others have reported that the stomach and upper small intestine of the critically ill patient similarly is colonized by the same spectrum of micro-organisms that predominate in nosocomial ICU-acquired infection and that proximal gut colonization is associated with systemic infection with the same organism [28,29]

An altered gut flora can produce systemic infection by one of two mechanisms: the aspiration of secretions from the oropharynx and stomach and the translocation of viable organisms across an anatomically intact intestinal mucosa, a process known as "bacterial translocation."[30] Best studied in animal models, the process of bacterial translocation has been documented in a wide variety of human conditions associated with one or more of alterations in the indigenous gut flora, splanchnic hypoperfusion, and local intestinal inflammation (**Table 1**) and probably accounts for many cases of primary bacteremia occurring in critically ill patients. Although the technique has not achieved popularity in North America, the extensive literature on selective digestive tract decontamination (SDD) provides compelling evidence of the importance of bacterial translocation as a mechanism for the acquisition of nosocomial infection in the critically ill patient. SDD entails the administration of oral, nonabsorbed antibiotics that are selectively active against aerobic gram-negative organisms and fungi, leaving the gram-positive and anaerobic flora intact. A systemic antimicrobial agent active against typical community-acquired gram-positive and gram-negative organisms (typically a cephalosporin or a quinolone) is administered for the first 3 or 4 days. The use of SDD is associated with a striking reduction in rates of infections—not only pneumonia, but also bacteremia and urinary tract infections—and a modest but statistically significant reduction in mortality.[31]

Finally, disease can result in changes in host–microbial homeostasis that benefit the bacterial pathogen. It has been reported, for example, that *Pseudomonas aeruginosa* colonizing the gastrointestinal tract up-regulates the virulence factor, Pseudomonas autoinducer, in response to stress in the host communicated through increased release of the host cytokine, hypoxia inducible factor-1α,[32] with the result that host mortality is increased.[33]

INNATE IMMUNITY

Innate immune mechanisms are those that do not require prior exposure to an antigen to elicit activation but instead are mediated by germ line–encoded proteins and by cells that respond to

Table 1
Disorders associated with bacterial translocation in humans

Disorder	Examples
Altered gut flora	*Candida* ingestion Cirrhosis Short bowel syndrome Critical illness
Altered intestinal physiology	Small bowel obstruction Obstructive jaundice
Intestinal inflammation	Inflammatory bowel disease
Intestinal ischemia	Aortic vascular disease Cardiac arrest Cardiopulmonary bypass
Miscellaneous	Trauma Elective laparotomy Home total parenteral nutrition Small bowel transplant

the presence of danger through the activation of a spectrum of nonspecific but potent defenses. These mechanisms have evolved over more than a billion years in response to a constantly changing external environment; as a result, the mechanisms of innate immunity are extraordinarily diverse and include, in addition to myeloid cells that are the primary cellular effectors of innate immunity, a broad spectrum of molecular mediators including the complement and coagulation cascades, eicosanoids, intermediates of oxygen and nitrogen, acute-phase reactants, cytokines, and a host of other proteins.

The human innate immune system is, in a sense, a living record of the history of our interactions with the environment, shaped because evolutionary changes that enable survival in the face of a particular threat became enriched in the human genome, whereas those that resulted in early death were not passed on. For example, the genetic variant of hemoglobin S responsible for sickle cell anemia provides protection against malaria in heterozygotes, accounting for its prevalence in populations of humans who evolved in areas where malaria is endemic. Similarly a variant in a key component of the signaling mechanism that enables cells of the innate immune system to recognize bacteria—a protein known as myelin and lymphocyte protein—is expressed differentially in human populations in relation to the prevalence of tuberculosis, pneumococcal disease, and malaria.[34]

Despite its diversity and complexity, the imperatives of the innate immune system can be summarized as supporting four specific needs:

1. To recognize the presence of a pathogen or other potential threat
2. To modulate the local environment to promote the containment of the threat
3. To eliminate the threat by (in the case of organisms) killing them and neutralizing their toxins
4. To limit the resulting tissue damage and promote the processes of tissue repair

Pathogen Recognition by the Innate Immune System

Multiple proteins of the innate immune system support the recognition of an invading pathogen or, more generally, the recognition of danger in the internal environment.[35] C-reactive protein, for example, was named because it binds specifically to the capsular polysaccharide of *Streptococcus pneumoniae*,[36] and mannose-binding lectin and related lectins bind a variety of pathogens and activate the complement cascade.[37] At least four

families of mammalian innate immune receptors are recognized: TLRs, nucleotide-binding oligomerization domain-like receptors, C-type lectin receptors, and triggering receptors expressed on myeloid cells.

The archetypal mechanism for the recognition of danger involves a family of 11 cell receptors known as TLRs.[38] (The somewhat unusual name for this family of pattern-recognition receptors arose because of their homology to *Toll*, a receptor in the fruit fly *Drosophila melanogaster* that plays a key role in dorsoventral patterning in the embryonic fly and a separate role in conferring antifungal immunity in the adult fly. Its discoverers at the Swiss laboratory where *Toll* was first identified found its role in embryologic development quite remarkable, so they designated this gene by the German word for "cool"—"toll.")[39]

The exquisite complexity of TLR recognition of danger is exemplified in the cellular response to endotoxin or lipopolysaccharide, a key constituent of the cell wall of all gram-negative bacteria (**Fig. 2**). Endotoxin is recognized initially by the plasma protein lipopolysaccharide-binding protein (LBP) and travels in the blood complexed with this protein. At the cell membrane, endotoxin is transferred from LBP to the receptors CD14 and TLR4, and its binding recruits an accessory protein, mystery domain 2 (MD2). This complex of bacterial lipid and host-recognition proteins induces the recruitment of intracellular proteins to the cytoplasmic tail of TLR4, initiating the signaling cascade that leads to new gene expression in the nucleus of the cell.

TLRs recognize conserved molecular patterns that are characteristic of bacteria and viruses (**Table 2**). It is increasingly apparent, however, that TLRs can be activated by endogenous ligands, typically proteins that normally are present intracellularly. Thus TLR activation is not specific for exogenous pathogens but is a more generic response to danger, and TLR ligands often are referred to as "danger-associated molecular patterns," or "DAMPs."

Invading micro-organisms also are recognized through interactions with the proteins of the complement cascade. Complement can be activated through one of three pathways: the classic pathway that is initiated by gram-negative bacteria, some viruses, and C-reactive protein; the alternate pathway initiated by a number of bacteria and fungi; and the mannose-binding lectin pathway that is activated specifically by organisms expressing mannose on the cell surface.[40] Activation of the complement cascade results in multiple effects, including the production of inflammatory mediators by C5a, opsonization of microbes by

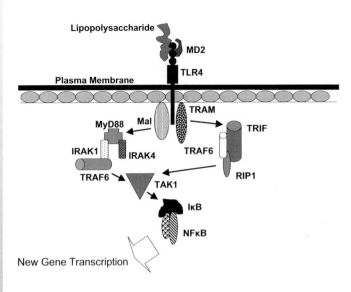

Fig. 2. Toll-like receptors interact with conserved molecular patterns characteristic of micro-organisms or of endogenous danger signals such as heat shock proteins. Their engagement results in the recruitment of adaptor proteins that activate MyD88-dependent and MyD88-independent intracellular signaling cascades. Ultimately these converge on the protein IκB, which maintains the transcription factor nuclear factor kappa B (NFκB) in an inactive state in the cytoplasm. Phosphorylation of IκB causes it to dissociate from NFκB, enabling NFκB to translocate from the cytoplasm to the nucleus and to initiate the increased transcription of key inflammatory genes. IκB, inhibitor of kappa β; IRAK1, interleukin-1 receptor-associated kinase; RIP1, receptor-interacting protein 1; TAK1, TGF-activated kinase 1; TRIF, TIR-domain-containing adapter inducing inteferon β; TRAM, TRIF-related adapter molecule.

C5b enabling their phagocytosis by macrophages and neutrophils, and the formation of membrane attack complex by the activation of C5 through C9 resulting in direct injury to the microbial cell wall.

The innate immune system uses a small number of germ line–encoded receptors to detect a limited set of highly conserved ligands. As a consequence, diverse insults can trigger similar cellular responses. Pattern recognition receptors rapidly detect pathogen molecules within the microenvironment of infection, and an innate response is initiated within minutes.

Optimizing the Local Environment to Support Host Defenses

Engagement of a TLR results in the recruitment of a number of adapter proteins and induces an intracellular signaling cascade that leads to the activation and nuclear translocation of key transcription

Table 2
Molecular patterns recognized by Toll-like receptors (TLRs) as being associated with danger

Danger Signal	Relevant TLR	Ligands
Gram-negative bacteria	TLR4	Endotoxin
	TLR2	Bacterial lipoprotein
	TLR5	Flagellin
Gram-positive bacteria	TLR2	Lipoteichoic acid
	TLR5	Peptidoglycan
		Flagellin
Mycobacteria	TLR2	Lipoarabinomannan
	TLR1	*Mycobacterium leprae* lipopeptide
Fungi	TLR4	Mannan
	TLR2	Zymosan
Bacterial DNA	TLR9	CpG DNA
Viruses	TLR3	Double-stranded RNA
	TLR7/8	Single-stranded RNA
	TLR4	Coxsackie virus
	TLR9	Herpes simplex
Endogenous ligands	TLR2	HSP60, HSP70, gp96
	TLR4	Oxidized phospholipids Heparan sulfate β defensin Surfactant protein A Heme HMGB1

Abbreviations: gp, glycoprotein; HMGBI, high mobility group box 1; HSP, heat shock protein.

factors such as nuclear factor kappa B (**Fig. 2**). The cellular consequences are profound. Exposure of a healthy human volunteer to lipopolysaccharide signaling through TLR4 results in the differential expression of more than 3700 genes in circulating leukocytes;[41] this response supports the localization of inflammatory cells at the site of the infectious challenge and the efficient killing and clearing of the invading micro-organisms.

The role in antibacterial immunity of each of the many hundreds of distinct host-derived compounds that are released following TLR activation is complex and poorly understood. For example, TNF has been shown to increase the growth of *Escherichia coli* in vitro,[42] whereas neutralization of TNF has variable effects on survival in experimental models of infectious challenge, increasing survival when the challenge is endotoxin or a gram-negative organism but reducing survival when the challenge species is *S. pneumoniae*, *Mycobacterium tuberculosis*, or *Candida*.[43] The activity of this network of endogenous mediators of innate immunity probably is understood more accurately as altering the local environment of infection—and the systemic response of the patient—to favor the activity of cellular host defenses.

Fixed tissue macrophages, found in abundance at sites of potential pathogen entry such as the lung, liver, peritoneum, or skin, play a central role in orchestrating the early host response to an invading pathogen. Macrophages release a number of pro-inflammatory mediators following TLR activation, in particular IL-1 and TNF. These products can act both locally and systemically. Upregulation of inducible nitric oxide synthase in the adjacent microvasculature results in increased synthesis and release of nitric oxide, and therefore in increased local vasodilatation, and produces the characteristic "rubor" of local inflammation. Cytokine-induced changes in endothelial permeability result in the interstitial leakage of protein-rich fluid, producing the "tumor" of inflammation and facilitating the passage of phagocytic cells from the vasculature into the site of microbial challenge. IL-8 from the macrophage is a potent neutrophil chemoattractant that aids in the directed migration of neutrophils into an infectious focus. Other macrophage products such as IL-10, vascular endothelial growth factor, and transforming growth factor-β (TGFβ) play an important role in the resolution of the local inflammatory response and in the initiation of tissue repair.

Host-derived cytokines also have potent effects on systemic homeostasis. A variety of cytokines can act on the hypothalamus to alter the thermoregulatory set point and induce fever, although fever also can be induced by the engagement of TLRs within the hypothalamus.[44] IL-6 acting on the liver induces an altered pattern of hepatocyte protein synthesis known as the "acute-phase response,"[45] whereas IL-1 induces hypoferremia,[46] depriving proliferating bacteria of a co-factor essential for growth.

Microbial Killing and Toxin Neutralization

The task of effectively overcoming the potentially deleterious consequences of an invading pathogen is accomplished primarily through the cellular effectors of innate immunity.

Polymorphonuclear neutrophils are the first cellular elements to be recruited to the site of an infectious challenge, exiting the circulation into the infected tissue in response to chemotactic signals generated by the invading bacteria and by macrophage products such as IL-8. Opsonization of a bacterium by complement or specific immunoglobulin enables it to interact with specific cell-surface receptors and leads to uptake of the organism by phagocytosis. Within the neutrophil, effective microbial killing is accomplished by both oxidative and nonoxidative systems.[47]

Oxidative killing occurs through the generation of highly reactive oxygen intermediates through the activity of nicotinamide adenine dinucleotide phosphate (NADPH) oxidase. NADPH oxidase is a complex of seven cytoplasmic proteins that is assembled at the membrane of the phagosome following neutrophil activation. The complex catalyzes the oxidation of NADPH to $NADP^+$ and the simultaneous reduction of molecular oxygen to superoxide anion (O_2^-). The superoxide anion, in turn, serves as the substrate for additional highly reactive molecular species including hydrogen peroxide, hydroxyl radical, hypochlorous acid, and, upon reaction with nitric oxide, peroxynitrite (**Fig. 3**).

Oxygen-independent antimicrobial mechanisms arise through the actions of preformed proteins contained in cytoplasmic granules. These proteins include proteolytic enzymes such a elastase, heparanase, myeloperoxidase, and proteinase 3; antimicrobial peptides such as defensins, cathepsins, and lysozyme; and membrane receptor proteins such as CD11b and the complement receptor, CR1.[48] The granule protein, bactericidal permeability-increasing protein, can bind and neutralize endotoxin.[49] Other plasma proteins, including high-density lipoprotein, can bind free endotoxin, and the enzymealkaline phosphatase has been shown to dephosphorylate the endotoxin molecule, reducing its intrinsic toxicity and so protecting the gut mucosa and liver from the high

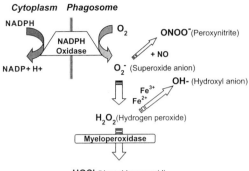

Fig. 3. Generation of reactive oxygen species by the NADPH oxidase. The seven-protein complex of the NADPH oxidase transfers an electron from NADPH to molecular oxygen, generating a superoxide anion. The superoxide anion, in turn, is converted into a series of reactive oxygen intermediates that kill microorganisms by causing structural damage to the cell membrane.

ambient levels of endotoxin within the gastrointestinal tract.[50]

An additional mechanism of bacterial killing by the neutrophil has been described recently. Following the death of the neutrophil by programmed cell death or apoptosis (a process that can be induced by the phagocytosis of a microorganism),[51] the DNA of the cell is extruded to create filamentous structures called "neutrophil extracellular traps" that ensnare and kill microorganisms.[52] Plasma from septic patients has been shown to induce platelet–neutrophil interactions through platelet TLR4 and, as a consequence, to induce the formation of neutrophil extracellular traps.[53]

Limiting Inadvertent Bystander Injury

Innate immunity is rapid in its activation and potent in its expression but nonspecific in its targets; as a consequence, bystander injury to host tissues is a common sequela.[54] Multiple mechanisms have evolved to limit this injury.

Activation of the coagulation cascade results in the expression of tissue factor and local deposition of fibrin, creating an abscess and walling off a focus of infection and the resulting host response from otherwise sterile body tissues.[55] Serine protease inhibitors such as α-1 antitrypsin block the effects of proteases produced by leukocytes.[56] Inhibitory M2 macrophages synthesize and release an array of anti-inflammatory mediators such as IL-10 and the IL-1 receptor antagonist that block or counteract the effects of pro-inflammatory cytokines.[57]

A neutrophil-mediated inflammatory response is limited by the programmed cell death (apoptosis) of the neutrophil. Circulating neutrophils in the healthy individual survive for no more than 6 to 8 hours before dying an apoptotic death and being removed by phagocytic cells of the reticuloendothelial system.[58] This constitutive apoptotic program can be subverted following exposure to a number of microbial products or host inflammatory mediators, with the result that the neutrophil survives longer in an activated state.[59] Intriguingly, the phagocytosis of bacteria by the neutrophil not only promotes the apoptotic death of the neutrophil but limits local tissue injury and, in an experimental model of lung injury produced by ischemia/reperfusion injury, improves survival.[60]

ADAPTIVE IMMUNITY

The adaptive immune system is an evolutionarily more recent development, appearing with the emergence of fishes more than 550 million years ago. Activated by products of cells of the innate immune system, adaptive immunity provides a measure of specificity that is not apparent in the adaptive immune response (**Table 3**). Moreover, in contrast to innate immunity, adaptive immunity can elicit either responsiveness or tolerance to an immunologic stimulus. The adaptive immune system has received more attention from immunologists.[61] Its role in antibacterial immunity is less well defined, and its contribution to the pathogenesis of sepsis—because of the high degree of specificity it shows toward its targets—is less compelling, although multiple derangements in adaptive immune responsiveness characteristically are encountered.

Adaptive immunity is induced following the processing of antigens that are not native to the host by antigen-presenting cells, in particular dendritic cells.[62] Dendritic cells, derived from circulating monocytes, take up proteins, degrading them into peptides that are expressed, in association with major histocompatibility complex molecules, on the dendritic cell surface. These processed antigens are capable of binding specific T-cell receptors, resulting in clonal expansion of the particular T-cell population.[63]

Several distinct subpopulations of T cells are recognized. T helper 1 (T_H1) cells are activated by IL-12 and express a panel of proinflammatory cytokines, including interferon-γ, TNF-β, and IL-2, that activate macrophages to enhanced antimicrobial activity. T_H2 cells, in contrast, are activated by IL-4, and release predominantly anti-inflammatory cytokines, including IL-10, IL-13, and TGFβ. Recently, an additional population of T cells,

Table 3
The innate and adaptive immune systems

Characteristic	Innate Immune System	Adaptive Immune System
Origins	Ancient	With evolution of bony fishes
Specificity	Nonspecific pattern recognition	Recognition of specific antigens
Activation	Rapid	Delayed
Consequences	Response to stimulus	Response or tolerance
Regulation	Cytokines and other host mediators	Cytokines and other host mediators
Soluble effectors	Complement, acute-phase reactants	Antibody
Cellular effectors	Myeloid cells: neutrophils and macrophages	T and B lymphocytes
Protection	Local	Systemic
Effects on host	Altered homeostasis Bystandertissue injury	No effects on homeostasis Minimal injury
Capacity for memory	None; encoded in genome	Key feature

designated "T$_H$17" cells, has been identified. T$_H$17 cells are induced by IL-6 and TGFβ and maintained by IL-23. They produce the cytokine, IL-17, that has been shown to play a central role in host responses to organisms such as *Klebsiella*, *Citrobacter*, and *Candida* and in the promotion of abscess formation.[64]

B lymphocytes express specific immunoglobulin as the B-cell receptor on their cell surfaces. Binding of an antigen to the expressed immunoglobulin triggers clonal expansion and secretion of specific antibody against the antigen. The immunoglobulin molecule is a glycoprotein consisting of a constant region that binds dedicated Fc receptors on phagocytic cells and a variable region that represents the antigen-recognition site of the molecule. Five classes of immunoglobulin are recognized on the basis of the structure of the constant region: IgG, IgM, IgA, IgE, and IgD.[65] Binding of an antigen by immunoglobulin serves to opsonize the antigen for phagocytosis by cells of the innate immune system.

ALTERED IMMUNITY IN THE CRITICALLY ILL PATIENT

Critical illness is associated with a broad spectrum of immunologic derangements that defy simple characterization. Competing conceptual models variously characterize the immune response of the critically ill patient as excessively activated or hyporesponsive;[66,67] in truth it is both simultaneously.

Physical barriers in the critically ill patient are breached by invasive devices, surgical or traumatic wounds, and iatrogenic factors such as pressure sores or ventilator-induced lung injury, facilitating invasive infection by the characteristic spectrum of ICU pathogens. Alterations in patterns of oropharyngeal and gut colonization, in concert with the disruption of mucosal barrier function, further support the acquisition of nosocomial infection through the process of bacterial translocation.

The innate immune system in sepsis shows evidence of both excessive activation and hyporesponsiveness. Levels of pro-inflammatory cytokines such as IL-6, TNF, and IL-1 are characteristically elevated,[68] but so are levels of anti-inflammatory cytokines such as IL-10[69] and the IL-1 receptor antagonist.[70] Circulating neutrophils show phenotypic features of activation including enhanced spontaneous respiratory burst activity and inhibition of apoptosis,[71,72] but they are less responsive to stimulation by microbial products[73] and manifest impaired chemotaxis in response to chemoattractant stimuli.[74]

Alterations in adaptive immune responses also are common in sepsis. Monocyte expression of HLA-DR is decreased,[75] and the number of circulating dendritic cells is reduced.[76] The number of dendritic cells in the spleen is reduced,[77] and the apoptosis of lymphocytes is increased.[78] Global T-cell responsiveness is typically reduced, reflected in impaired skin test reactivity to recall antigens in vivo[79] and in impaired lymphocyte proliferation to mitogens in vitro.[80] The generation of a specific antibody response to a T-cell–dependent antigen is impaired,[81] whereas the response to a T-cell–independent antigen is preserved or even enhanced.[82]

SUMMARY

The immune response to infection is an immensely complex process, shaped by more than 1 billion years of evolution and involving a diverse network of cells and molecular mediators. Life-threatening infection results in an equally complex series of derangements, whose evolution, at least in animal models, can be linked plausibly to adverse outcome. It is a tempting but egregious oversimplification to try to characterize these derangements as global defects of excessive or inadequate function; the very modest benefits associated with experimental interventions to modulate these defects attest to the inadequacy of such conceptual models.[83]

Altered immune responsiveness in the critically ill patient unquestionably shapes the clinical course of sepsis, however, and the possibility that unfolding biologic insights might be translated into treatments to reduce the morbidity and mortality of the most common complication of critical illness continues to tantalize.

REFERENCES

1. Matzinger P. The danger model: a renewed sense of self. Science 2002;296(5566):301–5.
2. Lederberg J. Infectious history. Science 2000; 288(5464):287–93.
3. Savage DC. Microbial ecology of the gastrointestinal tract. Annu Rev Med 1977;31:107–33.
4. Hudault S, Guignot J, Servin AL. Escherichia coli strains colonising the gastrointestinal tract protect germfree mice against Salmonella typhimurium infection. Gut 2001;49(1):47–55.
5. Charles PE, Dalle F, Aube H, et al. Candida spp. colonization significance in critically ill medical patients: a prospective study. Intensive Care Med 2005;31(3): 393–400.
6. Hooper LV, Gordon JI. Commensal host-bacterial relationships in the gut. Science 2001;292(5519): 1115–8.
7. Souza DG, Viera AT, Soares AC, et al. The essential role of the intestinal microbiota in facilitating acute inflammatory responses. J Immunol 2004;173(6): 4137–46.
8. O'Neill AJ, Doyle BT, Molloy E, et al. Gene expression profile of inflammatory neutrophils: alterations in the inhibitors of apoptosis proteins during spontaneous and delayed apoptosis. Shock 2004;21(6): 512–8.
9. Luk T, Malam Z, Marshall JC. Pre-B cell colony-enhancing factor (PBEF)/visfatin: a novel mediator of innate immunity. J Leukoc Biol 2008;83(4):804–16.
10. Netea MG, Van Der Graaf CA, Vonk AG, et al. The role of toll-like receptor (TLR) 2 and TLR4 in the host defense against disseminated candidiasis. J Infect Dis 2002;185(10):1483–9.
11. Marshall JC. Lipopolysaccharide: an endotoxin or an exogenous hormone? Clin Infect Dis 2005; 41(Suppl 7):S470–80.
12. Giannella RA, Broitman SA, Zamcheck N. Gastric acid barrier to ingested microorganisms in man: studies in vivo and in vitro. Gut 1972;13:251–6.
13. Begley M, Gahan GC, Hill C. The interaction between bacteria and bile. FEMS Microbiol Rev 2005; 29(4):625–51.
14. Young PJ, Pakeerathan S, Blunt MC, et al. A low-volume, low-pressure tracheal tube cuff reduces pulmonary aspiration. Crit Care Med 2006;34(3): 632–9.
15. Sackner MA, Hirsch J, Epstein S. Effect of cuffed endotracheal tubes on tracheal mucous velocity. Chest 1975;68(6):774–7.
16. Bassi GL, Zanella A, Cressoni M, et al. Following tracheal intubation, mucus flow is reversed in the semirecumbent position: possible role in the pathogenesis of ventilator-associated pneumonia. Crit Care Med 2008;36(2):518–25.
17. Adair CG, Gorman SP, Feron BM, et al. Implications of endotracheal tube biofilm for ventilator-associated pneumonia. Intensive Care Med 1999;25(10): 1072–6.
18. Pugin J, Dunn-Siegrist I, Dufour J, et al. Cyclic stretch of human lung cells induces an acidification and promotes bacterial growth. Am J Respir Cell Mol Biol 2008;38(3):362–70.
19. Lin CY, Zhang H, Cheng KC, et al. Mechanical ventilation may increase susceptibility to the development of bacteremia. Crit Care Med 2003;31(5): 1429–34.
20. Vincent JL, Sakr Y, Sprung CL, et al. Sepsis in European intensive care units: results of the SOAP study. Crit Care Med 2006;34(2):344–53.
21. Marshall JC. The gastrointestinal flora and its alterations in critical illness. Curr Opin Crit Care 1999; 5:119–25.
22. Van Der Waaij D. The ecology of the human intestine and its consequences for overgrowth by pathogens such as Clostridium difficile. Annu Rev Microbiol 1989;43:69–87.
23. Dann SM, Eckmann L. Innate immune defenses in the intestinal tract. Curr Opin Gastroenterol 2007; 23(2):115–20.
24. Lee J, Mo JH, Katakura K, et al. Maintenance of colonic homeostasis by distinctive apical TLR9 signalling in intestinal epithelial cells. Nat Cell Biol 2006; 8(12):1327–36.
25. Rescigno M, Urbano M, Valzasina B, et al. Dendritic cells express tight junction proteins and penetrate gut epithelial monolayers to sample bacteria. Nat Immunol 2001;2(4):361–7.
26. McCracken VJ, Lorenz RG. The gastrointestinal ecosystem: a precarious alliance among epithelium, immunity and microbiota. Cell Microbiol 2001;3(1):1–11.
27. Johanson WG, Pierce AK, Sanford JP. Changing pharyngeal bacterial flora of hospitalized patients. N Engl J Med 1969;281:1137–40.

28. Du Moulin GC, Hedley-Whyte J, Paterson DG, et al. Aspiration of gastric bacteria in antacid treated patients: a frequent cause of postoperative colonisation of the airway. Lancet 1982;1:242–5.

29. Marshall JC, Christou NV, Meakins JL. The gastrointestinal tract. The "undrained abscess" of multiple organ failure. Ann Surg 1993;218:111–9.

30. Wells CL, Maddaus MA, Simmons RL. Proposed mechanisms for the translocation of intestinal bacteria. Rev Infect Dis 1988;10:958–79.

31. Nathens AB, Marshall JC. Selective decontamination of the digestive tract in surgical patients. Arch Surg 1999;134:170–6.

32. Patel NJ, Zaborina O, Wu L, et al. Recognition of intestinal epithelial HIF-1alpha activation by Pseudomonas aeruginosa. Am J Physiol Gastrointest Liver Physiol 2007;292(1):G134–42.

33. Wu L, Estrada O, Zaborina O, et al. Recognition of host immune activation by Pseudomonas aeruginosa. Science 2005;309(5735):774–7.

34. Khor CC, Chapman SJ, Vannberg FO, et al. A Mal functional variant is associated with protection against invasive pneumococcal disease, bacteremia, malaria and tuberculosis. Nat Genet 2007; 39(4):523–8.

35. Akira S, Uematsu S, Takeuchi O. Pathogen recognition and innate immunity. Cell 2006;124(4): 783–801.

36. Mold C, Nakayama S, Holzer TJ, et al. C-reactive protein is protective against Streptococcus pneumoniae infection in mice. J Exp Med 1981; 154:1703–8.

37. Fujita T, Matsushita M, Endo Y. The lectin-complement pathway—its role in innate immunity and evolution. Immunol Rev 2004;198:185–202.

38. Akira S, Takeda K, Kaisho T. Toll-like receptors: critical proteins linking innate and acquired immunity. Nat Immunol 2001;2(8):675–80.

39. Anderson KV, Jürgens G, Nüsslein-Vollhard C. Establishment of dorsal-ventral polarity in the Drosophila embryo: genetic studies on the role of the Toll gene product. Cell 1985;42(3):779–89.

40. Walport MJ. Complement. N Engl J Med 2001; 344(14):1058–66.

41. Calvano SE, Xiao W, Richards DR, et al. A network-based analysis of systemic inflammation in humans. Nature 2005;437(7061):1032–7.

42. Lee JH, Del Sorbo L, Khine AA, et al. Modulation of bacterial growth by tumor necrosis factor-alpha in vitro and in vivo. Am J Respir Crit Care Med 2003; 168(12):1462–70.

43. Lorente JA, Marshall JC. Neutralization of tumor necrosis factor (TNF) in pre-clinical models of sepsis. Shock 2005;24(Suppl 1):107–19.

44. Dinarello CA. Infection, fever, and exogenous and endogenous pyrogens: some concepts have changed. J Endotoxin Res 2004;10(4):201–22.

45. Suffredini AF, Fantuzzi G, Badolato R, et al. New insights into the biology of the acute phase response. J Clin Immunol 1999;19(4):203–14.

46. Dinarello CA. Biological basis for interleukin-1 in disease. Blood 1996;87:2095–147.

47. Marshall JC. Neutrophils in the pathogenesis of sepsis. Crit Care Med 2005;33(Suppl 12):S502–5.

48. Faurschou M, Borregaard N. Neutrophil granules and secretory vesicles in inflammation. Microbes Infect 2003;5:1317–27.

49. Elsbach P. The bactericidal/permeability-increasing protein (BPI) in antibacterial host defense. J Leukoc Biol 1998;64(1):14–8.

50. Tuin A, Huizinga-Van der Vlag A, van Loenen-Weemaes AM, et al. On the role and fate of LPS-dephosphorylating activity in the rat liver. Am J Physiol Gastrointest Liver Physiol 2006;290(2): G377–85.

51. Watson RWG, Redmond HP, Wang JH, et al. Neutrophils undergo apoptosis following ingestion of Escherichia coli. J Immunol 1996;156:3986–92.

52. Brinkmann V, Zychlinsky A. Beneficial suicide: why neutrophils die to make NETs. Nat Rev Microbiol 2007;5(8):577–82.

53. Clark SR, Ma AC, Taverner SA, et al. Platelet TLR4 activates neutrophil extracellular traps to ensnare bacteria in septic blood. Nat Med 2007;13(4): 463–9.

54. Smith JA. Neutrophils, host defense, and inflammation: a double-edged sword. J Leukoc Biol 1994; 56:672–86.

55. Marshall JC. Inflammation, coagulopathy, and the pathogenesis of the multiple organ dysfunction syndrome. Crit Care Med 2001;29(Suppl):S99–106.

56. Könlein T, Welte T. Alpha-1 antitrypsin deficiency: pathogenesis, clinical presentation, diagnosis, and treatment. Am J Med 2008;121(1):3–9.

57. Meneghin A, Hogaboam CM. Infectious disease, the innate immune response, and fibrosis. J Clin Invest 2007;117(3):530–8.

58. Savill JS, Wyllie AH, Henson JE, et al. Macrophage phagocytosis of aging neutrophils in inflammation. J Clin Invest 1989;83:865–75.

59. Marshall JC, Malam Z, Jia SH. Modulating neutrophil apoptosis. Sepsis: new insights, new therapies. Chichester (UK): John Wiley & Sons; 2007. p. 53–72.

60. Sookhai S, Wang JJ, McCourt M, et al. A novel therapeutic strategy for attenuating neutrophil-mediated lung injury in vivo. Ann Surg 2002;235(2): 285–91.

61. Beutler B. Innate immunity: an overview. Mol Immunol 2004;40(12):845–59.

62. Steinman RM, Banchereau J. Taking dendritic cells into medicine. Nature 2007;449(7161):419–26.

63. Trombetta ES, Mellman I. Cell biology of antigen processing in vitro and in vivo. Annu Rev Immunol 2005; 23:975–1028.

64. Korn T, Oukka M, Kuchroo V, et al. Th17 cells: effector T cells with inflammatory properties. Semin Immunol 2007;19(6):362–71.

65. Delves PJ, Roitt IM. The immune system. First of two parts. N Engl J Med 2000;343(1):37–49.

66. Bone RC. Sir Isaac Newton, sepsis, SIRS, and CARS. Crit Care Med 1996;24(7):1125–8.

67. Hotchkiss RS, Karl IE. The pathophysiology and treatment of sepsis. N Engl J Med 2003;348(2):238–50.

68. Casey LC, Balk RA, Bone RC. Plasma cytokines and endotoxin levels correlate with survival in patients with the sepsis syndrome. Ann Intern Med 1993;119:771–8.

69. Taniguchi T, Koido Y, Aiboshi J, et al. Change in the ratio of interleukin-6 to interleukin-10 predicts a poor outcome in patients with systemic inflammatory response syndrome. Crit Care Med 1999;27(7):1262–4.

70. Marie C, Muret J, Fitting C, et al. Interleukin-1 receptor antagonist production during infectious and noninfectious systemic inflammatory response syndrome. Crit Care Med 2000;28(7):2277–82.

71. Jimenez MF, Watson RWG, Parodo J, et al. Dysregulated expression of neutrophil apoptosis in the systemic inflammatory response syndrome (SIRS). Arch Surg 1997;132:1263–70.

72. Taneja R, Parodo J, Kapus A, et al. Delayed neutrophil apoptosis in sepsis is associated with maintenance of mitochondrial transmembrane potential ($\Delta\Psi$M) and reduced caspase-9 activity. Crit Care Med 2004;32(7):1460–9.

73. Romaschin AD, Foster DM, Walker PM, et al. Let the cells speak: neutrophils as biologic markers of the inflammatory response. Sepsis 1998;2(2):119–25.

74. Arraes SM, Freitas MS, da Silva SV, et al. Impaired neutrophil chemotaxis in sepsis associates with GRK expression and inhibition of actin assembly and tyrosine phosphorylation. Blood 2006;108(9):2906–13.

75. Docke WD, Randow F, Syrbe U, et al. Monocyte deactivation in septic patients: restoration by IFN-gamma treatment. Nature Med 1997;3(6):678–81.

76. Guisset O, Dilhuydy MS, Thiébaut R, et al. Decrease in circulating dendritic cells predicts fatal outcome in septic shock. Intensive Care Med 2007;33(1):148–52.

77. Hotchkiss RS, Tinsley KW, Swanson PE, et al. Depletion of dendritic cells, but not macrophages, in patients with sepsis. J Immunol 2002;168(5):2493–500.

78. Hotchkiss RS, Swanson PE, Freeman BD, et al. Apoptotic cell death in patients with sepsis, shock, and multiple organ dysfunction. Crit Care Med 1999;27(7):1230–51.

79. Christou NV, Meakins JL, Gordon J, et al. The delayed hypersensitivity response and host resistance in surgical patients. Ann Surg 1995;222:534–48.

80. Keane RM, Birmingham W, Shatney CM, et al. Prediction of sepsis in the multitraumatic patient by assays of lymphocyte responsiveness. Surg Gynecol Obstet 1983;156:163–7.

81. Nohr CW, Christou NV, Broadhead M, et al. Failure of humoral immunity in surgical patients. Surg Forum 1983;34:127–9.

82. Nohr CW, Latter DA, Meakins JL, et al. In vivo and in vitro humoral immunity in surgical patients: antibody response to pneumococcal polysaccharide. Surgery 1986;100:229–38.

83. Marshall JC. Sepsis: rethinking the approach to clinical research. J Leukoc Biol 2008;83(3):471–82.

The Compensatory Anti-inflammatory Response Syndrome (CARS) in Critically Ill Patients

Nicholas S. Ward, MD[a],*, Brian Casserly, MD[a], Alfred Ayala, PhD[b]

KEYWORDS

- Sepsis
- Compensatory anti-inflammatory response syndrome
- Anergy • Systemic inflammatory response syndrome
- Anti-inflammatory • Human leukocyte antigen

The acronym CARS stands for the compensatory anti-inflammatory response syndrome and was coined in a 1996 paper by Bone to help describe an immunologic phenomenon that increasingly was noticed to occur in sepsis.[1] Like its precursor, the systemic inflammatory response syndrome (SIRS), CARS is a complex and incompletely defined pattern of immunologic responses to severe infection. The difference was that while SIRS was a proinflammatory syndrome that seemed tasked with killing infectious organisms through activation of the immune system, CARS was a systemic deactivation of the immune system tasked with restoring homeostasis from an inflammatory state. Moreover, it has become apparent that CARS is not simply the cessation of SIRS, it can exist separately from SIRS. Additionally, it has a distinct set of cytokines and cellular responses and may have a powerful influence on clinical outcomes in sepsis.

BACKGROUND/HISTORY

The studies that led to this concept came from two different streams of medical research, one that was new at the time of Bone's article and one quite old.

The new information to which Bone referred in his paper was the large set of data that recently had emerged from numerous studies in which agents that blocked inflammation were used in human sepsis patients.[2] In stark contrast to the animal data, the human studies showed poor efficacy of these agents and even suggested that harm could be done in some cases. Bone hypothesized that a powerful anti-inflammatory response already existed to balance the destructive killing of the proinflammatory response and that agents that upset the balance too far in either direction could lead to death, either through uncontrolled inflammation, or failure to defend against infectious organisms.

This concept of autoimmunosuppression was not new, however. It had existed in the medical literature for many decades, largely in the surgical and burn literature. Doctors in these fields long had observed that massive tissue injury such as that caused by burns or trauma made patients more susceptible to infections. It soon was recognized that many of these patients were anergic, indicating impaired lymphocyte function. Much research followed in the 1970s and 1980s trying to characterize the cause and nature of this impaired immunity.[3–7] In the decades that

[a] Division of Pulmonary, Critical Care, and Sleep Medicine, The Warren Alpert Medical School of Brown University, 593 Eddy Street, APC 707, Providence, RI 02912, USA
[b] Division of Surgical Research, Department of Surgery, The Warren Alpert Medical School of Brown University, Providence, RI 02912, USA
* Corresponding author.
E-mail address: nicholas_ward@brown.edu (N.S. Ward).

Clin Chest Med 29 (2008) 617–625
doi:10.1016/j.ccm.2008.06.010
0272-5231/08/$ – see front matter © 2008 Elsevier Inc. All rights reserved.

have followed, much has been learned about the mechanisms of the body's anti-inflammatory response, and it is clear that the immunosuppression of sepsis described by Bone is likely another form of that previously described. The term CARS, as used today, usually reflects all autoimmunosuppression caused by a major insult such as sepsis, burns, or tissue injury. This article reviews the literature on CARS, focusing on the major lines of inquiry in human and animal, research and discusses some of the possible therapeutic benefits this research may generate in the future.

WHAT DEFINES THE COMPENSATORY ANTI-INFLAMMATORY RESPONSE SYNDROME?

To better understand CARS, it is helpful to understand what responses characterize the proinflammatory state that precedes it. It now is known that inflammation can be triggered in two main ways, either by infections with pathogens like bacteria, or by the products of tissue destruction. The innate immune system describes a network of immune cells and their surface receptors designed to recognize and react to either dead tissue or pathogens. When elements of either of these encounter certain lymphocytes or monocytes, they bind to pre-existing receptors and cause activation (lymphocytes) or are ingested and then presented on cell surface receptors to activate other cells (monocytes). What follows is an expansion and activation of several immune cell lines such as polymorphonucleocytes (PMNs) and B lymphocytes stimulated by the proinflammatory cytokines interleukin (IL)-1 and tumor necrosis factor (TNF). The presence of these cytokines also leads to other clinical manifestations of infection such as fever, capillary leak, vasodilation, and the expression of heat shock proteins from the liver.[8]

The CARS response essentially reverses many of these processes and has been characterized over the last several decades to include:

> Cutaneous anergy
> Reduction of lymphocytes by means of apoptosis
> Decreased cytokine response of monocytes to stimulation
> Decreased numbers of human leukocyte antigen (HLA) antigen-presenting receptors on monocytes
> Expression of cytokines such as IL-10 that suppress TNF expression (**Box 1**)

Much research suggests that the clinical effect of this has a profound impact on patient outcomes. Indeed clinicians long have noted that

---

Box 1
Characterization of compensatory anti-inflammatory response syndrome

Cellular/molecular elements

Lymphocyte dysfunction (ie, reduced proliferative and/or type 1 helper T-cell [Th1] cytokine production in response-defined antigens or specific T-cell stimuli)

Lymphocyte Apoptosis

Down-regulation of monocyte HLA receptors

Monocyte deactivation (ie, reduced Th1/proinflammatory cytokine production in response stimuli)

IL-10 production

Transforming growth factor-beta production

Prostaglandin E2 production

Clinical elements

Cutaneous anergy

Hypothermia

Leukopenia

Susceptibility to infection

Failure to clear infection

---

many people who succumb from sepsis die after the initial proinflammatory insult has ceased, often from a second infection. Additionally, many patients who have sepsis, especially those who have poor pre-existing health, seem never to mount the inflammatory response that should characterize infection, instead presenting with low leukocyte counts and hypothermia (**Fig. 1**). This article discusses some of the major studies that led to current knowledge of CARS and what may be coming in the future.

Lymphocytes in Compensatory Anti-inflammatory Response Syndrome

Lymphocytes play a central role in modulating the sepsis response. This is highlighted by altered proinflammatory immune response and increased mortality, after polymicrobial septic challenge in mice lacking both T- and B-cells.[9] Their importance relates to their capacity to interact with the innate and adaptive immune responses and their ability to coordinate, amplify, and attenuate the inflammatory response. Lymphocyte anergy (the inability to respond to recall antigens in vivo, [eg, tetanus toxin]) or decreased responsiveness to mitogenic stimulus long has been demonstrated in patients following major surgery, blunt trauma, and thermal injury.[10–12] Further studies using

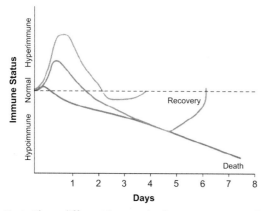

Fig.1. Three different immunologic responses to sepsis in three hypothetical patients of varying pre-existing health status. The relative magnitude of the anti-inflammatory (CARS) response in relation to the proinflammatory (SIRS) response is what is important in determining death in many sepsis patients. (*From* Hotchkiss RS, Karl IE. Medical progress: the pathophysiology and treatment of sepsis. N Engl J Med 2003;348(2):47; with permission.)

both animal and human in vitro models helped better characterize these lymphocyte alterations.

In 1985, Abraham and Chang[13] demonstrated reduced ability of T lymphocytes to respond to the mitogens concanavalin A and phytohemagglutinin following traumatic injury. Later, it was discovered that the period of immunoparalysis after trauma was characterized by increased expression of inhibitory coreceptors (PD-1, CD47, CTLA4) on T lymphocytes and decreased expression of coactivator receptors such as CD28 on lymphocytes.[14] This altered phenotype of lymphocytes correlated with diminished proliferation response contributing to anergy. Most significantly, a relationship between the loss of cell-mediated immunity in patients following traumatic injury, and the development of sepsis and late death had been established.[12,15]

As investigators began to look at lymphocyte function in sepsis (as opposed to trauma), it was clear that similar, if not identical patterns of dysfunction were occurring. For example, it was shown that patients who have sepsis exhibit defects in their T lymphocytes, because the cells fail to proliferate in response to mitogenic stimuli and also fail to produce IL-2 or -12.[16–18] Activated CD4 T-cells can be subdivided into two functionally distinct, highly polarized subsets, termed type 1 helper T-cell (Th1) and type 2 helper T-cell (Th2), depending on their pattern of lymphokine secretion and related functional activities. They secrete either cytokines with inflammatory Th1 properties, including TNF-α, interferon-γ, and IL-2,

or cytokines with more anti-inflammatory Th2 properties (eg, IL-4 and -10). Lymphocytes from patients with burns or sepsis have reduced levels of Th1 cytokines but increased levels of the Th2 cytokines IL-4 and -10, and reversal of the Th2 response improves survival among patients who have sepsis.[17,18]

Some newer studies, however, show a somewhat different picture. For example, global down-regulation of Th1 and Th2 responses in patients after sepsis or severe trauma also has been observed.[19,20] This suggests that there may be complete down-regulation of T-cell effector response rather than a shift to an anti-inflammatory response. Similarly, Heidecke and colleagues[16] examined T-cell function in patients who had peritonitis and found that they had decreased Th1 function without increased Th2 cytokine production. In this study, effective T-cell proliferation and cytokine secretion correlated with mortality.

More recent findings have been identified a role for other regulatory T-cell populations suppressing T-cell immunity, including natural killer T-cells (NKT) and Gamma delta T-cells ($\gamma\delta$). Blocking the activation of NKT cells by means of an anti-CD1d antibody prevented this immune suppression.[21] Using a model of burn injury on $\gamma\delta$ T-cell deficient mice, Schwacha and colleagues[22] demonstrated a reduced production of proinflammatory cytokines, suggesting that $\gamma\delta$ T-cells played an important role in postburn survival. The exact mechanisms by which these regulatory lymphocyte subsets affect the immune response remain subjects of controversy but may represent future therapeutic targets in the management of sepsis.

ANTIGEN-PRESENTING CELLS
Monocytes

Critical to the inflammatory response are the recognition and killing of invading organisms by monocytes. Equally important, monocytes present antigens by means of expression of HLA receptors and secrete proinflammatory cytokines to amplify the immune response.[23] Multiple studies have demonstrated clearly that following either trauma or sepsis, monocytes have diminished capacity for both these responses. Specifically, they secrete fewer cytokines when stimulated and down-regulate expression of HLA receptors.[24–30] Monocytes from septic patients who had decreased mHLA-DR produced low amounts of TNF-α and IL-1 in response to bacterial challenges.[31] This down-regulation of monocyte function generally predicts increased risk of secondary infection and poor prognosis. The role of this phenomenon in critically ill human patients is discussed in more detail in a later section.

DENDRITIC CELLS

Dendritic cells (DC) function as an important mediator in immune responses. Several investigators have found that their numbers decrease following the cecal ligation and puncture (CLP) model of sepsis in rodents.[32,33]

In people, Guisset and colleagues[34] have observed that septic patients who survived exhibited significantly higher circulating blood DC counts than those who died. In a postmortem study of spleen from 26 septic patients and 20 trauma patients, Hotchkiss and colleagues[35] observed that sepsis caused a dramatic reduction in the percentage area of spleen occupied by follicular DCs. The importance of DCs in mediating the immune response is emphasized further by murine studies showing improved outcome in sepsis by replenishing the DC population.[36] Also, Fujita and colleagues[37] have demonstrated improved survival in septic patients using the adoptive transfer of bone marrow-derived regulatory DCs (DCregs) in mice. These approaches may represent therapeutic modalities of the future.

Cytokines in Compensatory Anti-inflammatory Response Syndrome

Just as the SIRS response is characterized by many different and sometimes redundant cytokines, the CARS response also seems to involve many cytokines. The most important however is clearly IL10. IL10 first was characterized around 1990 and was shown to regulate T-cell populations.[38,39] It now has been established that IL-10 has multiple immunosuppressive roles,[40] with its most important being the downregulation of TNF. In animal models of sepsis, the administration of IL10 has been shown to have both positive[41–43] and negative[44,45] effects on outcome, which likely depend on the time of administration and the severity of the infection. In one carefully done animal model, Ashare and colleagues[46] followed levels of proinflammatory and anti-inflammatory cytokines throughout the whole course of sepsis in mice. They found that bacterial levels in tissue correlated with IL-10 levels and that if the complementary proinflammatory response was blocked by pretreatment with IL-1 receptor antagonist, bacterial levels were higher, as was mortality. Similarly, Song and colleagues[47] showed that blocking IL-10 activity early had no effect on mortality; blocking it late (12 hours) after sepsis, however, improved mortality. These studies help illustrate how IL-10 helps maintain

a careful balance of the immune system in inflammation; thus manipulation of it is so dangerous.

APOPTOSIS

Regulation of apoptosis of immune cell populations during sepsis and other traumatic states may play a crucial role balancing the hyperactive inflammatory state with excessive injury to the host. Several studies suggest this balance is critical to outcome of experimental animals and possibly septic patients.[48,49] The immunoparalysis that has been shown to be a hallmark of CARS response in sepsis may be a pathologic result of increased immune effector cell apoptosis. Additionally, it has been proposed that the clearance of increased numbers of apoptotic cells may drive immune suppression through the cells that handle them. Uptake of apoptotic cells by macrophages and DCs stimulates immune tolerance by inducing the release of anti-inflammatory cytokines, including IL-10 and transforming growth factor-β (TGF), and suppressing the release of proinflammatory cytokines.[50,51]

A key role of apoptosis in patients with sepsis was illustrated by Hotchkiss and colleagues[49,52] in two studies that compared patients who died of sepsis with patients who died of nonseptic etiologies. Autopsies of patients who had sepsis revealed extensive apoptosis of lymphocytes and gastrointestinal (GI) epithelial cells. These findings were similar to animal studies showing comparable widespread lymphocyte and GI epithelial cell death in sepsis.[53,54] Le Tulzo and colleagues[55] demonstrated exaggerated lymphocyte apoptosis is present in peripheral blood of patients with septic shock, contrary to those with simple sepsis or critically ill nonseptic patients. Additionally, lymphocyte apoptosis occurs rapidly, leads to a profound and persistent lymphocyte loss, and is associated with poor patient outcome. Evidence that apoptosis is a direct mediator of the immune dysfunction rather than just a marker of immune dysfunction comes from murine studies, where prevention of apoptosis improves survival in sepsis.[56,57]

CLINICAL SIGNIFICANCE OF UNDERSTANDING COMPENSATORY ANTI-INFLAMMATORY RESPONSE SYNDROME
Biomarkers

In addition to the studies mentioned previously, there have been many efforts to study the magnitude of the CARS response in relation to patient outcomes. This has led some to see CARS biomarkers as a possible tool for prognosis and therapy.[58] In an early study, Keane and colleagues[59] looked at lymphocytes removed and cultured from 31 patients who had severe trauma. They found that, overall, lymphocyte response to stimulation with mitogens was reduced markedly from controls. Furthermore, responses were lower, and the duration of suppression was longer in those patients who became infected. Additionally, the suppression of response preceded the onset of infection. Extremely low responses were found in three patients who later died.

A larger number of studies, however, have focused on monocytes and their apparent down-regulation of HLA receptors as a biomarker.[24,25,27,28,60–65] In 1995, Asadulla and colleagues[24] studied 57 neurosurgical patients and found that HLA-DR expression was lower in 14 patients who developed infection, compared with patients who had an uncomplicated postoperative course ($P < .0001$). Out of 10 patients who had less than 30% HLA-DR positive monocytes, nine developed infection. They hypothesized that the mechanism of this down-regulation was high levels of endogenous cortisol, as the effect coincided with high corticotropin (ACTH) and cortisol concentrations. Additionally, similar down-regulation was seen in other patients who received high doses of exogenous corticosteroids. Subsequent studies supported the theory that the magnitude of HLA-DR receptor down-regulation predicted various other poor outcomes such as sepsis in liver transplant patients.[28] That story, however, was confounded by exogenous steroids in some patients.[27] Allen and colleagues[66] found HLA levels predicted sepsis in pediatric cardiac surgery patients. In a small study of septic adults, Su and colleagues[64] found that levels of HLA-DR positive monocytes less than 30% were more predictive of mortality than Acute Physiology and Chronic Health Evaluation (APACHE) II scores.

More recent studies looking at the predicative power of HLA receptor have yielded different results. In 2003, three papers were published that yielded similar findings. Hynninen and colleagues[61] evaluated the HLA-DR expression of 61 patients who had sepsis at admission and showed no predictive power of HLA expression for survival. Another study of 70 septic patients also found no correlation between HLA expression and infectious or mortality outcomes.[63] Interestingly, this study showed that if patients' monocytes were stimulated with G-CSF ex-vivo, their HLA expression increased. The third study looked at 85 cardiac surgery patients. HLA expression was measured at presurgery, immediately after, and 1 day later. Their data showed that although all patients' HLA levels declined after surgery, the magnitude of the response did not correlate with sepsis/SIRS or other infectious complications.[62] Reasons for the different results still are being investigated but may be the result of small sample sizes, timing, or well-described variation caused by the different laboratory techniques used. In one study, the same samples were analyzed in two different laboratories and differed by as much as 20%.[62]

Other studies have looked at anti-inflammatory cytokine levels as predictors of poor outcomes; most of these studies have been on human patients and have borne mixed results. These data likely reflect the varied magnitudes and time courses of both pro- and anti-inflammatory cytokine expression in real patients. In 1998, Doughty and colleagues[67] sampled 53 pediatric ICU patients and found that high IL-10 levels correlated with three or more organ dysfunctions and mortality. Ahlstrom and colleagues[60] found no predictive value in IL-10 levels in patients who had SIRS, but Simmons and colleagues[68] found that IL-10 levels did correlate with mortality in a sample of 93 critically ill patients who had acute renal failure. Perhaps the most interesting data come from two studies that looked at the ratio of IL-10 to TNF. In a large study of over 400 patients admitted to the hospital for fever, van Dissel and colleagues[69] showed that a higher IL-10 to TNF ratio was predictive of mortality. A similar study by Gogos and colleagues[58] in a population of patients who had mixed sepsis showed the same results.

Potential Therapeutics

Given the still incomplete understanding of CARS response, it is not surprising that little has been done to use this knowledge as a point of therapeutic intervention in sepsis. Nevertheless, there have been several studies that have addressed therapeutics, and they can be grouped into two main categories: hormonal and cytokine therapies.

The hormonal therapy came from earlier studies showing that testosterone seemed to have a negative impact on sepsis and trauma outcomes and is believed to act through augmenting post-injury immunosuppression.[70] Two subsequent studies by the same investigators showed that administration of the estrogen-like drug dehydroepiandrosterone reduced the immunosuppression and improved mortality in septic mice.[71,72]

More research has focused on manipulation of cytokines to reverse the CARS immunosuppression. At least five studies have examined the use of gamma interferon, which has been shown in vivo to reverse monocyte deactivation.[73,74]

Two very similar small trials were done on human subjects who had sepsis.[75,76] In both studies, subjects who had sepsis and monocyte HLA-DR expression of 30% or less were given interferon-γ. Both groups reported increases in HLA-DR expression, usually after just one dose. One of the studies also examined the monocytes ex vivo and showed that interferon improved monocyte cytokine production also.[75] A third human trial was different, in that it sought study the effects of interferon-γ regionally.[77] In this study, the authors selected 21 patients who had severe trauma and alveolar macrophage dysfunction as determined by a bronchoalveolar lavage sample showing macrophage HLA-DR expression of 30% or less. Interferon-γ was the administered via inhalation. They found about 50% of the subjects had an increase in their alveolar macrophage HLA-DR expression. These patients had a lower incidence of pneumonia but no other differences in outcomes. The small numbers and lack of a control population in all three of these studies limit the conclusions that can be drawn, especially because HLA-DR expression is known to increase as patients recover.

SUMMARY

It has become clear that during sepsis or other major inflammatory stresses, there is a carefully orchestrated balance within the host organism. The proinflammatory forces rise to eliminate pathogens and dead tissue, and in doing so, often cause injury to the host. The timely arrival of anti-inflammatory responses such as the CARS response seeks to limit the damage while not interfering with the pathogen elimination. Just like its mirror image SIRS, however, the CARS response can be dangerous when its effects are unchecked or poorly timed, leaving the host too vulnerable to the next set of pathogens. Hopefully, further work in this field will allow one to manipulate this response favorably to improve outcomes in sepsis and related injuries.

REFERENCES

1. Bone RC. Sir Isaac Newton, sepsis, SIRS, and CARS. Crit Care Med 1996;24(7):1125–8.
2. Freeman BD, Natanson C. Anti-inflammatory therapies in sepsis and septic shock. Expert Opin Investig Drugs 2000;9(7):1651–63.
3. MacLean LD, Meakins JL, Taguchi K, et al. Host resistance in sepsis and trauma. Ann Surg 1975; 182(3):207–17.
4. Munster AM. Post-traumatic immunosuppression is due to activation of suppressor T cells. Lancet 1976;1(7973):1329–30.
5. Meakins JL, Pietsch JB, Bubenick O, et al. Delayed hypersensitivity: indicator of acquired failure of host defenses in sepsis and trauma. Ann Surg 1977; 186(3):241–50.
6. Miller CL, Baker CC. Changes in lymphocyte activity after thermal injury. The role of suppressor cells. J Clin Invest 1979;63(2):202–10.
7. Wolfe JH, Wu AV, O'Connor NE, et al. Anergy, immunosuppressive serum, and impaired lymphocyte blastogenesis in burn patients. Arch Surg 1982; 117(10):1266–71.
8. Oberholzer A, Oberholzer C, Moldawer LL. Sepsis syndromes: understanding the role of innate and acquired immunity. Shock 2001;16(2):83–96.
9. Shelley O, Murphy T, Paterson H, et al. Interaction between the innate and adaptive immune systems is required to survive sepsis and control inflammation after injury. Shock 2003;20(2):123–9.
10. Daniels JC, Sakai H, Cobb EK, et al. Evaluation of lymphocyte reactivity studies in patients with thermal burns. J Trauma 1971;11(7):595–601.
11. Hensler T, Hecker H, Heeg K, et al. Distinct mechanisms of immunosuppression as a consequence of major surgery. Infect Immun 1997;65(6):2283–91.
12. O'Mahony JB, Wood JJ, Rodrick ML, et al. Changes in T lymphocyte subsets following injury. Assessment by flow cytometry and relationship to sepsis. Ann Surg 1985;202(5):580–6.
13. Abraham E, Chang YH. The effects of hemorrhage on mitogen-induced lymphocyte proliferation. Circ Shock 1985;15(2):141–9.
14. Bandyopadhyay G, De A, Laudanski K, et al. Negative signaling contributes to T-cell anergy in trauma patients. Crit Care Med 2007;35(3):794–801.
15. Stephan RN, Kupper TS, Geha AS, et al. Hemorrhage without tissue trauma produces immunosuppression and enhances susceptibility to sepsis. Arch Surg 1987;122(1):62–8.
16. Heidecke CD, Hensler T, Weighardt H, et al. Selective defects of T lymphocyte function in patients with lethal intraabdominal infection. Am J Surg 1999;178(4):288–92.
17. O'Sullivan ST, Lederer JA, Horgan AF, et al. Major injury leads to predominance of the T helper-2 lymphocyte phenotype and diminished interleukin-12 production associated with decreased resistance to infection. Ann Surg 1995;222(4):482–90 discussion 490–482.
18. Rodrick ML, Wood JJ, Grbic JT, et al. Defective IL-2 production in patients with severe burns and sepsis. Lymphokine Res 1986;5(Suppl 1):S75–80.
19. Puyana JC, Pellegrini JD, De AK, et al. Both T-helper-1- and T-helper-2-type lymphokines are depressed in posttrauma anergy. J Trauma 1998; 44(6):1037–45 discussion 1045–1036.

20. Wick M, Kollig E, Muhr G, et al. The potential pattern of circulating lymphocytes TH1/TH2 is not altered after multiple injuries. Arch Surg 2000;135(11): 1309–14.

21. Palmer JL, Tulley JM, Kovacs EJ, et al. Injury-induced suppression of effector T cell immunity requires CD1d-positive APCs and CD1d-restricted NKT cells. J Immunol 2006;177(1):92–9.

22. Schwacha MG, Ayala A, Chaudry IH. Insights into the role of gammadelta T lymphocytes in the immunopathogenic response to thermal injury. J Leukoc Biol 2000;67(5):644–50.

23. Krakauer T, Oppenheim JJ. IL-1 and tumor necrosis factor-alpha each up-regulate both the expression of IFN-gamma receptors and enhance IFN-gamma-induced HLA-DR expression on human monocytes and a human monocytic cell line (THP-1). J Immunol 1993;150(4):1205–11.

24. Fumeaux T, Pugin J. Is the measurement of monocytes HLA-DR expression useful in patients with sepsis? Intensive Care Med 2006;32(8):1106–8.

25. Volk HD, Reinke P, Docke WD. Immunological monitoring of the inflammatory process: Which variables? When to assess? Eur J Surg Suppl 1999;(584):70–2.

26. Volk HD, Reinke P, Krausch D, et al. Monocyte deactivation–rationale for a new therapeutic strategy in sepsis. Intensive Care Med 1996;22(Suppl 4): S474–81.

27. Asadullah K, Woiciechowsky C, Docke WD, et al. Very low monocytic HLA-DR expression indicates high risk of infection–immunomonitoring for patients after neurosurgery and patients during high dose steroid therapy. Eur J Emerg Med 1995;2(4): 184–90.

28. van den Berk JM, Oldenburger RH, van den Berg AP, et al. Low HLA-DR expression on monocytes as a prognostic marker for bacterial sepsis after liver transplantation. Transplantation 1997; 63(12):1846–8.

29. Denzel C, Riese J, Hohenberger W, et al. Monitoring of immunotherapy by measuring monocyte HLA-DR expression and stimulated TNFalpha production during sepsis after liver transplantation. Intensive Care Med 1998;24(12):1343–4.

30. Haveman JW, van den Berg AP, van den Berk JM, et al. Low HLA-DR expression on peripheral blood monocytes predicts bacterial sepsis after liver transplantation: relation with prednisolone intake. Transpl Infect Dis 1999;1(3):146–52.

31. Astiz M, Saha D, Lustbader D, et al. Monocyte response to bacterial toxins, expression of cell surface receptors, and release of anti-inflammatory cytokines during sepsis. J Lab Clin Med 1996;128(6): 594–600.

32. Ding Y, Chung CS, Newton S, et al. Polymicrobial sepsis induces divergent effects on splenic and peritoneal dendritic cell function in mice. Shock 2004;22(2):137–44.

33. Flohe SB, Agrawal H, Schmitz D, et al. Dendritic cells during polymicrobial sepsis rapidly mature but fail to initiate a protective Th1-type immune response. J Leukoc Biol 2006;79(3):473–81.

34. Guisset O, Dilhuydy MS, Thiebaut R, et al. Decrease in circulating dendritic cells predicts fatal outcome in septic shock. Intensive Care Med 2007;33(1): 148–52.

35. Hotchkiss RS, Tinsley KW, Swanson PE, et al. Depletion of dendritic cells, but not macrophages, in patients with sepsis. J Immunol 2002;168(5): 2493–500.

36. Toliver-Kinsky TE, Cui W, Murphey ED, et al. Enhancement of dendritic cell production by fms-like tyrosine kinase-3 ligand increases the resistance of mice to a burn wound infection. J Immunol 2005; 174(1):404–10.

37. Fujita S, Seino K, Sato K, et al. Regulatory dendritic cells act as regulators of acute lethal systemic inflammatory response. Blood 2006;107(9):3656–64.

38. MacNeil IA, Suda T, Moore KW, et al. IL-10, a novel growth cofactor for mature and immature T cells. J Immunol 1990;145(12):4167–73.

39. O'Garra A, Stapleton G, Dhar V, et al. Production of cytokines by mouse B cells: B lymphomas and normal B cells produce interleukin 10. Int Immunol 1990;2(9):821–32.

40. Oberholzer A, Oberholzer C, Moldawer LL. Interleukin-10: A complex role in the pathogenesis of sepsis syndromes and its potential as an anti-inflammatory drug. Crit Care Med 2002;30(1 Supp):S58–63.

41. Berg DJ, Kuhn R, Rajewsky K, et al. Interleukin-10 is a central regulator of the response to LPS in murine models of endotoxic shock and the Shwartzman reaction but not endotoxin tolerance. J Clin Invest 1995;96(5):2339–47.

42. Howard M, Muchamuel T, Andrade S, et al. Interleukin 10 protects mice from lethal endotoxemia. J Exp Med 1993;177(4):1205–8.

43. van der Poll T, Jansen PM, Montegut WJ, et al. Effects of IL-10 on systemic inflammatory responses during sublethal primate endotoxemia. J Immunol 1997;158(4):1971–5.

44. Remick DG, Garg SJ, Newcomb DE, et al. Exogenous interleukin-10 fails to decrease the mortality or morbidity of sepsis. Crit Care Med 1998;26(5): 895–904.

45. Steinhauser ML, Hogaboam CM, Kunkel SL, et al. IL-10 is a major mediator of sepsis-induced impairment in lung antibacterial host defense. J Immunol 1999;162(1):392–9.

46. Ashare A, Powers LS, Butler NS, et al. Anti-inflammatory response is associated with mortality and severity of infection in sepsis. Am J Physiol Lung Cell Mol Physiol 2005;288(4):L633–40.

47. Song GY, Chung CS, Chaudry IH, et al. What is the role of interleukin 10 in polymicrobial sepsis: anti-inflammatory agent or immunosuppressant? Surgery 1999;126(2):378–83.

48. Ayala A, Xin Xu Y, Ayala CA, et al. Increased mucosal B-lymphocyte apoptosis during polymicrobial sepsis is a Fas ligand but not an endotoxin-mediated process. Blood 1998;91(4):1362–72.

49. Hotchkiss RS, Swanson PE, Freeman BD, et al. Apoptotic cell death in patients with sepsis, shock, and multiple organ dysfunction. Crit Care Med 1999;27(7):1230–51.

50. Fadok VA, Bratton DL, Konowal A, et al. Macrophages that have ingested apoptotic cells in vitro inhibit proinflammatory cytokine production through autocrine/paracrine mechanisms involving TGF-beta, PGE2, and PAF. J Clin Invest 1998;101(4):890–8.

51. Voll RE, Herrmann M, Roth EA, et al. Immunosuppressive effects of apoptotic cells. Nature 1997;390(6658):350–1.

52. Hotchkiss RS, Tinsley KW, Swanson PE, et al. Sepsis-induced apoptosis causes progressive profound depletion of B and CD4+ T lymphocytes in humans. J Immunol 2001;166(11):6952–63.

53. Hiramatsu M, Hotchkiss RS, Karl IE, Buchman TG. Cecal ligation and puncture (CLP) induces apoptosis in thymus, spleen, lung, and gut by an endotoxin and TNF-independent pathway. Shock 1997;7(4):247–53.

54. Hotchkiss RS, Swanson PE, Cobb JP, et al. Apoptosis in lymphoid and parenchymal cells during sepsis: findings in normal and T- and B-cell-deficient mice. Crit Care Med 1997;25(8):1298–307.

55. Le Tulzo Y, Pangault C, Gacouin A, et al. Early circulating lymphocyte apoptosis in human septic shock is associated with poor outcome. Shock 2002;18(6):487–94.

56. Hotchkiss RS, Swanson PE, Knudson CM, et al. Overexpression of Bcl-2 in transgenic mice decreases apoptosis and improves survival in sepsis. J Immunol 1999;162(7):4148–56.

57. Hotchkiss RS, Tinsley KW, Swanson PE, et al. Prevention of lymphocyte cell death in sepsis improves survival in mice. Proc Natl Acad Sci U S A 1999;96(25):14541–6.

58. Gogos CA, Drosou E, Bassaris HP, Skoutelis A. Pro- versus anti-inflammatory cytokine profile in patients with severe sepsis: a marker for prognosis and future therapeutic options. J Infect Dis 2000;181(1):176–80.

59. Keane RM, Birmingham W, Shatney CM, et al. Prediction of sepsis in the multitraumatic patient by assays of lymphocyte responsiveness. Surg Gynecol Obstet 1983;156(2):163–7.

60. Hynninen M, Pettila V, Takkunen O, et al. Predictive value of monocyte histocompatibility leukocyte antigen-DR expression and plasma interleukin-4 and -10 levels in critically ill patients with sepsis. Shock 2003;20(1):1–4.

61. Oczenski W, Krenn H, Jilch R, et al. HLA-DR as a marker for increased risk for systemic inflammation and septic complications after cardiac surgery. Intensive Care Med 2003;29(8):1253–7.

62. Perry SE, Mostafa SM, Wenstone R, et al. Is low monocyte HLA-DR expression helpful to predict outcome in severe sepsis? Intensive Care Med 2003;29(8):1245–52.

63. Ahlstrom A, Hynninen M, Tallgren M, et al. Predictive value of interleukins 6, 8 and 10, and low HLA-DR expression in acute renal failure. Clin Nephrol 2004;61(2):103–10.

64. Su L, Zhou DY, Tang YQ, et al. [Clinical value of monitoring CD14+ monocyte human leukocyte antigen (locus) DR levels in the early stage of sepsis]. Zhongguo Wei Zhong Bing Ji Jiu Yi Xue 2006;18(11):677–9.

65. Zhang YT, Fang Q. [Study on monocyte HLA-DR expression in critically ill patients after surgery]. Zhonghua Wai Ke Za Zhi 2006;44(21):1480–2.

66. Allen ML, Peters MJ, Goldman A, et al. Early postoperative monocyte deactivation predicts systemic inflammation and prolonged stay in pediatric cardiac intensive care. Crit Care Med 2002;30(5):1140–5.

67. Doughty L, Carcillo JA, Kaplan S, et al. The compensatory anti-inflammatory cytokine interleukin 10 response in pediatric sepsis-induced multiple organ failure. Chest 1998;113(6):1625–31.

68. Simmons EM, Himmelfarb J, Sezer MT, et al. Plasma cytokine levels predict mortality in patients with acute renal failure. Kidney Int 2004;65(4):1357–65.

69. van Dissel JT, van Langevelde P, Westendorp RG, et al. Anti-inflammatory cytokine profile and mortality in febrile patients. Lancet 1998;351(9107):950–3.

70. Angele MK, Wichmann MW, Ayala A, et al. Testosterone receptor blockade after hemorrhage in males. Restoration of the depressed immune functions and improved survival following subsequent sepsis. Arch Surg 1997;132(11):1207–14.

71. Angele MK, Catania RA, Ayala A, et al. Dehydroepiandrosterone: an inexpensive steroid hormone that decreases the mortality due to sepsis following trauma-induced hemorrhage. Arch Surg 1998;133(12):1281–8.

72. Catania RA, Angele MK, Ayala A, et al. Dehydroepiandrosterone restores immune function following trauma-haemorrhage by a direct effect on T lymphocytes. Cytokine 1999;11(6):443–50.

73. Hershman MJ, Appel SH, Wellhausen SR. Interferon-gamma treatment increases HLA-DR expression on monocytes in severely injured patients. Clin Exp Immunol 1989;77(1):67–70.

74. Bundschuh DS, Barsig J, Hartung T, et al. Granulo-cyte-macrophage colony-stimulating factor and IFN-gamma restore the systemic TNF-alpha response to endotoxin in lipopolysaccharide-desensitized mice. J Immunol 1997;158(6):2862–71.

75. Docke WD, Randow F, Syrbe U, et al. Monocyte deactivation in septic patients: restoration by IFN-gamma treatment. Nat Med 1997;3(6):678–81.

76. Kox WJ, Bone RC, Krausch D, et al. Interferon gamma-1b in the treatment of compensatory anti-inflammatory response syndrome. A new approach: proof of principle. Arch Intern Med 1997;157(4):389–93.

77. Nakos G, Malamou-Mitsi VD, Lachana A, et al. Immunoparalysis in patients with severe trauma and the effect of inhaled interferon-gamma. Crit Care Med 2002;30(7):1488–94.

The Coagulant Response in Sepsis

Marcel Levi, MD

KEYWORDS

- Sepsis • Coagulation • Inflammation
- Disseminated intravascular coagulation
- Tissue factor • Antithrombin • Protein C

Virtually all patients with sepsis have coagulation abnormalities.[1] These abnormalities range from subtle activation of coagulation, which can only be detected by sensitive markers for coagulation factor activation, to somewhat stronger coagulation activation, which may be detectable by a small decrease in platelet count and subclinical prolongation of global clotting times, to fulminant disseminated intravascular coagulation (DIC), characterized by simultaneous widespread microvascular thrombosis and profuse bleeding from various sites.[2] Septic patients with severe forms of DIC may present with manifest thromboembolic disease or clinically less apparent microvascular fibrin deposition, which predominantly presents as multiple organ dysfunction.[3,4] Alternatively, severe bleeding may be the leading symptom.[5] However, a patient with DIC quite often has simultaneous thrombosis and bleeding. Bleeding is caused by consumption and subsequent exhaustion of coagulation proteins and platelets resulting from the ongoing activation of the coagulation system.[6]

Clinically relevant coagulation abnormalities may occur in 50% to 70% of patients with sepsis, whereas about 35% of patients meet the criteria for DIC.[7,8] In general, the incidence of thrombocytopenia (platelet count $<150 \times 10^9/L$) in critically ill medical patients is 35% to 50%.[9–11] Typically, the platelet count decreases during the first 4 days in the intensive care unit (ICU).[12] Sepsis is a clear risk factor for thrombocytopenia in critically ill patients, and the severity of sepsis correlates with the decrease in platelet count.[13] The main factors that contribute to thrombocytopenia in patients with sepsis are impaired platelet production, increased consumption or destruction, and

sequestration in the spleen or at the endothelial level.[14] Impaired production of platelets in the bone marrow may seem contradictory in light of the high levels of platelet production–stimulating proinflammatory cytokines, such as tumor necrosis factor (TNF)-α and IL-6, and the high concentration of circulating thrombopoietin in patients with sepsis, which theoretically should stimulate megakaryopoiesis in the bone marrow.[15] However, in a substantial number of patients with sepsis, marked hemophagocytosis may occur, consisting of active phagocytosis of megakaryocytes and other hematopietic cells by monocytes and macrophages, hypothetically due to stimulation with high levels of macrophage colony-stimulating factor in sepsis.[16] Due to ongoing generation of thrombin, platelet consumption probably also plays an important role in patients with sepsis. Platelet activation, consumption, and destruction may also occur at the endothelial site as a result of the extensive endothelial cell–platelet interaction in sepsis, which may vary among different vascular beds in various organs.[17] A prolonged global coagulation time (such as the prothrombin time (PT) or the activated partial thromboplastin time (aPTT)) occurs in 14% to 28% of patients.[18,19] Other coagulation test abnormalities include high fibrin split products (in 99% of patients with sepsis)[20–22] and low levels of coagulation inhibitors, such as antithrombin and protein C (90% of sepsis patients).[22,23]

RELEVANCE OF COAGULATION ABNORMALITIES IN PATIENTS WITH SEPSIS

Ample evidence shows that activation of coagulation in concert with inflammatory activation can

Department of Medicine (F4-219), Academic Medical Center, University of Amsterdam, Meibergdreef 9, 1105 AZ Amsterdam, The Netherlands
E-mail address: m.m.levi@amc.uva.nl

Clin Chest Med 29 (2008) 627–642
doi:10.1016/j.ccm.2008.06.006

result in microvascular thrombosis and thereby contributes to multiple organ failure in patients with severe sepsis.[24] First, extensive data have been reported on postmortem findings of patients with coagulation abnormalities and DIC in patients with severe infectious diseases.[25,26] These autopsy findings include diffuse bleeding at various sites, hemorraghic necrosis of tissue, microthrombi in small blood vessels, and thrombi in midsize and larger arteries and veins. Fibrin deposition in small and midsize vessels of various organs has invariably resulted in ischemia and necrosis.[27] The presence of these intravascular thrombi appears to be clearly and specifically related to the clinical dysfunction of the organ. Second, experimental animal studies of DIC show fibrin deposition in various organs. Experimental bacteremia or endotoxemia causes intra- and extravascular fibrin deposition in kidneys, lungs, liver, brain, and various other organs. Amelioration of the hemostatic defect by various interventions in these experimental models appears to restore organs to normal functioning and, in some but not all cases, reduce mortality.[28–31] Interestingly, some studies indicate that amelioration of the systemic coagulation activation has profound benefits in resolving local fibrin deposition and improving functions of failing organs.[5,32] Last, clinical studies support the notion of coagulation as an important denominator of clinical outcome. DIC has been shown to be an independent predictor of organ failure and mortality in patients with sepsis.[3,33] In a consecutive series of patients with severe sepsis, the mortality of patients with DIC was 43%, as compared with 27% in those without DIC.[34] In this study, the severity of the coagulopathy was also directly related to mortality in septic patients.

Coagulation abnormalities may have other harmful consequences apart from microvascular thrombosis and organ dysfunction. The relevance of thrombocytopenia in patients with sepsis is in the first place related to an increased risk of bleeding. Indeed, in particular critically ill patients with a platelet count of less than 50×10^9/L have a four- to fivefold greater risk for bleeding as compared with patients with a higher platelet count.[9,11] The risk of intracerebral bleeding in patients with sepsis during ICU admission is relatively low (0.3%–0.5%), but in 88% of patients with this complication the platelet count is less than 100×10^9/L.[35] Regardless of the cause, thrombocytopenia is an independent predictor of ICU mortality in multivariate analyses with a relative risk of 1.9 to 4.2 in various studies.[9,11,36] A sustained thrombocytopenia over more than 4 days after ICU admission or a drop in platelet count of greater than 50% during ICU stay is related to a four- to

sixfold increase in mortality.[9,12] The platelet count was shown to be a stronger predictor for ICU mortality than composite scoring systems, such as the Acute Physiology and Chronic Evaluation II score or the Multiple Organ Dysfunction Score. Also, low levels of coagulation factors in patients with sepsis, as reflected by prolonged global coagulation times, may be a risk factor for bleeding and mortality. A PT or aPTT ratio greater than 1.5 in critically ill patients was found to predict excessive bleeding and increased mortality.[18,19]

PATHOGENETIC PATHWAYS IN THE COAGULOPATHY OF SEPSIS

In recent years, the mechanisms involved in the pathologic derangement of coagulation in patients with sepsis have become increasingly clear. Apparently various mechanisms at different sites in the hemostatic balance act simultaneously toward a procoagulant state (**Fig. 1**). The most important mediators orchestrating this imbalance of the coagulation system during sepsis are cytokines.[37] Increasing evidence points to extensive cross talk between the coagulation system and the system related to inflammation. Through this cross talk, inflammation promotes coagulation while coagulation considerably affects inflammatory activity.[38] Interestingly, systemic activation of coagulation and inflammation in sepsis can have some organ-specific manifestations relevant for the specific organ dysfunction as a consequence of severe sepsis.[39]

Initiation of Coagulation Activation via the Tissue Factor Pathway

It was initially thought that the systemic activation of coagulation in patients with sepsis was a result of direct activation of the contact system by microorganisms or endotoxin.[40] However, in the 1990s it became apparent that the principal initiator of thrombin generation in sepsis is tissue factor and that the contact system is not involved. The evidence that points to a pivotal role of the tissue factor–factor VIIa system in the initiation of thrombin generation comes from studies of human endotoxemia or cytokinemia, which did not show any change in markers for activation of the contact system.[41,42] Furthermore, abrogation of the tissue factor–factor VII(a) pathway by monoclonal antibodies specifically directed against tissue factor or factor VIIa activity resulted in a complete inhibition of thrombin generation in endotoxin-challenged chimpanzees and prevented the occurrence of DIC and mortality in baboons infused with *Escherichia coli*.[30,43,44]

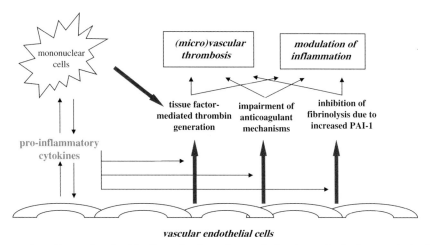

Fig. 1. Pathogenetic pathways involved in the activation of coagulation in sepsis. During sepsis, both perturbed endothelial cells and activated mononuclear cells may produce proinflammatory cytokines that mediate coagulation activation. Activation of coagulation is initiated by tissue factor expression on activated mononuclear cells and endothelial cells. In addition, down-regulation of physiologic anticoagulant mechanisms and inhibition of fibrinolysis by endothelial cells further promote intravascular fibrin deposition. PAI-1, plasminogen activator inhibitor–1.

Tissue factor, a transmembrane 45 kD protein, is constitutively expressed on a number of cells throughout the body.[45] The majority of these cells are in tissues not in direct contact with blood, such as the adventitial layer of large blood vessels. However, tissue factor makes contact with blood when vascular integrity is disrupted or when cells present in the circulation start expressing tissue factor. In sepsis, circulating mononuclear cells, stimulated by proinflammatory cytokines, express tissue factor, which leads to systemic activation of coagulation. However, other than in severe meningococcemia,[46] it has proved difficult to demonstrate ex vivo tissue factor expression on monocytes of septic patients or experimental animals systemically exposed to microorganisms. It has been shown, however, that low-dose endotoxemia in healthy subjects results in a 125-fold increase in tissue factor mRNA levels in blood monocytes.[47] Another source of tissue factor may be polymorphonuclear cells,[48] although it is unlikely that these cells actually synthesize tissue factor in substantial quantities.[49] Based on the observation that tissue factor from leukocytes transfers to activated platelets on a collagen surface in an ex vivo perfusion system, it is hypothesized that this "blood borne" tissue factor is transferred between cells through microparticles derived from activated mononuclear cells.[50]

Platelets play a pivotal role in the pathogenesis of coagulation abnormalities in sepsis. Platelets can be activated directly by, for example, proinflammatory mediators, such as platelet activating factor.[51] Thrombin, once formed, activates

additional platelets. Activation of platelets may also accelerate fibrin formation by another mechanism. The expression of P-selectin on the platelet membrane not only mediates the adherence of platelets to leukocytes and endothelial cells but also enhances the expression of tissue factor on monocytes.[52] The molecular mechanism of this effect relies on nuclear factor kappa-B (NFκB) activation, induced by binding of activated platelets to neutrophils and mononuclear cells. P-selectin can be easily shed from the surface of the platelet membrane. Soluble P-selectin levels have been shown to increase during systemic inflammation.[52]

Impairment of Physiologic Anticoagulant Pathways in Sepsis

In general, three major anticoagulant pathways regulate activation of coagulation: antithrombin, the protein C system, and tissue factor pathway inhibitor (TFPI). During sepsis-induced activation of coagulation, the function of all three pathways can be impaired (**Fig. 2**).

Antithrombin is a serine protease inhibitor and the main inhibitor of thrombin and factor Xa. During severe inflammatory responses, antithrombin levels are markedly decreased because of consumption (as a result of ongoing thrombin generation), impaired synthesis (as a result of a negative acute phase response), and degradation by elastase from activated neutrophils.[53,54] A reduction in glycosaminoglycan availability at the endothelial surface (due to the influence of

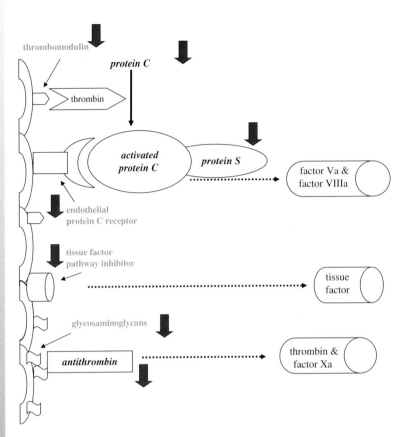

Fig. 2. The three important physiologic antiocoagulant mechanisms and their points of impact in the coagulation system. In sepsis, these mechanisms are impaired by various mechanisms (*thick arrows*). The protein C system is dysfunctional because of low levels of zymogen protein C, down-regulation of thrombomodulin and the endothelial protein C receptor, and low levels of free protein S due to acute phase-induced high levels of its binding protein (ie, C4b-binding protein). There is a relative insufficiency of the endothelial cell–associated tissue factor pathway inhibitor. The antithrombin system is defective because of low levels of antithrombin and impaired glycosaminoglycan expression on perturbed endothelial cells.

proinflammatory cytokines on endothelial synthesis) also contributes to reduced antithrombin function, since glycosaminoglycans act as physiologic heparinlike cofactors of antithrombin. Binding of glycosaminoglycans to antithrombin induces a conformational change at the reactive center of the antithrombin molecule, thereby transforming this protease inhibitor from a slow to a very efficient inhibitor of thrombin and other active coagulation factors.[55] Prospective clinical studies in patients at high risk for sepsis have shown that a marked decrease in levels of antithrombin precedes the clinical manifestation of the infection, which may indicate that antithrombin is involved in the early stages of coagulation activation during sepsis.[56]

Endothelial dysfunction is even more important in the impairment of the protein C system during inflammation. Under physiologic conditions, protein C is activated by thrombin bound to the endothelial cell membrane–associated thrombomodulin. Thrombomodulin is a membrane protein with several domains, including a lectinlike domain, six epidermal growth factor (EGF)–like repeats, a transmembrane domain, and a short cytoplasmatic tail.[57] The binding of thrombin to thrombomodulin occurs at the site of the EGF-like

repeats.[58] This binding not only results in an increase of about 100-fold in the activation of protein C, but also blocks the thrombin-mediated conversion of fibrinogen into fibrin and inhibits the binding of thrombin to other cellular receptors on platelets and inflammatory cells. In addition, thrombomodulin accelerates the activation of the plasma carboxypeptidase thrombin-activatable fibrinolysis inhibitor, an important inhibitor of fibrinolysis.[59] Activated protein C regulates coagulation activation by proteolytic cleavage of the essential cofactors Va and VIIIa. Binding of protein C to the EPCR results in a fivefold augmentation of the activation of protein C by the thrombomodulin-thrombin complex.[60] However, during severe inflammation, such as occurs in sepsis, in addition to low levels of protein C due to impaired synthesis[53] and degradation by neutrophil elastase (which has been described at least in vitro),[61] the protein C system is defective because of down-regulation of thrombomodulin at the endothelial surface, mediated by the proinflammatory cytokines TNF-α and IL-1β.[62] Observations in patients with severe gram-negative septicemia indeed confirm the down-regulation of thrombomodulin in vivo and impaired activation of protein C.[63] In this study, histologic analysis of skin biopsies from patients with meningococcal sepsis showed decreased endothelial expression of thrombomodulin, both in vessels with thrombosis and those without. Low levels of free protein S (the cofactor of activated protein C) may further compromise adequate functioning of the protein C system. In plasma, 60% of protein S is complexed to a complement regulatory protein, C4b binding protein (C4bBP). Increased plasma levels of C4bBP as a consequence of the acute phase reaction in inflammatory diseases may result in a relative free protein S deficiency. The β-chain of C4bBP (which mainly governs the binding to protein S) is not significantly affected during the acute phase response,[64] according to studies involving septic baboons that showed that infusion of C4bBP increases organ dysfunction and mortality.[65] Animal experiments of severe inflammation-induced coagulation activation convincingly show that compromising the protein C system results in increased morbidity and mortality, whereas restoring an adequate function of activated protein C improves survival and organ failure.[66] Interestingly, experiments in mice with a one-allele targeted deletion of the protein C gene (resulting in heterozygous protein C deficiency) have more severe DIC and organ dysfunction and a higher mortality than their wild-type littermates.[67]

A third inhibitory mechanism of thrombin generation involves TFPI, the main inhibitor of the tissue factor–factor VIIa complex. TFPI is a complex multidomain Kunitz-type protease inhibitor that binds to the tissue factor–factor VIIa complex and factor Xa.[68] The TFPI–factor Xa complex may bind to negatively charged membrane surfaces, which may increase the local concentration of TFPI at cellular sites and facilitate inhibition of membrane-bound tissue factor–factor VIIa complex. The role of TFPI in the regulation of inflammation-induced coagulation activation is not completely clear. Experiments show that administration of recombinant TFPI (providing higher than normal plasma concentrations of TFPI) blocks inflammation-induced thrombin generation in humans. Meanwhile, observations have confirmed that pharmacologic doses of TFPI are capable of preventing mortality during systemic infection and inflammation. Such experiments and observations suggest that high concentrations of TFPI are capable of significantly modulating tissue factor–mediated coagulation.[28,69] However, the endogenous concentration of TFPI is presumably insufficiently capable of regulating coagulation activation and downstream consequences during systemic inflammation, as has been confirmed in a clinical study of patients with sepsis.[70,71]

Plasminogen Activator Inhibitor–1–Mediated Inhibition of Endogenous Fibrinolysis in Sepsis

Experimental models indicate that at the time of maximal activation of coagulation in sepsis, the fibrinolytic system is largely shut off. The acute fibrinolytic response to inflammation is the release of plasminogen activators, in particular tissue-type plasminogen activator and urokinase-type plasminogen activator, from storage sites in vascular endothelial cells. However, this increase in plasminogen activation and subsequent plasmin generation is counteracted by a delayed but sustained increase in plasminogen activator inhibitor-1 (PAI-1).[72,73] The resulting effect on fibrinolysis is complete inhibition and, as a consequence, inadequate fibrin removal, thereby contributing to microvascular thrombosis. Experiments in mice with targeted disruptions of genes' encoding components of the plasminogen-plasmin system confirm that fibrinolysis plays a major role in inflammation-induced coagulation. Mice with a deficiency of plasminogen activators have more extensive fibrin deposition in organs when challenged with endotoxin, whereas PAI-1 knockout mice, in contrast to wild-type controls, have no microvascular thrombosis upon endotoxin challenge.[74,75] Studies have shown that a functional mutation in the PAI-1 gene, the 4G/5G polymorphism, not only influences the plasma levels of PAI-1, but is also linked to clinical outcome of meningococcal septicemia. Patients with the 4G/4G genotype have significantly higher PAI-1 concentrations in plasma and an increased risk of death.[76] Further investigations demonstrate that the PAI-1 polymorphism does not influence the risk of contracting meningitis as such, but probably increases the likelihood of developing septic shock from meningococcal infection.[77]

Interaction Between Inflammatory and Coagulant Pathways

Similar to almost all systemic inflammatory responses to infection, several cytokines mediate the derangement of coagulation and fibrinolysis in sepsis. It was initially thought that, because TNF is the first cytokine to appear in the circulation after infusion of bacteria or endotoxin and because TNF exerts potent procoagulant effects in vitro, TNF mediates activation of coagulation.[42,78] Following the injection of TNF, the observed activation of the coagulation system was virtually identical to the endotoxin-induced effects on coagulation. However, in studies using various strategies to block TNF activity, it has become clear that the endotoxin-induced increase in TNF could be completely abolished without affecting activation of coagulation, although TNF seems to drive the effects on anticoagulant pathways and fibrinolysis.[79,80] Also, in baboons infused with a lethal dose of *E coli*, treatment with an anti-TNF antibody had little or no effect on fibrinogen consumption.[81] In subsequent studies, the role of IL-6 was investigated. It could be shown that infusion of a monoclonal anti–IL-6 antibody resulted in the complete abrogation of endotoxin-induced activation of coagulation in chimpanzees.[82] In addition, studies in cancer patients receiving recombinant IL-6 indicated that thrombin is indeed generated following the injection of this cytokine.[83] Thus, these data suggest that IL-6 rather than TNF is relevant as a mediator for the induction of the procoagulant response in DIC. While IL-1 is a potent agonist of tissue factor expression in vitro, its role has not been clarified in vivo. Administration of an IL-1 receptor antagonist partly blocked the procoagulant response in a sepsis model in baboons, and patients treated with an IL-1 receptor inhibitor showed reduced thrombin generation.[84–86] However, most of the procoagulant changes after an endotoxin challenge occur well before IL-1 becomes detectable in the circulation, leaving unresolved the question of IL-1's potential direct role in coagulation activation in sepsis. Anti-inflammatory cytokines, such as IL-10, may modulate the activation of coagulation.[87] However, the relevance of this regulatory role of anti-inflammatory cytokines in the pathogenesis of the sepsis-associated coagulopathy remains to be established.

Coagulation proteases and protease inhibitors not only interact with coagulation protein zymogens, but also with specific cell receptors to induce signaling pathways. In particular, protease interactions that affect inflammatory processes may be important in sepsis. Coagulation of whole blood in vitro results in a detectable expression of IL-1β mRNA in blood cells,[88] and thrombin markedly enhances endotoxin-induced IL-1 activity in culture supernatants of guinea pig macrophages.[89] Similarly, clotting blood produces IL-8 in vitro.[90] Factor Xa, thrombin, and fibrin can also activate endothelial cells, eliciting the synthesis of IL-6, IL-8, or both.[91,92] The most important mechanisms by which coagulation proteases influence inflammation is by binding to protease-activated receptors (PARs), of which four types (PAR 1–4) have been identified, all belonging to the family of transmembrane-domain, G-protein–coupled receptors.[93] A peculiar feature of PARs (in contrast to most other receptors of the superfamily) is that they serve as their own ligand. Proteolytic cleavage by an activated coagulation factor leads to exposure of a neoamino terminus, which activates the same receptor (and possibly adjacent receptors), initiating transmembrane signaling. PAR-1, -3, and -4 are thrombin receptors whereas PAR-2 cannot bind thrombin but can be activated by the tissue factor–factor VIIa complex, factor Xa, and trypsin. PAR-1 can also serve as receptor of the tissue factor–factor VIIa complex and factor Xa. PARs are localized in the vasculature on endothelial cells, mononuclear cells, platelets, fibroblasts, and smooth muscle cells.[93] Binding of thrombin to thrombin's cellular receptor may induce the production of several cytokines and growth factors, as mentioned above. Binding of tissue factor–factor VIIa to PAR-2 also results in up-regulation of inflammatory responses (production of reactive oxygen species and expression of major histocompatibility complex class II and cell adhesion molecules) in macrophages and affects neutrophil infiltration and proinflammatory cytokine (TNF-α, IL-1β) expression.[94,95] In vivo evidence for a role of coagulation-protease stimulation of inflammation comes from recent experiments showing that the administration of recombinant factor VIIa to healthy human subjects causes a small but significant three- to fourfold rise in plasma levels of IL-6 and IL-8.[96]

Fibrinogen and fibrin can directly stimulate expression of proinflammatory cytokines (such as TNF-α and IL-1β) on mononuclear cells and induce production of chemokines (including IL-8 and monocyte chemoattractant protein–1) by endothelial cells and fibroblasts.[97] The effects of fibrin and fibrinogen on mononuclear cells are at least in part mediated by Toll-like receptor–4.[98] Fibrinogen-deficient mice indeed show inhibition of macrophage adhesion and less thrombin-mediated cytokine production in vivo.[97]

Considerable cross talk also exists between physiologic anticoagulant pathways and inflammatory mediators. Antithrombin can act as a mediator of inflammation by, for example, direct binding to neutrophils and other leucocytes and thereby attenuating cytokine and chemokine receptor expression.[99] In addition, there is mounting evidence that the protein C system also has an important function in modulating inflammation.[57,100] Indeed, activated protein C has been found to inhibit endotoxin-induced production of TNF-α, IL-1β, IL-6, and IL-8 by cultured monocytes/macrophages.[101,102] Further, activated protein C abrogates endotoxin-induced cytokine release and leukocyte activation in rats in vivo.[103] Blocking the protein C pathway by a monoclonal antibody in septic baboons exacerbates the inflammatory response, as evidenced by increased levels of proinflammatory cytokines and more leukocyte infiltration and tissue destruction at histologic analysis.[104,105] Conversely, administration of activated protein C ameliorates the inflammatory activation in various models of severe systemic inflammation.[66,100] Infusion of activated protein C abrogates inflammatory activity and improves organ function and survival in an experimental E coli sepsis model in baboons.[66] Furthermore, in models of endotoxin-induced shock and lung and kidney injury in rats, administration of activated protein C resulted in a significant improvement of organ function, associated with lower levels of inflammatory cytokines and less leucocyte infiltration.[100] Mice with a one-allele targeted disruption of the protein C gene (resulting in heterozygous protein C deficiency) have not only a more severe coagulation response to endotoxin but also demonstrate significant differences in inflammatory responses, as shown by higher levels of circulating proinflammatory cytokines.[67] It is likely that the effects of activated protein C on inflammation are mediated by the endothelial protein C receptor (EPCR), which may mediate downstream inflammatory processes.[57] Binding of activated protein C to the EPCR was shown to affect gene expression profiles of cells by inhibiting endotoxin-induced calcium fluxes in the cell and by blocking NFκB nuclear translocation, which is a prerequisite for increases in proinflammatory cytokines and adhesion molecules.[106,107] Recent experiments also suggest that EPCR binding of activated protein C can result in activation of PAR-1.[108] Like activated protein C, EPCR itself may have anti-inflammatory properties. Soluble EPCR, the extracellular domain of the cell-associated EPCR shed from the cell surface by the action of an inducible metalloproteinase,[109] can bind to proteinase 3, an elastaselike enzyme. The resulting complex binds to the adhesion integrin macrophage 1 antigen.[110] Blocking the EPCR with a specific monoclonal antibody aggravates both the coagulation and the inflammatory response to E coli infusion.[105] Lastly, activated protein C is capable of inhibiting endothelial cell apoptosis, which also seems to be mediated by binding of activated protein C to the endothelial protein C receptor and seems to require PAR-1.[111,112]

The Glycocalyx as an Interface for Inflammation and Coagulation

Recent research points to an important role of the inner layer of the endothelium (ie, the glycocalyx) in the interaction between inflammation and coagulation. In sepsis, glycosaminoglycans are downregulated as a result of proinflammatory cytokines, which can thereby have an impact on the function

of antithrombin and TFPI and on leukocyte adhesion and transmigration. Besides glycosaminoglycans and highly sulphated polysaccharides, the glycocalyx consists of glycoproteins, hyaluronic acid, and membrane-associated proteins. The glycocalyx plays a role not only in coagulation but also in other endothelial functions, including antioxidant functions, functions related to maintaining a vascular barrier, and nitric oxide–mediated vasodilation—all processes known to be involved in sepsis.[113,114] It was shown recently that specific disruption of the glycocalyx results in thrombin generation and platelet adhesion within a few minutes.[115,116] Moreover, loss of glycocalyx in vivo has been associated with subendothelial edema formation.[117] It seems conceivable that the glycocalyx is disturbed in sepsis also, although evidence for this is still preliminary. Further research is needed to more precisely understand the role of the glycocalyx in modulating endothelial function, including anticoagulation, and the role of the endothelium in modulating glycocalyx in sepsis.

DIAGNOSTIC APPROACH TO COAGULATION ABNORMALITIES IN SEPSIS

Apart from DIC, several other reasons exist for coagulation abnormalities in patients with sepsis.[118] While severe sepsis often causes thrombocytopenia, and while thrombocytopenia is common in patients with severe sepsis, other diseases also may cause thrombocytopenia. Sometimes these diseases may occur alongside sepsis. Such diseases include immune thrombocytopenia, medication-induced bone marrow depression, heparin-induced thrombocytopenia, and thrombotic microangiopathies.[10,119] It is important to properly diagnose these causes of thrombocytopenia because each may require a distinctive treatment strategy.[17,120] Laboratory tests can be helpful in differentiating the coagulopathy in sepsis from various other hemostatic disorders, such as vitamin K deficiency or liver failure.

Specific Markers for Intravascular Thrombin Generation and Fibrin Turnover

According to the current understanding of sepsis-associated coagulation abnormalities, the determination of soluble fibrin in plasma appears to be crucial.[121,122] In general, the sensitivity of these assays for severe coagulation activation or DIC is higher than the specificity. Indeed, initial clinical studies indicate that if the concentration of soluble fibrin has increased above a defined threshold, a diagnosis of DIC can be made.[20,123] Most of the clinical studies show a sensitivity of 90% to

100% for the diagnosis of DIC, but a rather low specificity.[124]

Fibrin degradation products (FDPs) may be detected by specific ELISAs or by latex agglutination assays, enabling rapid and bedside determination in emergency cases.[125] None of the available assays for FDPs discriminates between degradation products of cross-linked fibrin and fibrinogen degradation, which may cause spuriously high results.[126,127] The specificity of high levels of FDPs is therefore limited and many other conditions, such as trauma, recent surgery, inflammation, or venous thromboembolism, are associated with elevated FDPs. More recently developed tests are specifically aimed at the detection of neoantigens on degraded cross-linked fibrin, such as fragment D-dimer. These tests better differentiate degradation of cross-linked fibrin from fibrinogen or FDPs.[128] D-dimer levels are high in patients with DIC, but also poorly distinguish patients with DIC from patients with venous thromboembolism, patients who have had recent surgery, or patients with inflammatory conditions.[125,129]

Activation peptides released upon the conversion of a coagulation factor zymogen to an active protease are sensitive markers for coagulation activation. Examples of such markers are prothrombin activation fragment F1 + 2 and the activation peptides of factors IX and X.[130–132] Indeed, these markers are markedly elevated in most patients with sepsis. Elevated plasma concentrations of thrombin-antithrombin complexes may well reflect the increased generation of thrombin, and thrombin-mediated fibrinogen-to-fibrin conversion can be monitored by increased levels of fibrinogen activation peptide fibrinopeptide-A.[133,134] All these markers are increased in most patients with sepsis and their high sensitivity may be helpful in detecting even low-grade activation of coagulation. Because many other conditions may lead to elevated plasma levels, the specificity of high levels of markers for coagulation factor activation is probably limited.

Diagnostic Management in a Routine Setting

Most of the newer, more sensitive tests described in the previous section are presently available only in specialized laboratories. Thus, although these tests may be very helpful in clinical trials and in other research, they are rarely available for use in routine settings. In these circumstances, a diagnosis of DIC may be made by a combination of platelet count, measurement of global clotting times (aPTT and PT), measurement of antithrombin III

or one or two clotting factors, and a test for FDPs.[135]

A scoring system, as proposed by the International Society of Thrombosis and Haemostasis, has recently been developed using simple laboratory tests available in almost all hospital laboratories (**Box 1**).[136] Intial prospective studies show that the sensitivity of the DIC score is 93%, whereas the specificity is 98%.[137] Interestingly, the severity of DIC according to this scoring system is related to the mortality in patients with sepsis (**Fig. 3**).[34]

SUPPORTIVE TREATMENT OF COAGULATION ABNORMALITIES IN SEPSIS

In addressing hemostatic abnormalities in patients with sepsis, the key measures are to specifically treat the sepsis by appropriate antibiotics and to control the infectious source. However, many

---

Box 1
Diagnostic algorithm for the diagnosis of overt DIC

1. Risk assessment: Does the patient have an underlying disorder known to be associated with overt DIC? If yes, proceed. If no, do not use this algorithm.

2. Order global coagulation tests (platelet count, PT, fibrinogen, soluble fibrin monomers, or FDPs).

3. Score global coagulation test results:

   Platelet count

   >100 = 0

   <100 = 1

   <50 = 2

   Elevated fibrin-related marker (eg, d-dimer)

   No increase = 0

   Moderate increase (<5× upper limit) = 2

   Strong increase (>5× upper limit) = 3

   Prolonged PT

   <3 seconds = 0

   >3 seconds but <6 seconds = 1

   >6 seconds = 2

   Fibrinogen level

   >1.0 g/L = 0

   <1.0 g/L = 1

4. Calculate score.

5. If ≥5: compatible with overt DIC; if <5: suggestive (not affirmative) for nonovert DIC; repeat next 1–2 days.

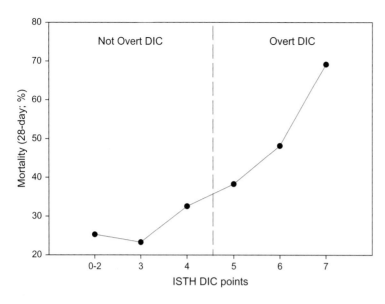

Fig. 3. Number of points on the International Society on Thrombosis and Haemostasis (ISTH) DIC score and 28-day mortality in patients with severe sepsis. Data were derived from the placebo group (n = 840) in the Recombinant Human Activated Protein C Worldwide Evaluation in Severe Sepsis (Prowess) trial on the efficacy of activated protein C in sepsis.

cases require additional supportive treatment for circulatory and respiratory support and to replace organ function. Coagulation abnormalities may proceed, even after proper treatment has been initiated. In those cases, supportive measures to manage the coagulation disorder may be considered and may positively affect morbidity and mortality. The development of such supportive management strategies has benefited from insights into the various mechanisms that play roles in the coagulation abnormalities associated with sepsis.

Plasma and Platelet Substitution Therapy

Low levels of platelets and coagulation factors may increase the risk of bleeding. However, plasma or platelet substitution therapy should not be instituted on the basis of laboratory results alone; it is indicated only in patients with active bleeding and in those requiring an invasive procedure or in those who are otherwise at risk for bleeding complications.[138] The suggestion that administration of blood components might "add fuel to the fire" has never been proven in clinical or experimental studies. The presumed efficacy of treatment with plasma, fibrinogen, cryoprecipitate, or platelets is not based on randomized controlled trials but appears to be rational therapy in bleeding patients or in patients at risk for bleeding because of a significant depletion of these hemostatic factors.[139] It may be necessary to use large volumes of plasma to correct the coagulation defect. Coagulation factor concentrates, such as prothrombin complex concentrate, may overcome this obstacle, but these compounds may lack essential factors, such as factor V. Moreover, older

literature advocated caution with the use of prothrombin complex concentrates in DIC because small traces of activated factors may worsen the coagulopathy. It is, however, not clear whether this caution is still relevant for the concentrates that are currently in use. Specific deficiencies in coagulation factors, such as fibrinogen, may be corrected by administration of purified coagulation factor concentrates.

Anticoagulants

Experimental studies have shown that heparin can at least partly inhibit the activation of coagulation in sepsis.[140] Uncontrolled case series in patients with sepsis and DIC have claimed to be successful. However, a beneficial effect of heparin on clinically important outcome events in patients with DIC has never been demonstrated in controlled clinical trials.[141] Experimental studies have shown that heparin can at least partly inhibit the activation of coagulation in DIC.[142] A recent large trial in patients with severe sepsis showed a slight (nonsignificant) benefit of low-dose heparin on 28-day mortality in patients with severe sepsis. However, the trial mostly underscored the importance of not stopping heparin in patients with DIC and abnormal coagulation parameters.[143] Therapeutic doses of heparin are indicated in patients with clinically overt thromboembolism or extensive fibrin deposition, such as purpura fulminans or acral ischemia. Patients with sepsis may benefit from prophylaxis to prevent venous thromboembolism, which may not be achieved with standard low-dose subcutaneous heparin.[144] Theoretically, the most logical anticoagulant agent to use in DIC is directed against tissue factor activity. Potential agents include recombinant tissue factor pathway inhibitor, inactivated factor VIIa, and recombinant NAPc2, a potent and specific inhibitor of the ternary complex between tissue factor–factor VIIa and factor Xa.[145] Phase II trials of recombinant TFPI showed promising results but a phase III trial did not show an overall survival benefit in patients treated with TFPI.[146,147]

Restoration of Anticoagulant Pathways

In view of the deficient state of physiologic anticoagulant pathways in patients with sepsis, restoration of these inhibitors may be a rational approach.[148] Since antithrombin is one of the most important physiologic inhibitors of coagulation, the use of antithrombin III concentrates in patients with DIC has been intensively studied on the basis of successful preclinical results. Most of the randomized controlled trials concern patients with sepsis, septic shock, or both. All trials show some beneficial effect in terms of improvement of laboratory parameters, shortening the duration of DIC, or even improvement in organ function.[6] A large-scale, multicenter, randomized controlled trial to directly address this issue showed no significant reduction in mortality of patients with sepsis who were treated with antithrombin concentrate.[149] Interestingly, post hoc subgroup analyses indicated some benefit in patients who did not receive concomitant heparin and who fulfilled the diagnostic criteria for DIC, but this observation needs prospective validation.[150]

Based on the notion that depression of the protein C system may significantly contribute to the pathophysiology of DIC, supplementation of (activated) protein C might be beneficial.[148] A beneficial effect of recombinant human activated protein C was demonstrated in a phase III trial of activated protein C concentrate in patients with sepsis. This trial was prematurely stopped because of efficacy in reducing mortality in these patients.[22] All-cause mortality at 28 days after inclusion was 24.7% in the activated protein C group versus 30.8% in the control group (19.4% relative risk reduction). The administration of activated protein C ameliorated coagulation abnormalities and resulted in fewer cases of organ failure.[151] In view of the above-described effects that activated protein C has on inflammation, part of the success may have been caused by a beneficial effect on inflammatory pathways. Interestingly, a post hoc analysis of this trial demonstrated that patients classified with DIC, according to the DIC scoring system of the International Society on Thrombosis and Haemostasis, benefited more from activated protein C treatment than did patients who did not have overt DIC.[34] The relative risk reduction in mortality of patients with sepsis and DIC who received activated protein C was 38%, in comparison with a relative risk reduction of 18% in patients with sepsis who did not have DIC. This seems to underscore the importance of the coagulation derangement in the pathogenesis of sepsis and of the impact that restoration of microvascular anticoagulant pathways may provide in the treatment of sepsis. Recombinant human-activated protein C has been licensed in most countries for treatment of patients with severe sepsis and two or more organ failures. It was shown not to be effective in patients with less severe sepsis.[152] The most frequently encountered adverse effect of activated protein C is bleeding. In the phase III study in patients with severe sepsis, the incidence of major bleeding (ie, bleeding reported as a serious adverse event) during the infusion period was 2.4% in the activated protein C group, as compared with 1.0% in the control group ($P = .02$).[22] During the 28-day study period, the incidence of major bleeding was 3.5% in the activated protein C group and 2.0% in the placebo group ($P = .06$).

SUMMARY

Sepsis often is associated with systemic intravascular activation of coagulation, potentially leading to widespread microvascular deposition of fibrin, thereby contributing to multiple organ dysfunction. A complex interaction exists between activation of inflammatory systems and the initiating and regulating pathways of coagulation. A diagnosis of sepsis-associated DIC can be made by a combination of routinely available laboratory tests, for which simple diagnostic algorithms have become available. Strategies aimed at the inhibition of coagulation activation may theoretically be justified and are being evaluated in clinical studies.

REFERENCES

1. Levi M, Marder VJ. Coagulation abnormalities in sepsis. In: Colman RW, Marder VJ, Clowes AW, et al, editors. Hemostasis and thrombosis: basic principles and clinical practice. 5th edition. Philadelphia: Lippincott William and Wilkins; 2006. p. 1601–13.
2. Levi M, ten Cate H, van der Poll T, et al. Pathogenesis of disseminated intravascular coagulation in sepsis. JAMA 1993;270(8):975–9.
3. Levi M, ten Cate H. Disseminated intravascular coagulation. N Engl J Med 1999;341(8):586–92.
4. Colman RW, Robboy SJ, Minna JD. Disseminated intravascular coagulation: a reappraisal. Annu Rev Med 1979;30:359–74.

5. Miller DL, Welty-Wolf K, Carraway MS, et al. Extrinsic coagulation blockade attenuates lung injury and proinflammatory cytokine release after intratracheal lipopolysaccharide. Am J Respir Cell Mol Biol 2002; 26(6):650–8.

6. Levi M, ten Cate H, van der Poll T. Disseminated intravascular coagulation: state of the art. Thromb Haemost 1999;82:695–705.

7. Wheeler AP, Bernard GR. Treating patients with severe sepsis. N Engl J Med 1999;340(3):207–14.

8. Levi M, de Jonge E, van der Poll T. Sepsis and disseminated intravascular coagulation. J Thromb Thrombolysis 2003;16(1–2):43–7.

9. Vanderschueren S, De Weerdt A, Malbrain M, et al. Thrombocytopenia and prognosis in intensive care. Crit Care Med 2000;28(6):1871–6.

10. Baughman RP, Lower EE, Flessa HC, et al. Thrombocytopenia in the intensive care unit. Chest 1993; 104(4):1243–7.

11. Strauss R, Wehler M, Mehler K, et al. Thrombocytopenia in patients in the medical intensive care unit: bleeding prevalence, transfusion requirements, and outcome. Crit Care Med 2002;30(8):1765–71.

12. Akca S, Haji Michael P, de Medonca A, et al. The time course of platelet counts in critically ill patients. Crit Care Med 2002;30:753–6.

13. Mavrommatis AC, Theodoridis T, Orfanidou A, et al. Coagulation system and platelets are fully activated in uncomplicated sepsis. Crit Care Med 2000;28(2):451–7.

14. Levi M. Platelets. Crit Care Med 2005;33(Suppl 12): S523–5.

15. Folman CC, Linthorst GE, van Mourik J, et al. Platelets release thrombopoietin (Tpo) upon activation: another regulatory loop in thrombocytopoiesis? Thromb Haemost 2000;83(6):923–30.

16. Francois B, Trimoreau F, Vignon P, et al. Thrombocytopenia in the sepsis syndrome: role of hemophagocytosis and macrophage colony-stimulating factor. Am J Med 1997;103(2):114–20.

17. Warkentin TE, Aird WC, Rand JH. Platelet-endothelial interactions: sepsis, HIT, and antiphospholipid syndrome. Hematology Am Soc Hematol Educ Program 2003;7:497–519.

18. Chakraverty R, Davidson S, Peggs K, et al. The incidence and cause of coagulopathies in an intensive care population. Br J Haematol 1996;93(2): 460–3.

19. MacLeod JB, Lynn M, McKenney MG, et al. Early coagulopathy predicts mortality in trauma. J Trauma 2003;55(1):39–44.

20. Shorr AF, Thomas SJ, Alkins SA, et al. D-dimer correlates with proinflammatory cytokine levels and outcomes in critically ill patients. Chest 2002; 121(4):1262–8.

21. Owings JT, Gosselin RC, Anderson JT, et al. Practical utility of the D-dimer assay for excluding thromboembolism in severely injured trauma patients. J Trauma 2001;51(3):425–9.

22. Bernard GR, Vincent JL, Laterre PF, et al. Efficacy and safety of recombinant human activated protein C for severe sepsis. N Engl J Med 2001;344(10): 699–709.

23. Gando S, Nanzaki S, Sasaki S, et al. Significant correlations between tissue factor and thrombin markers in trauma and septic patients with disseminated intravascular coagulation. Thromb Haemost 1998;79(6):1111–5.

24. Levi M, Keller TT, van Gorp E, et al. Infection and inflammation and the coagulation system. Cardiovasc Res 2003;60(1):26–39.

25. Robboy SJ, Major MC, Colman RW, et al. Pathology of disseminated intravascular coagulation (DIC). Analysis of 26 cases. Hum Pathol 1972;3(3): 327–43.

26. Shimamura K, Oka K, Nakazawa M, et al. Distribution patterns of microthrombi in disseminated intravascular coagulation. Arch Pathol Lab Med 1983; 107(10):543–7.

27. Coalson JJ. Pathology of sepsis, septic shock, and multiple organ failure. Perspective on sepsis and septic shock. Fullerton (CA): Society of Critical Care Medicine; 1986. p. 27–59.

28. Creasey AA, Chang AC, Feigen L, et al. Tissue factor pathway inhibitor reduces mortality from Escherichia coli septic shock. J Clin Invest 1993; 91(6):2850–6.

29. Kessler CM, Tang Z, Jacobs HM, et al. The suprapharmacologic dosing of antithrombin concentrate for Staphylococcus aureus–induced disseminated intravascular coagulation in guinea pigs: substantial reduction in mortality and morbidity. Blood 1997;89(12):4393–401.

30. Taylor FB Jr, Chang A, Ruf W, et al. Lethal E. coli septic shock is prevented by blocking tissue factor with monoclonal antibody. Circ Shock 1991;33(3): 127–34.

31. Taylor FB Jr, Chang A, Esmon CT, et al. Protein C prevents the coagulopathic and lethal effects of Escherichia coli infusion in the baboon. J Clin Invest 1987;79(3):918–25.

32. Welty-Wolf KE, Carraway MS, Miller DL, et al. Coagulation blockade prevents sepsis-induced respiratory and renal failure in baboons. Am J Respir Crit Care Med 2001;164(10 Pt 1):1988–96.

33. Fourrier F, Chopin C, Goudemand J, et al. Septic shock, multiple organ failure, and disseminated intravascular coagulation. Compared patterns of antithrombin III, protein C, and protein S deficiencies [see comments]. Chest 1992;101(3): 816–23.

34. Dhainaut JF, Yan SB, Joyce DE, et al. Treatment effects of drotrecogin alfa (activated) in patients with severe sepsis with or without overt

disseminated intravascular coagulation. J Thromb Haemost 2004;2:1924–33.

35. Oppenheim-Eden A, Glantz L, Eidelman LA, et al. Spontaneous intracerebral hemorrhage in critically ill patients: incidence over six years and associated factors. Intensive Care Med 1999;25(1):63–7.

36. Stephan F, Hollande J, Richard O, et al. Thrombocytopenia in a surgical ICU. Chest 1999;115(5):1363–70.

37. Levi M, van der Poll T, ten Cate H, et al. The cytokine-mediated imbalance between coagulant and anticoagulant mechanisms in sepsis and endotoxaemia. Eur J Clin Invest 1997;27(1):3–9.

38. Levi M, van der Poll T, Buller HR. The bidirectional relationshiop between coagulation and inflammation. Circulation 2004;109(22):2698–704.

39. Aird WC. Vascular bed–specific hemostasis: role of endothelium in sepsis pathogenesis. Crit Care Med 2001;29(Suppl 7):S28–34.

40. Kalter ES, Daha MR, ten CJ, et al. Activation and inhibition of Hageman factor–dependent pathways and the complement system in uncomplicated bacteremia or bacterial shock. J Infect Dis 1985;151(6):1019–27.

41. van Deventer SJ, Buller HR, ten Cate JW, et al. Experimental endotoxemia in humans: analysis of cytokine release and coagulation, fibrinolytic, and complement pathways. Blood 1990;76(12):2520–6.

42. van der Poll T, Buller HR, ten Cate H, et al. Activation of coagulation after administration of tumor necrosis factor to normal subjects. N Engl J Med 1990;322(23):1622–7.

43. Levi M, ten Cate H, Bauer KA, et al. Inhibition of endotoxin-induced activation of coagulation and fibrinolysis by pentoxifylline or by a monoclonal anti-tissue factor antibody in chimpanzees. J Clin Invest 1994;93(1):114–20.

44. Biemond BJ, Levi M, ten Cate H, et al. Complete inhibition of endotoxin-induced coagulation activation in chimpanzees with a monoclonal Fab fragment against factor VII/VIIa. Thromb Haemost 1995;73(2):223–30.

45. Ruf W, Edgington TS. Structural biology of tissue factor, the initiator of thrombogenesis in vivo. FASEB J 1994;8(6):385–90.

46. Osterud B, Flaegstad T. Increased tissue thromboplastin activity in monocytes of patients with meningococcal infection: related to an unfavourable prognosis. Thromb Haemost 1983;49(1):5–7.

47. Franco RF, de JE, Dekkers PE, et al. The in vivo kinetics of tissue factor messenger RNA expression during human endotoxemia: relationship with activation of coagulation. Blood 2000;96(2):554–9.

48. Giesen PL, Rauch U, Bohrmann B, et al. Blood-borne tissue factor: another view of thrombosis. Proc Natl Acad Sci U S A 1999;96(5):2311–5.

49. Osterud B, Rao LV, Olsen JO. Induction of tissue factor expression in whole blood—lack of evidence for the presence of tissue factor expression on granulocytes. Thromb Haemost 2000;83:861–7.

50. Rauch U, Bonderman D, Bohrmann B, et al. Transfer of tissue factor from leukocytes to platelets is mediated by CD15 and tissue factor. Blood 2000;96(1):170–5.

51. Zimmerman GA, McIntyre TM, Prescott SM, et al. The platelet-activating factor signaling system and its regulators in syndromes of inflammation and thrombosis. Crit Care Med 2002;30(Suppl 5):S294–301.

52. Shebuski RJ, Kilgore KS. Role of inflammatory mediators in thrombogenesis. J Pharmacol Exp Ther 2002;300(3):729–35.

53. Vary TC, Kimball SR. Regulation of hepatic protein synthesis in chronic inflammation and sepsis. Am J Physiol 1992;262(2 Pt 1):C445–52.

54. Seitz R, Wolf M, Egbring R, et al. The disturbance of hemostasis in septic shock: role of neutrophil elastase and thrombin, effects of antithrombin III and plasma substitution. Eur J Haematol 1989;43(1):22–8.

55. Opal SM, Kessler CM, Roemisch J, et al. Antithrombin, heparin, and heparan sulfate. Crit Care Med 2002;30(Suppl 5):S325–31.

56. Mesters RM, Mannucci PM, Coppola R, et al. Factor VIIa and activity during severe sepsis and septic shock in neutropenic patients. Blood 1996;88(3):881–6.

57. Esmon CT. New mechanisms for vascular control of inflammation mediated by natural anticoagulant proteins. J Exp Med 2002;196(5):561–4.

58. Zushi M, Gomi K, Yamamoto S, et al. The last three consecutive epidermal growth factor–like structures of human thrombomodulin comprise the minimum functional domain for protein C-activating cofactor activity and anticoagulant activity. J Biol Chem 1989;264(18):10351–3.

59. Bajzar L, Morser J, Nesheim M. TAFI, or plasma procarboxypeptidase B, couples the coagulation and fibrinolytic cascades through the thrombin-thrombomodulin complex. J Biol Chem 1996;271(28):16603–8.

60. Taylor FB Jr, Peer GT, Lockhart MS, et al. Endothelial cell protein C receptor plays an important role in protein C activation in vivo. Blood 2001;97(6):1685–8.

61. Eckle I, Seitz R, Egbring R, et al. Protein C degradation in vitro by neutrophil elastase. Biol Chem Hoppe Seyler 1991;372(11):1007–13.

62. Nawroth PP, Stern DM. Modulation of endothelial cell hemostatic properties by tumor necrosis factor. J Exp Med 1986;163(3):740–5.

63. Faust SN, Levin M, Harrison OB, et al. Dysfunction of endothelial protein C activation in severe

meningococcal sepsis. N Engl J Med 2001;345(6): 408–16.

64. Garcia de Frutos P, Alim RI, Hardig Y, et al. Differential regulation of alpha and beta chains of C4b-binding protein during acute-phase response resulting in stable plasma levels of free anticoagulant protein S. Blood 1994;84(3):815–22.

65. Taylor F, Chang A, Ferrell G, et al. C4b-binding protein exacerbates the host response to Escherichia coli. Blood 1991;78(2):357–63.

66. Taylor FB Jr, Dahlback B, Chang AC, et al. Role of free protein S and C4b binding protein in regulating the coagulant response to Escherichia coli. Blood 1995;86(7):2642–52.

67. Levi M, Dorffler-Melly J, Reitsma PH, et al. Aggravation of endotoxin-induced disseminated intravascular coagulation and cytokine activation in heterozygous protein C deficient mice. Blood 2003;101:4823–7.

68. Broze GJ Jr, Girard TJ, Novotny WF. Regulation of coagulation by a multivalent Kunitz-type inhibitor. Biochemistry 1990;29(33):7539–46.

69. de Jonge E, Dekkers PE, Creasey AA, et al. Tissue factor pathway inhibitor (TFPI) dose-dependently inhibits coagulation activation without influencing the fibrinolytic and cytokine response during human endotoxemia. Blood 2000;95:1124–9.

70. Gando S, Kameue T, Morimoto Y, et al. Tissue factor production not balanced by tissue factor pathway inhibitor in sepsis promotes poor prognosis. Crit Care Med 2002;30:1729–34.

71. Levi M. The imbalance between tissue factor and tissue factor pathway inhibitor in sepsis. Crit Care Med 2002;30(8):1914–5.

72. van der Poll T, Levi M, Buller HR, et al. Fibrinolytic response to tumor necrosis factor in healthy subjects. J Exp Med 1991;174(3):729–32.

73. Biemond BJ, Levi M, ten CH, et al. Plasminogen activator and plasminogen activator inhibitor I release during experimental endotoxaemia in chimpanzees: effect of interventions in the cytokine and coagulation cascades. Clin Sci (Lond) 1995;88(5): 587–94.

74. Yamamoto K, Loskutoff DJ. Fibrin deposition in tissues from endotoxin-treated mice correlates with decreases in the expression of urokinase-type but not tissue-type plasminogen activator. J Clin Invest 1996;97(11):2440–51.

75. Pinsky DJ, Liao H, Lawson CA, et al. Coordinated induction of plasminogen activator inhibitor–1 (PAI-1) and inhibition of plasminogen activator gene expression by hypoxia promotes pulmonary vascular fibrin deposition. J Clin Invest 1998; 102(5):919–28.

76. Hermans PW, Hibberd ML, Booy R, et al. 4G/5G promoter polymorphism in the plasminogen-activator-inhibitor-1 gene and outcome of meningococcal disease. Meningococcal Research Group. Lancet 1999;354(9178):556–60.

77. Westendorp RG, Hottenga JJ, Slagboom PE. Variation in plasminogen-activator-inhibitor-1 gene and risk of meningococcal septic shock. Lancet 1999; 354(9178):561–3.

78. Bauer KA, ten CH, Barzegar S, et al. Tumor necrosis factor infusions have a procoagulant effect on the hemostatic mechanism of humans. Blood 1989;74(1):165–72.

79. van der Poll T, Levi M, van Deventer SJ, et al. Differential effects of anti–tumor necrosis factor monoclonal antibodies on systemic inflammatory responses in experimental endotoxemia in chimpanzees. Blood 1994;83(2):446–51.

80. van der Poll T, Coyle SM, Levi M, et al. Effect of a recombinant dimeric tumor necrosis factor receptor on inflammatory responses to intravenous endotoxin in normal humans. Blood 1997;89(10): 3727–34.

81. Hinshaw LB, Tekamp-Olson P, Chang AC, et al. Survival of primates in LD100 septic shock following therapy with antibody to tumor necrosis factor (TNF alpha). Circ Shock 1990;30(3):279–92.

82. van der Poll T, Levi M, Hack CE, et al. Elimination of interleukin 6 attenuates coagulation activation in experimental endotoxemia in chimpanzees. J Exp Med 1994;179(4):1253–9.

83. Stouthard JM, Levi M, Hack CE, et al. Interleukin-6 stimulates coagulation, not fibrinolysis, in humans. Thromb Haemost 1996;76(5):738–42.

84. Fischer E, Marano MA, Van Zee KJ, et al. Interleukin-1 receptor blockade improves survival and hemodynamic performance in Escherichia coli septic shock, but fails to alter host responses to sublethal endotoxemia. J Clin Invest 1992;89(5):1551–7.

85. Jansen PM, Boermeester MA, Fischer E, et al. Contribution of interleukin-1 to activation of coagulation and fibrinolysis, neutrophil degranulation, and the release of secretory-type phospholipase A2 in sepsis: studies in nonhuman primates after interleukin-1 alpha administration and during lethal bacteremia. Blood 1995;86(3):1027–34.

86. Boermeester MA, van LP, Coyle SM, et al. Interleukin-1 blockade attenuates mediator release and dysregulation of the hemostatic mechanism during human sepsis. Arch Surg 1995;130(7):739–48.

87. Pajkrt D, van der Poll T, Levi M, et al. Interleukin-10 inhibits activation of coagulation and fibrinolysis during human endotoxemia. Blood 1997;89(8): 2701–5.

88. Mileno MD, Margolis NH, Clark BD, et al. Coagulation of whole blood stimulates interleukin-1 beta gene expression. J Infect Dis 1995;172(1):308–11.

89. Jones A, Geczy CL. Thrombin and factor Xa enhance the production of interleukin-1. Immunology 1990;71(2):236–41.

90. Johnson K, Choi Y, DeGroot E, et al. Potential mechanisms for a proinflammatory vascular cytokine response to coagulation activation. J Immunol 1998;160(10):5130–5.

91. Sower LE, Froelich CJ, Carney DH, et al. Thrombin induces IL-6 production in fibroblasts and epithelial cells. Evidence for the involvement of the seven-transmembrane domain (STD) receptor for alpha-thrombin. J Immunol 1995;155(2):895–901.

92. van der Poll T, de Jonge E, Levi M. Regulatory role of cytokines in disseminated intravascular coagulation. Semin Thromb Hemost 2001;27(6):639–51.

93. Coughlin SR. Thrombin signalling and protease-activated receptors. Nature 2000;407(6801):258–64.

94. Cunningham MA, Romas P, Hutchinson P, et al. Tissue factor and factor VIIa receptor/ligand interactions induce proinflammatory effects in macrophages. Blood 1999;94(10):3413–20.

95. Cenac N, Coelho AM, Nguyen C, et al. Induction of intestinal inflammation in mouse by activation of proteinase-activated receptor-2. Am J Pathol 2002;161(5):1903–15.

96. de Jonge E, Friederich PW, Levi M, et al. Activation of coagulation by administration of recombinant factor VIIa elicits interleukin-6 and interleukin-8 release in healthy human subjects. Clin Diagn Lab Immunol 2003;10:495–7.

97. Szaba FM, Smiley ST. Roles for thrombin and fibrin(ogen) in cytokine/chemokine production and macrophage adhesion in vivo. Blood 2002;99(3):1053–9.

98. Smiley ST, King JA, Hancock WW. Fibrinogen stimulates macrophage chemokine secretion through Toll-like receptor 4. J Immunol 2001;167(5):2887–94.

99. Kaneider NC, Forster E, Mosheimer B, et al. Syndecan-4–dependent signaling in the inhibition of endotoxin-induced endothelial adherence of neutrophils by antithrombin. Thromb Haemost 2003;90(6):1150–7.

100. Okajima K. Regulation of inflammatory responses by natural anticoagulants. Immunol Rev 2001;184:258–74.

101. Grey ST, Tsuchida A, Hau H, et al. Selective inhibitory effects of the anticoagulant activated protein C on the responses of human mononuclear phagocytes to LPS, IFN-gamma, or phorbol ester. J Immunol 1994;153(8):3664–72.

102. Yuksel M, Okajima K, Uchiba M, et al. Activated protein C inhibits lipopolysaccharide-induced tumor necrosis factor-alpha production by inhibiting activation of both nuclear factor-kappa B and activator protein-1 in human monocytes. Thromb Haemost 2002;88(2):267–73.

103. Murakami K, Okajima K, Uchiba M, et al. Activated protein C attenuates endotoxin-induced pulmonary vascular injury by inhibiting activated leukocytes in rats. Blood 1996;87(2):642–7.

104. Taylor FB Jr. Studies on the inflammatory-coagulant axis in the baboon response to E. coli: regulatory roles of proteins C, S, C4bBP and of inhibitors of tissue factor. [review] [13 refs]. Prog Clin Biol Res 1994;381:175–94.

105. Taylor FB Jr, Stearns-Kurosawa DJ, Kurosawa S, et al. The endothelial cell protein C receptor aids in host defense against Escherichia coli sepsis. Blood 2000;95(5):1680–6.

106. White B, Schmidt M, Murphy C, et al. Activated protein C inhibits lipopolysaccharide-induced nuclear translocation of nuclear factor kappaB (NF-kappaB) and tumour necrosis factor alpha (TNF-alpha) production in the THP-1 monocytic cell line. Br J Haematol 2000;110(1):130–4.

107. Hancock WW, Grey ST, Hau L, et al. Binding of activated protein C to a specific receptor on human mononuclear phagocytes inhibits intracellular calcium signaling and monocyte-dependent proliferative responses. Transplantation 1995;60(12):1525–32.

108. Riewald M, Petrovan RJ, Donner A, et al. Activation of endothelial cell protease activated receptor 1 by the protein C pathway. Science 2002;296(5574):1880–2.

109. Xu J, Qu D, Esmon NL, et al. Metalloproteolytic release of endothelial cell protein C receptor. J Biol Chem 2000;275(8):6038–44.

110. Kurosawa S, Esmon CT, Stearns-Kurosawa DJ. The soluble endothelial protein C receptor binds to activated neutrophils: involvement of proteinase-3 and CD11b/CD18. J Immunol 2000;165(8):4697–703.

111. Cheng T, Liu D, Griffin JH, et al. Activated protein C blocks p53-mediated apoptosis in ischemic human brain endothelium and is neuroprotective. Nat Med 2003;9:338–42.

112. Mosnier LO, Griffin JH. Inhibition of staurosporine-induced apoptosis of endothelial cells by activated protein C requires protease activated receptor-1 and endothelial cell protein C receptor. Biochem J 2003;373:65–70.

113. Weinbaum S, Zhang X, Han Y, et al. Mechanotransduction and flow across the endothelial glycocalyx. Proc Natl Acad Sci U S A 2003;100(13):7988–95.

114. Maczewski M, Duda M, Pawlak W, et al. Endothelial protection from reperfusion injury by ischemic preconditioning and diazoxide involves a SOD-like anti-O2- mechanism. J Physiol Pharmacol 2004;55(3):537–50.

115. Vink H, Constantinescu AA, Spaan JA. Oxidized lipoproteins degrade the endothelial surface layer: implications for platelet-endothelial cell adhesion. Circulation 2000;101(13):1500–2.

116. Nieuwdorp M, van Haeften TW, Gouverneur MC, et al. Loss of endothelial glycocalyx during acute hyperglycemia coincides with endothelial dysfunction and coagulation activation in vivo. Diabetes 2006;55(2):480–6.

117. van den Berg BM, Vink H, Spaan JA. The endothelial glycocalyx protects against myocardial edema. Circ Res 2003;92(6):592–4.

118. Levi M, Opal SM. Coagulation abnormalities in critically ill patients. Crit Care 2006;10(4):222–8.

119. Neame PB, Kelton JG, Walker IR, et al. Thrombocytopenia in septicemia: the role of disseminated intravascular coagulation. Blood 1980;56(1):88–92.

120. Levi M. Platelets in sepsis. Hematology 2005; 10(Suppl):1129–31.

121. Dempfle CE, Pfitzner SA, Dollman M, et al. Comparison of immunological and functional assays for measurement of soluble fibrin. Thromb Haemost 1995;74(2):673–9.

122. McCarron BI, Marder VJ, Kanouse JJ, et al. A soluble fibrin standard: comparable dose-response with immunologic and functional assays. Thromb Haemost 1999;82(1):145–8.

123. Dempfle CE. The use of soluble fibrin in evaluating the acute and chronic hypercoagulable state [review] [147 refs]. Thromb Haemost 1999;82(2):673–83.

124. Horan JT, Francis CW. Fibrin degradation products, fibrin monomer and soluble fibrin in disseminated intravascular coagulation. Semin Thromb Hemost 2001;27(6):657–66.

125. Carr JM, McKinney M, McDonagh J. Diagnosis of disseminated intravascular coagulation. Role of D-dimer. Am J Clin Pathol 1989;91(3):280–7.

126. Boisclair MD, Ireland H, Lane DA. Assessment of hypercoagulable states by measurement of activation fragments and peptides [review] [113 refs]. Blood Rev 1990;4(1):25–40.

127. Prisco D, Paniccia R, Bonechi F, et al. Evaluation of new methods for the selective measurement of fibrin and fibrinogen degradation products. Thromb Res 1989;56(4):547–51.

128. Shorr AF, Trotta RF, Alkins SA, et al. D-dimer assay predicts mortality in critically ill patients without disseminated intravascular coagulation or venous thromboembolic disease. Intensive Care Med 1999;25(2):207–10.

129. Greenberg CS, Devine DV, McCrae KM. Measurement of plasma fibrin D-dimer levels with the use of a monoclonal antibody coupled to latex beads. Am J Clin Pathol 1987;87(1):94–100.

130. Teitel JM, Bauer KA, Lau HK, et al. Studies of the prothrombin activation pathway utilizing radioimmunoassays for the F2/F1 + 2 fragment and thrombin–antithrombin complex. Blood 1982;59(5):1086–97.

131. Bauer KA, Kass BL, ten CH, et al. Detection of factor X activation in humans. Blood 1989;74(6):2007–15.

132. ten Cate H, Bauer KA, Levi M, et al. The activation of factor X and prothrombin by recombinant factor VIIa in vivo is mediated by tissue factor. J Clin Invest 1993;92(3):1207–12.

133. Takahashi H, Wada K, Niwano H, et al. Comparison of prothrombin fragment 1 + 2 with thrombin-antithrombin III complex in plasma of patients with disseminated intravascular coagulation. Blood Coagul Fibrinolysis 1992;3(6):813–8.

134. Kario K, Matsuo T, Kodama K, et al. Imbalance between thrombin and plasmin activity in disseminated intravascular coagulation. Assessment by the thrombin-antithrombin-III complex/plasmin-alpha-2-antiplasmin complex ratio. Haemostasis 1992;22(4):179–86.

135. Levi M, de Jonge E, Meijers J. The diagnosis of disseminated intravascular coagulation. Blood Rev 2002;16(4):217–23.

136. Taylor FBJ, Toh CH, Hoots WK, et al. Towards definition, clinical and laboratory criteria, and a scoring system for disseminated intravascular coagulation. Thromb Haemost 2001;86(5):1327–30.

137. Bakhtiari K, Meijers JC, de Jonge E, et al. Prospective validation of the International Society of Thrombosis and Haemostasis scoring system for disseminated intravascular coagulation. Crit Care Med 2004;32:2416–21.

138. Alving BM, Spivak JL, DeLoughery TG. Consultative hematology: hemostasis and transfusion issues in surgery and critical care medicine. In: McArthur JR, Schechter GP, Schrier SL, editors. Hematology 1998 (The American Society of Hematology Education Program Book) American Society of Hematology; 1998. p. 320–341.

139. de Jonge E, Levi M, Stoutenbeek CP, et al. Current drug treatment strategies for disseminated intravascular coagulation. Drugs 1998;55(6):767–77.

140. du Toit H, Coetzee AR, Chalton DO. Heparin treatment in thrombin-induced disseminated intravascular coagulation in the baboon. Crit Care Med 1991;19(9):1195–200.

141. Feinstein DI. Diagnosis and management of disseminated intravascular coagulation: the role of heparin therapy. Blood 1982;60(2):284–7.

142. Pernerstorfer T, Hollenstein U, Hansen J, et al. Heparin blunts endotoxin-induced coagulation activation. Circulation 1999;100(25):2485–90.

143. Levi M, Levy M, Williams MD, et al. Prophylactic heparin in patients with severe sepsis treated with drotrecogin alfa (activated). Am J Respir Crit Care Med 2007;176(5):483–90.

144. Dorffler-Melly J, de Jonge E, Pont AC, et al. Bioavailability of subcutaneous low-molecular-weight heparin to patients on vasopressors. Lancet 2002;359(9309):849–50.

145. Vlasuk GP, Bergum PW, Bradbury AE, et al. Clinical evaluation of rNAPc2, an inhibitor of the fVIIa/tissue

factor coagulation complex. Am J Cardiol 1997;80:
66S–71S.

146. Abraham E, Reinhart K, Svoboda P, et al. Assessment of the safety of recombinant tissue factor pathway inhibitor in patients with severe sepsis: a multicenter, randomized, placebo-controlled, single-blind, dose escalation study. Crit Care Med 2001;29(11):2081–9.

147. Abraham E, Reinhart K, Opal S, et al. Efficacy and safety of tifacogin (recombinant tissue factor pathway inhibitor) in severe sepsis: a randomized controlled trial. JAMA 2003;290(2):238–47.

148. Levi M, de Jonge E, van der Poll T. Rationale for restoration of physiological anticoagulant pathways in patients with sepsis and disseminated intravascular coagulation. Crit Care Med 2001;429(Suppl 7): S90–4.

149. Warren BL, Eid A, Singer P, et al. Caring for the critically ill patient. High-dose antithrombin III in severe sepsis: a randomized controlled trial. JAMA 2001;286(15):1869–78.

150. Kienast J, Juers M, Wiedermann CJ, et al. Treatment effects of high-dose antithrombin without concomitant heparin in patients with severe sepsis with or without disseminated intravascular coagulation. J Thromb Haemost 2006;4(1):90–7.

151. Vincent JL, Angus DC, Artigas A, et al. Effects of drotrecogin alfa (activated) on organ dysfunction in the PROWESS trial. Crit Care Med 2003;31(3): 834–40.

152. Abraham E, Laterre PF, Garg R, et al. Drotrecogin alfa (activated) for adults with severe sepsis and a low risk of death. N Engl J Med 2005;353(13): 1332–41.

The Heterogeneity of the Microcirculation in Critical Illness

Eva Klijn, MD[a], C.A. Den Uil, MD[b], Jan Bakker, MD, PhD[a], Can Ince, PhD[a],*

KEYWORDS

- Critical illness • Microcirculation • Multi organ failure
- Orthogonal polarization spectral imaging
- Sidestream dark field imaging • Sepsis • Shock

In recent years, interest in the role of microcirculation in critical illness has grown. This seems logical because microcirculation is ultimately responsible for providing oxygen to the tissues. Microcirculation is a complex network, with special morphologic features tailored for the specific function of the tissues it supplies. Recently, new imaging techniques and clinical investigations have identified microcirculation as a pivotal element in the pathogenesis of sepsis.

Although major progress has been made in the treatment of sepsis, mortality and morbidity rates associated with sepsis remain high.[1,2] Hemodynamic treatment is primarily aimed at correcting global hemodynamic and oxygen-derived variables.[2] Despite aggressive correction of global parameters with volume resuscitation and vasoactive agents, some patients progress into multiorgan failure and die.[3,4] The ultimate aim of resuscitation is to correct and avoid tissue hypoxia. However, the end points used to evaluate the achievements of resuscitation therapy (eg, lactate levels, venous oxygen saturation, and mean arterial pressure) are not sensitive enough to detect regional hypoxia. This lack of sensitivity is primarily due to the distributive defect associated with septic shock, in which a defect in the distribution of normal cardiac output (or even increased cardiac output) results in regional hypoxia that is not detected by conventional hemodynamic monitoring of systemic circulation. This occult hypoxia highlights the necessity of finding new end points for the treatment of severe sepsis and septic shock.

This review first explores the characteristic features of several microvascular beds that can be visualized at the bedside. Second, the distinctive abnormalities occurring during sepsis are discussed in relation to different types of shock. In addition, we review the response of microcirculation to available therapeutic modalities frequently used to treat septic shock patients. Although many methods exist to study microcirculation, either directly or indirectly, this review mainly focuses on the use of either orthogonal polarization spectral (OPS) imaging or sidestream dark field (SDF) imaging[5,6] for direct clinical visualization of microcirculation with bedside vital microscopy. Because the heterogeneity of microvascular alterations among different organs and within individual organs is a key characteristic of the pathophysiology of hemodynamic dysfunction in sepsis, the preferred technique for identifying these alterations is direct visualization.

THE ANATOMY AND FUNCTION OF DIFFERENT MICROCIRCULATORY BEDS

Microcirculation has evolved from being a hypothesized necessary link between the arteries and veins, in Harvey's theory of circulation, to a possible end point of resuscitation in critical illness. In 1661, Malpighi demonstrated, for the first time in vivo, long,

[a] Department of Intensive Care, Erasmus MC University Medical Center, PO Box 2040, Room H 627, 3000 CA Rotterdam, The Netherlands
[b] Department of Cardiology, Erasmus MC University Medical Center, 3000 CA Rotterdam, The Netherlands
* Corresponding author.
E-mail address: c.ince@erasmusmc.nl (C. Ince).

Clin Chest Med 29 (2008) 643–654
doi:10.1016/j.ccm.2008.06.008
0272-5231/08/$ – see front matter © 2008 Elsevier Inc. All rights reserved.

thin-walled tubes, which he termed capillaries. Technical advances made in recent years have made it possible to directly or indirectly study micro-circulation in different pathologic states. Most of the information concerning the functional morphology of microcirculation has been obtained from extensive studies involving experimental animals.

Microvasculature consists of arterioles, capillaries, and postcapillary venules, of which the arterioles are the major determinant of vascular resistance. Blood flow depends on a pressure gradient along the vascular tree, as well as the amount and distribution of resistance across the microvasculature bed. Circular smooth muscle cells surround the arteriolar walls. By alternately contracting and relaxing, these muscle cells control microvascular flow and its distribution. In specific microcirculatory beds, such as those of the brain pericytes, surrounding arterioles can also cause constriction and regulate blood flow.[7] This vascular tone controls the diameter of the vessels because, as described by the law of Poiseuille, the resistance to flow is primarily determined by the radius. The proximal arteriole determines the total blood flow to the capillaries, whereas the terminal arterioles and precapillary sphincters control the distribution of blood within the capillaries. Capillary walls, which consist of a single layer of endothelium and basement membranes, represent the principal site of oxygen and nutrient exchange between blood and tissue. Changes in systemic blood pressure lead to a corresponding change in microcirculatory flow, which is then compensated for by local readjustments. These changes ensure that the microcirculatory blood flow is adequate to meet the oxygen requirements of the parenchymal cells, a mechanism called autoregulation.

The microvasculature characteristics of each organ system are closely related to the functional role played by the organ as a whole. The number of capillaries per unit mass of organ or tissue (capillary density) may be related to the organ's metabolic requirements (muscles, heart, brain) or to other functional requirements (skin, intestinal mucosa, kidney).[8] Oxygen transport to the tissues occurs via passive diffusion from the capillaries, as was first described by Krogh early in the 20th century.[9] The diffusion of oxygen in this manner is considered to be the main rate-limiting process in oxygen transport to tissue. Besides diffusion from the capillaries, diffusion of oxygen to the parenchymal cells also occurs from the larger vessels, such as the arterioles and venules. Although the microvascular beds of most organs and tissues clearly have both metabolic and functional components, one or the other usually predominates. In this way, the morphology of each microcirculatory bed is designed to fit the function and oxygen requirements of each organ.

Regarding critical illness, skeletal muscle has been the most extensively studied tissue in experimental studies. This is due to its easy accessibility and to the technical limitations of intravital microscopes, the main instruments used in such studies. Interest later shifted to other microvascular beds, such as those of the intestine and brain. Upon the introduction of OPS and SDF imaging, microcirculation could be observed in humans, and the location most often studied with these techniques has, to date, been the sublingual region. This is because this region is easily accessible and its vascularization is close to the brain and heart. The extent to which studies of this region can be extrapolated to other microvascular beds is uncertain. However, sublingual microcirculatory alterations do have clinical significance. The superior sensitivity of sublingual microcirculation as an indicator linking the severity of disease to systemic hemodynamic and oxygen-derived variables (demonstrated in several clinical studies) makes tissue in the sublingual region clinically relevant for detecting microcirculatory alterations.

ORTHOGONAL POLARIZATION SPECTRAL AND SIDESTREAM DARK FIELD IMAGING FOR CLINICAL MONITORING OF MICROCIRCULATION

The intravital microscope has provided much insight into the physiology and pathophysiology of microcirculation in several models of disease. However, the microscope's technical limitations have limited its impact. The main limitation of this technique is the need for transillumination of the microcirculatory bed from below for visualization. Observing the microcirculation of organ surfaces using epi-illumination causes surface reflection of the incident light, resulting in poor visualization of the underlying microcirculatory bed. Therefore, the intravital microscope has been used mainly for the study of organs that permit transillumination, such as the mesenteric, cremaster, and hind limb muscles. Fluorescence microscopy (illumination from above), in combination with the infusion of fluorescence indicator dyes, has facilitated the study of other organs. Not being able to apply these types of techniques to clinically relevant, large animal models has limited the clinical relevance in studying the microcirculation. In small-animal studies, the relation between macro- and microcirculation, an essential link needed to understand the role of microcirculation in functional hemodynamics, had not been sufficiently elucidated. This limited their translational applicability to clinical scenarios. The technical limitations of transillumination were finally overcome with the introduction of the OPS imaging technique.

OPS imaging illuminates tissues with polarized green light and measures the reflected light from the tissue surface after filtering out the polarized portion of the reflected light.[6] OPS imaging thus makes it possible to visualize microcirculation without transillumination. This modality filters out the surface reflection and permits visualization of subsurface structures. Green light is absorbed by hemoglobin in red blood cells, thereby tracking the movement of red blood cells, which appear in microcirculation as moving dark globules. However, due to its inadequate imaging, the OPS technique has only limited sensitivity for studying capillary kinetics and morphology in detail. An improved optical modality to address this shortcoming was introduced with SDF imaging.[5] Covered by a disposable cap, the SDF probe is placed directly on tissue surfaces. The light from the concentrically positioned light-emitting diodes (530-nm wavelength) penetrates 1 mm into the tissue, thus illuminating the microcirculation and its components. Because hemoglobin absorbs this wavelength, erythrocytes can be clearly observed as flowing cells. Also, because there is no direct optical contact with the sensing central core of the probe, surface reflections do not interfere with image collection. Therefore, remarkably clear images of microcirculation can be captured. The resulting improved image quality allows for better automatic analysis of the images, and the low energy requirement of SDF imaging further enhances its utility by allowing battery or portable computer operation. Using these techniques, brain, sublingual, cutaneous, and conjunctival microcirculation have been studied during surgery and intensive care.

CLINICAL EVALUATION OF MICROCIRCULATION DURING SURGERY AND INTENSIVE CARE

Both OPS and SDF imaging can be used to investigate the microcirculation of organ surfaces. OPS imaging has been used to visualize human brain microcirculation during neurosurgery.[6] Given its embryologic association with the gastrointestinal tract and its easy accessibility, sublingual microcirculation has been extensively studied, especially in intensive care medicine. In addition, these techniques have been applied to the study of microcirculation in the nail fold.[10,11] From a historic perspective, however, the study of the human brain during surgery represents a new, uncharted area of clinical research.[6] **Figs. 1–4** illustrate several microcirculatory beds described below, as well as their corresponding microcirculatory images, acquired using OPS and SDF imaging.

Brain Microcirculation

The microvascular bed of the cerebral cortex consists of a dense, highly interconnected network that arises from pial arteries. Irregular tortuous capillaries characterize this cerebrocortical capillary bed, and these capillaries are supplied by branches of cortical penetrating arteries, which cannot be visualized in vivo.[12] The arteriolar system is composed of three main vasculature zones: the pial, cortical, and subcortical vascular networks. When the brain surface is examined with intravital microscopy, the capillaries appear to have no preferential orientation or characteristic length. Also, the capillaries cannot usually be traced back to their pial arteries. On the brain surface, the arterial microanastomoses characterize the pial microarterial network.[13] The capillaries drain into postcapillary venules that give rise to the pial veins. It is still unclear whether arteriovenous anastomoses are present in the cerebral microvasculature. Capillary density in the brain is related to the average metabolic rate at steady state.[14] In addition to the classical factors that control microcirculatory blood flow (myogenic, metabolic, and neurohumoral mechanisms), evidence suggests that pericytes located around the capillaries regulate cerebral blood flow in both normal and pathologic states.[7]

The initial observation of normal brain microcirculation using OPS imaging was followed by several other reports on the structure of cerebral cortical microcirculation in different disease states. First, it was shown that, during surgery for subarachnoid hemorrhage, the cortical microvasculature response to hypocapnia was different between patients prone to vasospasm and patients who did not develop vasospasm.[15] In addition, excision of arteriovenous malformations in the brain resulted in increased microcirculatory flow and functional capillary density in the perinidal brain tissue.[16]

Conjunctival Microcirculation

Direct access to brain microvasculature is impossible outside the operating room. However, a recent study suggests that the microcirculation of the conjunctiva might function as an indicator of the cerebral microcirculation.[17] At the bedside, the most accessible part of the eye for evaluating microcirculation is the bulbar conjunctiva, which offers a complete vascular bed with arterioles, capillaries, and small collecting venules. Earlier studies using intravital microscopy have reported on the behavior of the conjunctival microcirculation in sickle cell

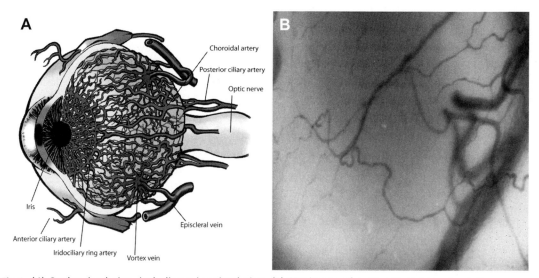

Fig. 1. (A) Ocular circulation, including microcirculation. (B) SDF image of conjunctival microcirculation.

patients.[18,19] The anterior segment of the human eye is supplied by the anterior ciliary arteries, which supply the anterior conjunctival, anterior episcleral, and limbal circulation. The episcleral arterial circle broadly resolves into superficial and deep components.[20] With intravital microscopy or OPS and SDF imaging, collecting venules are visualized as heavy, prominent, dark vessels situated parallel to narrower, straighter vessels, which comprise the accompanying terminal arterioles.[21] Capillaries arise at intervals from the end arterioles and form an irregular network of vessels that come together to form the venular system. The arterioles frequently terminate in main arteriovenous channels that communicate directly to the venular tree. This is most notable near the corneoscleral junction.[22]

The bulbar conjunctiva has been most extensively studied in diabetes and hypertensive patients. In these patient groups, several alterations in microcirculatory morphology and flow have been demonstrated. Microcirculatory alterations in the conjunctiva, however, have not yet been investigated in sepsis.

Sublingual Microcirculation

The sublingual area is one of the most easily accessible human mucosal surfaces, which is why it has been extensively investigated. The external carotid artery, the lingual artery, and the sublingual artery supply blood to the sublingual area. Only a limited number of sublingual arterioles are

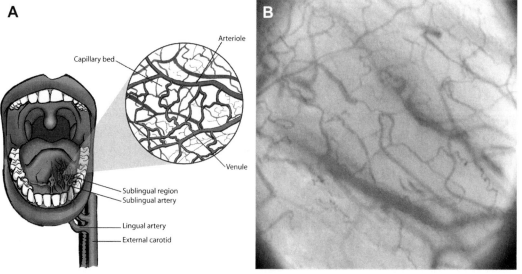

Fig. 2. (A) Sublingual circulation, including microcirculation. (B) OPS image of sublingual microcirculation.

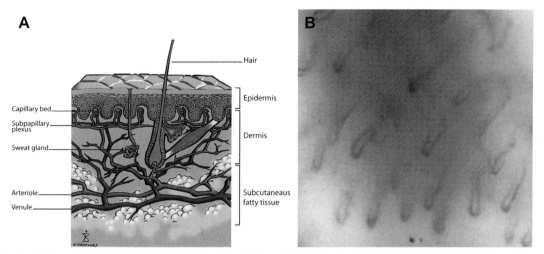

Fig. 3. (*A*) Dermal circulation, including microcirculation. (*B*) SDF image of nail fold microcirculation.

present, whereas numerous capillaries (diameter <20 μm) and venules (diameter 20–100 μm) are present in the sublingual area. Because perfusion of the sublingual mucosa is related to blood flow in the external carotid artery, sublingual perfusion may, in part, reflect cerebral blood flow. However, only a few studies have taken the cerebral and sublingual perfusion measurements simultaneously. Perfusion of the sublingual area could represent blood flow in the splanchnic region for two major reasons. First, this is suspected because the tongue shares a common embryogenic origin with the gut. Second, studies in critically ill patients reported good correlations between sublingual and gastric mucosal carbon dioxide pressures, as measured with sublingual capnometry and gastric tonometry, respectively, further strengthening the hypothesis.[23,24]

Intestinal Microcirculation

Branches from a common submucosal vasculature supply blood to the muscle, submucosal layer, and mucosal layer of the gut. Small arteries that branch extensively in the submucosal layer penetrate the muscularis layer of the intestinal wall. The branches all lead to capillary beds and, though diffusive shunting is thought to occur at the base of the villi, there is no evidence for arteriovenous shunts in the intestinal circulation.[25] Several submucosal arteries that transport blood back to the muscularis layer form a network of arterioles and capillaries around the intestinal smooth muscle cells. Other submucosal arteries supply blood to the mucosa and to each intestinal villus, where dense capillary networks exist. Veins leaving the villi join veins from the mucosal and muscularis layers, and they

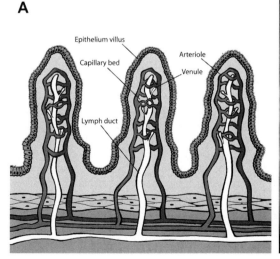
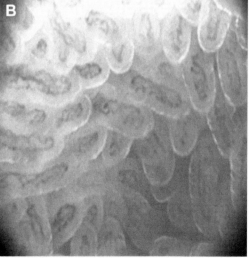

Fig. 4. (*A*) Intestinal microcirculation. (*B*) OPS image of villus microcirculation.

exit the intestinal wall alongside the mesenteric arteries that supply blood. Because absorption of water and solutes is one of the primary functions of the villi, the capillaries in the mucosal villi are very dense. A critical feature that may facilitate reabsorption of water is that the vessels carrying blood into and out of the villus lie close together, in parallel paths. Because the afferent and efferent blood vessels in the villi are close together, oxygen could diffuse from the arterioles to the venules at the base of the villus.[26] It is probably this organization that makes the tip of the villus the part most vulnerable to shock. The integrity of the intestinal mucosa is important to preventing the translocation of bacteria and toxins into systemic circulation. Hypoperfusion of the gut mucosa may contribute to mucosal injury.[27,28] In this context, experimental studies have evaluated the effect of sepsis and also hemorrhagic shock on the intestinal microcirculatory blood flow.[29–31] A recent study by Dubin and colleagues[31] demonstrated that endotoxic shock in a sheep rapidly induced alterations in intestinal and sublingual microcirculation. Fluid resuscitation normalized the systemic and intestinal hemodynamics, while also restoring the microvascular flow at the sublingual and intestinal serosal levels. However, the microvascular flow and percentage of perfused vessels in the intestinal mucosa were not effectively restored after fluid resuscitation. Human data are scarce, and they are limited to the observations in stomas of patients with abdominal sepsis. Boerma and colleagues,[32] after comparing the microcirculatory alterations between the sublingual region and stomas in patients admitted with abdominal sepsis, reported no correlation between sublingual and intestinal microcirculatory alterations on day 1 of sepsis. After 3 days of sepsis, however, these regional alterations became more systemic and correlations were found between the sublingual and intestinal microcirculatory alterations. The alterations in one microcirculatory bed, therefore, do not necessary reflect alterations in other microvascular beds. However, although microcirculatory beds may differ substantially in different organs, studies have clearly demonstrated the clinical significance of sublingual microcirculatory alterations in sepsis. These alterations indicate the response to treatment and resuscitation and serve as sensitive and specific indicators of bad outcome.

Cutaneous Microcirculation

The study of cutaneous microvascularization with OPS, SDF, and intravital microscopy has been limited to the nail fold area because of the distinctive construction of its skin, which is a thick epidermal layer. Other techniques have also been used to study skin microcirculatory blood flow in illness. Using laser Doppler flowmetry, Young and Cameron[33] demonstrated an impaired microcirculatory blood flow response of the forearm after transient ischemia. Using intravital microscopy, the blood flow velocity in the capillary bed of the nail fold was found to be decreased in normotensive febrile patients.[34] In investigating cutaneous microcirculation, the question remains: To what extent is microcirculatory flow of the skin important in critical illness? This question arises mainly because of the role thermoregulatory properties play in governing and interfering with the skin microvasculature. Because the major role of cutaneous circulation is thermoregulation, blood flow to the skin typically exceeds metabolic requirements. In the deep dermis, branches from subcutaneous arteries that penetrate the dermis form an arterial plexus.[35] The vessels within this plexus generally run parallel to the surface. Arterioles penetrating from the dermal plexus to the subpapillary region form a subpapillary plexus. Capillaries connect to the subpapillary venous plexus, and single capillary loops ascend to each papilla. The descending portion of the capillary joins the subpapillary venous plexus, which drains into the deeper cutaneous venous plexus. Due to the numerous arteriovenous shunts (only in apical regions) and because many cutaneous veins run close to parallel arteries, the resulting countercurrent heat exchange conserves heat. The combination of the richly sympathetic innervations of the cutaneous arterioles with the high blood flow relative to oxygen demand allows a primary control of reflexes.

Other Microcirculatory Beds

In addition to these areas of investigation, other microcirculatory beds have been studied using OPS and SDF imaging. While these applications have been limited to single studies, such studies have demonstrated the applicability of these techniques to other organ surfaces if they can be exposed for investigation. For instance, rectal microcirculation was studied in patients with malaria.[36] During maxillofacial surgery and especially for assessing wound healing, these techniques have also been used to explore additional areas of the oral cavity.[37] Finally, during surgery in which several organ surfaces are exposed, investigations have examined microcirculation in the liver, pancreas, and kidney.[38–40]

MICROCIRCULATION IN SEPSIS

Observational studies of sublingual microcirculation in sepsis have contributed to the understanding of the pathophysiology of acute circulatory failure and multiple organ dysfunction.[41] Both clinical and experimental studies have previously indicated that sepsis and septic shock are disorders of microcirculation. In the early phases of sepsis, a persistent deficit in microcirculatory perfusion is associated with poor outcome, as was demonstrated by De Backer and colleagues.[42] These investigators compared the sublingual microcirculation in septic patients versus that of healthy volunteers and detected a significant decrease in the proportion and density of small perfused vessels during sepsis. In addition, the alterations were more severe in nonsurvivors than in survivors. Meanwhile, Sakr and colleagues[3] observed that the recovery of microcirculatory alterations within the first 24 hours indicated survival outcome. In this study, the persistent loss of capillary perfusion was one of the most sensitive and specific hemodynamic predictors of survival from septic shock. Trzeciak and colleagues[4] studied the effects of an early goal-directed protocol on indices of microcirculatory perfusion in early sepsis. They demonstrated that, even in the context of early goal-directed therapy, microcirculatory flow was more markedly impaired and more heterogeneous in septic nonsurvivors than in survivors. Interestingly, the investigators found a correlation between microcirculatory and macrocirculatory parameters in early sepsis, but this correlation was weaker in later sepsis. This finding emphasizes the importance of early resuscitation, since time is one of the most important factors affecting therapeutic strategies for improving microcirculation.[43]

Many pathogenic mechanisms contribute to the microcirculatory abnormalities that occur during sepsis. In this context, microcirculation can be regarded as the integrative compartment in which all of these factors come together. Left uncorrected, microcirculatory abnormalities can lead to multiorgan failure and death. The most challenging septic patients are those who have received treatment but remain resistant to improvement. Here, the initial hit, in combination with therapy, time, comorbidity, and genetic background, all contribute to the complex pathogenesis of sepsis that leads to organ failure. Together, these are referred to as the microcirculatory and mitochondrial distress syndrome.[41]

Significant increases in leukocyte rigidity are observed during sepsis. This rigidity subsequently decreases with an improvement in the clinical condition.[44] A significant role has also been attributed to the mechanical behavior of white blood cells in microcirculatory alterations.[45] During sepsis, red blood cells are less likely to become deformed and more likely to aggregate.[46–48] The vasodilatory effects of several mediators released during sepsis, in combination with the excessive amounts of fluids given (which reduce viscosity), result in a low systemic resistance and low arterial pressure. The capillary leakage caused by endothelial injury of the capillaries results in hypovolemia and tissue edema, both of which result in larger diffusion distances between oxygen-carrying red blood cells and parenchymal cells. A possible initial contributing factor to the disruption of the barrier function of the microcirculatory milieu could lie in the disruption of the glycocalyx, which covers the endothelium and forms an important barrier and transduction system.[49] As was previously observed, this layer of the glycocalyx can be disrupted during inflammation and cardiovascular disease. It can also be measured using OPS or SDF imaging.[50,51] Recently, in a volunteer study, administration of endotoxin resulted in a shedding of the glycocalyx detected sublingually using OPS imaging. The shedding could be partially prevented by administration of a tumor necrosis factor scavenger.[52] In addition to metabolic, myogenic, and neurohumoral regulatory mechanisms that control microcirculatory blood flow, other regulatory factors can alter vascular tone and affect blood flow. Over the last decade, it has been demonstrated that red blood cells play an important role in the regulation of vascular tone through their ability to sense hypoxia and respond by releasing vasodilatory substances, such as nitric oxide (NO) and ATP.[53] It has been suggested that excessive NO production plays a key role in the pathology of microcirculatory abnormalities in sepsis. Excessive NO induced by inducible NO synthase (iNOS) has deleterious effects on red blood cell function because it overrides the naturally occurring regulatory mechanisms of vasodilation and vasoconstriction associated with autoregulation. The iNOS induction caused by cytokine release during bacteremia results in excessive NO formation during inflammation and infection,[54] resulting in the loss of vascular tone due to the reduced responsiveness to vasoconstrictors.[55] The inhomogeneous expression of iNOS between different organ compartments could represent the underlying cause of the shunting of the microcirculation in various organ segments.[56] The heterogeneity caused by shunting results in local areas of hypoxia and impairs oxygen extraction. The shunting theory of sepsis could explain why resuscitation strategies based on the correction of upstream hemodynamic variables do not correct the downstream indicators of hypoxia because they are unable to recruit shunted microcirculatory units.[57] The functionally vulnerable microcirculatory units are bypassed, and oxygen is shunted from the arteriole to the venous compartment. As described above, various mechanisms in sepsis could contribute to microcirculatory dysfunction and promote shunting. In sepsis, the perfusion in the capillaries is more severely altered, even while the flow in larger microvessels is preserved in septic shock patients, which represents direct evidence of shunting pathways in resuscitated sepsis.[58] Direct evidence of functional shunting pathways is derived from microcirculatory PO_2 measurements using palladium porphyrin phosphorescence. During various conditions of shock and resuscitation, microcirculatory PO_2 levels become lower than the PO_2 of the venous effluent of an organ, demonstrating the action of functional shunting.[57]

Several experimental studies have been performed to elucidate the differences in microcirculatory response to different types of shock. Particular focus has been placed on differentiating between the effects that distributive (eg, sepsis) and hypovolemic (eg, hemorrhage) types of shock have on microcirculation.[59] Collectively, these studies have shown that the microcirculatory abnormalities in sepsis can occur in the presence of normal (or even supranormal) systemic hemodynamics. In contrast, with hypovolemic shock, the microcirculation and systemic hemodynamics seem to follow each other more closely.

This difference is probably due to the fact that autoregulatory mechanisms still function in hypovolemic shock, whereas these mechanisms are severely impaired in septic shock. In addition, the differing courses of shock could be the result of differing responses from various microvascular beds. At the arteriolar level, the cremaster muscle and diaphragm respond differently from the small intestine.[60–62] In the intestine, arteriolar constriction occurs at all levels of the arteriolar network. In contrast, in the cremaster muscle and diaphragm, larger arterioles constrict and smaller ones dilate. Therefore, there appears to be heterogeneity not only between organs but also within a single organ. Experimental studies have thus demonstrated that an increase in heterogeneity is associated with a decrease in functional capillary density and diminished red blood cell velocity in models of sepsis.[63]

Several studies have reported that global hemodynamics do not necessarily reflect regional blood flow during sepsis and septic shock.[4,64] Farquhar and colleagues,[29] using a subacute model of sepsis, found that capillary density in the distal small bowel mucosa decreases during normotension. Lam and colleagues[63] used a skeletal muscle preparation in the same subacute sepsis

model to observe the distributions of perfused capillaries and red blood cell flow. They demonstrated an increase in capillaries with stopped flow and a decrease in the total number of capillaries. In addition, they demonstrated an increase in the spatial heterogeneity of red blood cell–perfused capillaries, similar to what later was demonstrated in clinical sepsis.[4] To underscore the dissociation of the presence of shock and microcirculatory abnormalities in sepsis, Nakajima and colleagues [30] compared the effects of hemorrhage and endotoxin shock at the microvascular level in a rat model. They found that, in the intestinal villi, the capillary density, red blood cell velocity, and flux all decreased. Yet, at the same level of hypotension, only moderate changes were detected during hemorrhagic shock. Boczkowski and colleagues[60] showed similar results in the microvascular bed of the diaphragm by comparing an acute model of sepsis with hypotensive hypovolemic controls. Fang and colleagues[65] demonstrated similar findings for buccal microcirculation in a subacute model of septic shock compared with hemorrhagic shock. Additionally, they demonstrated that when both models where matched according to the cardiac index, the microcirculatory alterations were similarly altered. After resuscitation, the improved global hemodynamics were not effective in improving the buccal capillary blood flow in septic shock, in contrast to those in hemorrhagic shock, where improved global hemodynamics were found to be effective.

Thus, in shock profiles other than distributive shock, microcirculatory alteration seems to be effectively corrected by resuscitating global hemodynamical variables. In septic shock, however, therapeutic modalities aimed at recruiting systemic variables do not always seem to be effective in recruiting microcirculation. Therefore, more specific therapies may be required.[56] These experimental studies have contributed to the view that sepsis is a disease of microcirculation.

RESUSCITATING THE MICROCIRCULATION

Clinical investigations are currently being conducted to determine whether treatment modalities aimed at recruiting microcirculation provide a beneficial therapeutic target. Several agents and resuscitation strategies have been studied in single center intensive care populations and experimental models. Various animal studies have demonstrated that, under conditions in which autoregulatory mechanisms have not been affected, fluid resuscitation successfully improves the microcirculatory abnormalities and oxygen transport to baseline values.[30,65] In septic shock, however, fluid resuscitation alone is ineffective in improving microcirculatory function. Even when the systemic variables have been normalized, microcirculatory alterations can persist.[3,42] Nevertheless, in a fraction of preload-dependent intensive care patients, a fluid loading of 500 mL within a 15-minute period was found to significantly improve microcirculatory parameters,[66] although it was not clear in that study whether the patients were treated for severe sepsis or septic shock.

In the clinical setting, several therapeutic agents have been demonstrated to effectively improve microcirculatory abnormalities in septic shock patients. One of the important findings from these studies is that the microvasculature, specifically endothelial function, is still responsive in sepsis. This was demonstrated elegantly by De Backer and colleagues,[42] who found that sublingual topical application of acetylcholine was able to recruit microcirculatory units in resuscitated septic patients. The topical sublingual application of acetylcholine reversed the local microcirculation in sepsis shock patients to normal values. Spronk and colleagues[58] demonstrated that intravenous infusion of an NO donor (nitroglycerin) improved sublingual microcirculation in normovolemic, pressure-resuscitated patients. Whether such therapeutic approaches will improve outcome has yet to be determined. De Backer and colleagues[64] also tested the effect of dobutamine, used at a fixed dosage, on microcirculation of the sublingual region of septic patients. Dobutamine improved the sublingual microcirculatory flow, with acetylcholine-induced reserve being preserved. They also found that lactate levels correlated with the degree of microcirculatory improvement, but not to changes in systemic hemodynamic parameters, such as cardiac output and blood pressure. These studies demonstrate that, in sepsis, microcirculatory alterations can persist independent of resolving macroscopic systemic hemodynamic variables, and that these alterations predict poor outcome.

Since the heterogeneous expression of iNOS is one of the factors contributing to the inflammation-induced autoregulatory dysfunction of microcirculatory flow, iNOS inhibition was hypothesized to improve microcirculatory function in sepsis. It has been demonstrated in several animal studies that a combined therapy of fluid and iNOS inhibitors can resuscitate weak microcirculatory units.[67] Interestingly, in a clinical study, although the mean arterial pressure was improved, the mortality in the group treated with nonselective iNOS inhibitors was significantly greater due to cardiovascular failure, resulting in an early termination of the trial.[68] Clearly, inhibition of the harmful effects of NO requires a more specific approach.

Although several questions remain concerning the mode of action of activated protein C (APC), there is evidence that it improves the microcirculatory flow indices in experimental models.[69,70] In humans, improvement in the microcirculatory flow observed with OPS imaging was reported during treatment with APC, which decreased after cessation of the APC treatment.[71] The latter finding may suggest that the timing and length of treatment with APC may be an essential component in its application.

SUMMARY

One of the key features of both experimental and human sepsis is the distributive alteration of microvascular blood flow. These distributive alterations have been demonstrated by a heterogeneous microvascular blood flow between different vascular beds, as has been clearly visualized through the use of such imaging techniques as OPS and SDF. Using these techniques, microhemodynamic alterations have been demonstrated to be associated with organ dysfunction and impaired outcome in sepsis. In light of the central role of microcirculatory alterations in the pathogenesis of sepsis, it seems logical to hypothesize that restoring microcirculatory function contributes to the treatment of sepsis. However, several questions remain unanswered. First, what is the clinical impact of sublingual monitoring of microcirculation in terms of clinical benefit and response to conventional therapy? Second, what are the best therapeutic interventions to recruit microcirculation, and how do these differ from conventional therapeutic modalities, in terms of monitoring? Finally, will the outcome of patients with sepsis improve when microcirculation is effectively resuscitated? To answer these questions, more evidence must be gathered. In answering these questions, it is clear that monitoring microcirculation will be an important component in the functional hemodynamic monitoring of critically ill patients.

REFERENCES

1. Dellinger RP. Cardiovascular management of septic shock. Crit Care Med 2003;31(3):946–55.
2. Rivers E, Nguyen B, Havstad S, et al. Early goal-directed therapy in the treatment of severe sepsis and septic shock. N Engl J Med 2001;345(19):1368–77.
3. Sakr Y, Dubois MJ, De Backer D, et al. Persistent microcirculatory alterations are associated with organ failure and death in patients with septic shock. Crit Care Med 2004;32(9):1825–31.
4. Trzeciak S, Dellinger RP, Parrillo JE, et al. Early microcirculatory perfusion derangements in patients

with severe sepsis and septic shock: relationship to hemodynamics, oxygen transport, and survival. Ann Emerg Med 2007;49(1):88–98, 98.

5. Goedhart P, Khalilzada M, Bezemer R, et al. Side-stream dark field (SDF) imaging: a novel strobo-scopic LED ring-based imaging modality for clinical assessment of the microcirculation. Opt Express 2007;15:15101–14.

6. Groner W, Winkelman JW, Harris AG, et al. Orthogonal polarization spectral imaging: a new method for study of the microcirculation. Nat Med 1999;5(10):1209–12.

7. Peppiatt CM, Howarth C, Mobbs P, et al. Bidirectional control of CNS capillary diameter by pericytes. Nature 2006;443(7112):700–4.

8. Sobin SS, Tremer HM. Three-dimensional organization of microvascular beds as related to function. In: Kaley G, Altura BM, editors. Microcirculation. Baltimore (MD): University Park Press; 1977. p. 43–67.

9. Krogh A. The number and the distribution of capillaries in muscle with the calculation of the oxygen pressure necessary for supplying tissue. J Physiol 1919; 52:409–515.

10. Mathura KR, Vollebregt KC, Boer K, et al. Comparison of OPS imaging and conventional capillary microscopy to study the human microcirculation. J Appl Physiol 2001;91(1):74–8.

11. Vollebregt KC, Boer K, Mathura KR, et al. Impaired vascular function in women with pre-eclampsia observed with orthogonal polarisation spectral imaging. BJOG 2001;108(11):1148–53.

12. Hudetz AG. Blood flow in the cerebral capillary network: a review emphasizing observations with intravital microscopy. Microcirculation 1997;4(2):233–52.

13. Duvernoy HM, Delon S, Vannson JL. Cortical blood vessels of the human brain. Brain Res Bull 1981; 7(5):519–79.

14. Gjedde A. The pathways of oxygen in brain. I. Delivery and metabolism of oxygen. Adv Exp Med Biol 2005; 566:269–75.

15. Pennings FA, Bouma GJ, Ince C. Direct observation of the human cerebral microcirculation during aneurysm surgery reveals increased arteriolar contractility. Stroke 2004;35(6):1284–8.

16. Pennings FA, Ince C, Bouma GJ. Continuous real-time visualization of the human cerebral microcirculation during arteriovenous malformation surgery using orthogonal polarization spectral imaging. Neurosurgery 2006;59(1):167–71.

17. Schaser KD, Settmacher U, Puhl G, et al. Noninvasive analysis of conjunctival microcirculation during carotid artery surgery reveals microvascular evidence of collateral compensation and stenosis-dependent adaptation. J Vasc Surg 2003;37(4):789–97.

18. Cheung AT, Harmatz P, Wun T, et al. Correlation of abnormal intracranial vessel velocity, measured by transcranial Doppler ultrasonography, with abnormal conjunctival vessel velocity, measured by computer-assisted intravital microscopy, in sickle cell disease. Blood 2001;97(11):3401–4.

19. Cheung AT, Chen PC, Larkin EC, et al. Microvascular abnormalities in sickle cell disease: a computer-assisted intravital microscopy study. Blood 2002; 99(11):3999–4005.

20. Meyer PA, Watson PG. Low dose fluorescein angiography of the conjunctiva and episclera. Br J Ophthalmol 1987;71(1):2–10.

21. Lee RE. Anatomical and physiological aspects of the capillary bed in the bulbar conjunctiva of man in health and disease. Angiology 1955;6(4): 369–82.

22. Lee RE, Holze EA. The peripheral vascular system in the bulbar conjunctiva of young normotensive adults at rest. J Clin Invest 1950;29(2):146–50.

23. Creteur J, De Backer D, Sakr Y, et al. Sublingual capnometry tracks microcirculatory changes in septic patients. Intensive Care Med 2006;32(4):516–23.

24. Marik PE. Sublingual capnography: a clinical validation study. Chest 2001;120(3):923–7.

25. Guth PH, Ross G, Smith E. Changes in intestinal vascular diameter during norepinephrine vasoconstrictor escape. Am J Physiol 1976;230(6):1466–8.

26. Stephenson RB. The splanchnic circulation. In: Patton HD, Fuchs AF, Hille B, et al, editors. Textbook of physiology. Philadelphia: W.B. Saunders Company; 1989. p. 911–23.

27. Fink MP, Antonsson JB, Wang HL, et al. Increased intestinal permeability in endotoxic pigs. Mesenteric hypoperfusion as an etiologic factor. Arch Surg 1991;126(2):211–8.

28. Deitch EA. The role of intestinal barrier failure and bacterial translocation in the development of systemic infection and multiple organ failure. Arch Surg 1990;125(3):403–4.

29. Farquhar I, Martin CM, Lam C, et al. Decreased capillary density in vivo in bowel mucosa of rats with normotensive sepsis. J Surg Res 1996;61(1):190–6.

30. Nakajima Y, Baudry N, Duranteau J, et al. Microcirculation in intestinal villi: a comparison between hemorrhagic and endotoxin shock. Am J Respir Crit Care Med 2001;164(8 Pt 1):1526–30.

31. Dubin A, Edul VS, Pozo MO, et al. Persistent villi hypoperfusion explains intramucosal acidosis in sheep endotoxemia. Crit Care Med 2008;36(2):535–42.

32. Boerma EC, van der Voort PH, Spronk PE, et al. Relationship between sublingual and intestinal microcirculatory perfusion in patients with abdominal sepsis. Crit Care Med 2007;35(4):1055–60.

33. Young JD, Cameron EM. Dynamics of skin blood flow in human sepsis. Intensive Care Med 1995; 21(8):669–74.

34. Weinberg JR, Boyle P, Thomas K, et al. Capillary blood cell velocity is reduced in fever without hypotension. Int J Microcirc Clin Exp 1991;10(1):13–9.

35. Roddie IC. Peripheral circulation and organ flow. Handbook of physiology. The cardiovascular system. Bethesda (MD): The American Physiological Society; 1983. p. 285–317.

36. Dondorp AM, Ince C, Charunwatthana P, et al. Direct in vivo assessment of microcirculatory dysfunction in severe falciparum malaria. J Infect Dis 2008;197(1): 79–84.

37. Lindeboom JA, Mathura KR, Aartman IH, et al. Influence of the application of platelet-enriched plasma in oral mucosal wound healing. Clin Oral Implants Res 2007;18(1):133–9.

38. Puhl G, Schaser KD, Vollmar B, et al. Noninvasive in vivo analysis of the human hepatic microcirculation using orthogonal polarization spectral imaging. Transplantation 2003;75(6):756–61.

39. Schmitz V, Schaser KD, Olschewski P, et al. In vivo visualization of early microcirculatory changes following ischemia/reperfusion injury in human kidney transplantation. Eur Surg Res 2008;40(1):19–25.

40. von Dobschuetz E, Biberthaler P, Mussack T, et al. Noninvasive in vivo assessment of the pancreatic microcirculation: orthogonal polarization spectral imaging. Pancreas 2003;26(2):139–43.

41. Ince C. The microcirculation is the motor of sepsis. Crit Care 2005;9(Suppl 4):S13–9.

42. De Backer D, Creteur J, Preiser JC, et al. Microvascular blood flow is altered in patients with sepsis. Am J Respir Crit Care Med 2002;166(1):98–104.

43. Dellinger RP, Levy MM, Carlet JM, et al. Surviving Sepsis Campaign: international guidelines for management of severe sepsis and septic shock: 2008. Intensive Care Med 2008;34(1):17–60.

44. Drost EM, Kassabian G, Meiselman HJ, et al. Increased rigidity and priming of polymorphonuclear leukocytes in sepsis. Am J Respir Crit Care Med 1999;159(6):1696–702.

45. Eppihimer MJ, Lipowsky HH. Leukocyte sequestration in the microvasculature in normal and low flow states. Am J Physiol 1994;267(3 Pt 2): H1122–34.

46. Baskurt OK, Gelmont D, Meiselman HJ. Red blood cell deformability in sepsis. Am J Respir Crit Care Med 1998;157(2):421–7.

47. Bateman RM, Jagger JE, Sharpe MD, et al. Erythrocyte deformability is a nitric oxide–mediated factor in decreased capillary density during sepsis. Am J Physiol Heart Circ Physiol 2001;280(6):H2848–56.

48. Piagnerelli M, Boudjeltia KZ, Vanhaeverbeek M, et al. Red blood cell rheology in sepsis. Intensive Care Med 2003;29(7):1052–61.

49. Cabrales P, Vazquez BY, Tsai AG, et al. Microvascular and capillary perfusion following glycocalyx degradation. J Appl Physiol 2007;102(6):2251–9.

50. Nieuwdorp M, Mooij HL, Kroon J, et al. Endothelial glycocalyx damage coincides with microalbuminuria in type 1 diabetes. Diabetes 2006;55(4):1127–32.

51. Nieuwdorp M, van Haeften TW, Gouverneur MC, et al. Loss of endothelial glycocalyx during acute hyperglycemia coincides with endothelial dysfunction and coagulation activation in vivo. Diabetes 2006;55(2):480–6.

52. Nieuwdorp M, Meuwese MC, Mooj HL, et al. Tumor necrosis factor-alpha inhibition protects against endotoxin-induced endothelial glycocalyx perturbation. Arteriosclerosis 2008; Epub ahead of print.

53. Ellsworth ML. The red blood cell as an oxygen sensor: What is the evidence? Acta Physiol Scand 2000;168(4):551–9.

54. Gocan NC, Scott JA, Tyml K. Nitric oxide produced via neuronal NOS may impair vasodilatation in septic rat skeletal muscle. Am J Physiol Heart Circ Physiol 2000;278(5):H1480–9.

55. Hollenberg SM, Cunnion RE, Zimmerberg J. Nitric oxide synthase inhibition reverses arteriolar hyporesponsiveness to catecholamines in septic rats. Am J Physiol 1993;264(2 Pt 2):H660–3.

56. Almac E, Siegemund M, Demirci C, et al. Microcirculatory recruitment maneuvers correct tissue CO2 abnormalities in sepsis. Minerva Anestesiol 2006; 72(6):507–19.

57. Ince C, Sinaasappel M. Microcirculatory oxygenation and shunting in sepsis and shock. Crit Care Med 1999;27(7):1369–77.

58. Spronk PE, Ince C, Gardien MJ, et al. Nitroglycerin in septic shock after intravascular volume resuscitation. Lancet 2002;360(9343):1395–6.

59. Weil MH, Shubin H. Proposed reclassification of shock states with special reference to distributive defects. Adv Exp Med Biol 1971;23(0):13–23.

60. Boczkowski J, Vicaut E, Aubier M. In vivo effects of Escherichia coli endotoxemia on diaphragmatic microcirculation in rats. J Appl Physiol 1992;72(6): 2219–24.

61. Cryer HM, Garrison RN, Kaebnick HW, et al. Skeletal microcirculatory responses to hyperdynamic Escherichia coli sepsis in unanesthetized rats. Arch Surg 1987;122(1):86–92.

62. Whitworth PW, Cryer HM, Garrison RN, et al. Hypoperfusion of the intestinal microcirculation without decreased cardiac output during live Escherichia coli sepsis in rats. Circ Shock 1989;27(2):111–22.

63. Lam C, Tyml K, Martin C, et al. Microvascular perfusion is impaired in a rat model of normotensive sepsis. J Clin Invest 1994;94(5):2077–83.

64. De Backer D, Creteur J, Dubois MJ, et al. The effects of dobutamine on microcirculatory alterations in patients with septic shock are independent of its systemic effects. Crit Care Med 2006;34(2):403–8.

65. Fang X, Tang W, Sun S, et al. Comparison of buccal microcirculation between septic and hemorrhagic shock. Crit Care Med 2006;34(Suppl 12):S447–53.

66. Deruddre S, Pottecher J, Georger J, et al. Sublingual microcirculatory improvement with fluid loading in

preload-dependent ICU patients. Intensive Care Med 2007;33(Suppl 2):S253.

67. Siegemund M, van Bommel J, Schwarte LA, et al. Inducible nitric oxide synthase inhibition improves intestinal microcirculatory oxygenation and CO_2 balance during endotoxemia in pigs. Intensive Care Med 2005;31(7):985–92.

68. Lopez A, Lorente JA, Steingrub J, et al. Multiple-center, randomized, placebo-controlled, double-blind study of the nitric oxide synthase inhibitor 546C88: effect on survival in patients with septic shock. Crit Care Med 2004;32(1):21–30.

69. Iba T, Kidokoro A, Fukunaga M, et al. Activated protein C improves the visceral microcirculation by attenuating the leukocyte-endothelial interaction in a rat lipopolysaccharide model. Crit Care Med 2005;33(2):368–72.

70. Lehmann C, Meissner K, Knock A, et al. Activated protein C improves intestinal microcirculation in experimental endotoxaemia in the rat. Crit Care 2006;10(6):R157.

71. De Backer D, Verdant C, Chierego M, et al. Effects of drotrecogin alfa activated on microcirculatory alterations in patients with severe sepsis. Crit Care Med 2006;34(7):1918–24.

Cellular Dysfunction in Sepsis

Mervyn Singer, MBBS, MD, FRCP

KEYWORDS

• Sepsis • Multiple organ failure • Mitochondria • Nitric oxide

Sepsis-induced multiple organ failure is a significant worldwide cause of mortality and morbidity. Unlike most other major killer conditions, its incidence is on the rise.[1] In the most recent United States mortality data (from 2003), septicemia ranked as the 10th most common cause of death after cancer, myocardial infarction, and so forth.[2] When combined with mortality related to influenza and pneumonia, death related to infection ranked 6th overall. Yet, despite billions of dollars and billions of hours poured into related research and into the development of novel therapies, little progress has been made toward producing significant outcome improvements in septic patient populations. Only one commercially developed agent, drotrecogin-alfa (activated protein C), has a current licensed indication for the treatment of severe sepsis, and even the efficacy of this product has been recently challenged by the European Medicines Agency, which has mandated another pivotal trial.[3] A raft of other noncommercial approaches, including corticosteroids, immunoglobulins, and early goal-directed therapy, have all generated a combination of promise, conflicting data, and persisting uncertainty due in large part to the relatively small numbers of patients and the disparate populations enrolled. I have argued that the greatest outcome benefits achieved in contemporary critical care have involved reductions in the degree of iatrogenic intervention, be it tidal volume, sedation dosing, or blood transfusion.[4] The covert harm potentially induced by virtually every drug, fluid, or mechanical procedure used in critical care practice on immune, hormonal, and metabolic systems should not be underestimated.[5]

This preamble suggests three important points. First, despite increasing understanding of mechanisms underlying inflammation-induced multiple organ failure, we still have an uncertain grasp of various fundamental questions. For example, how does the inflammatory process actually result in organ failure? How and why do these dysfunctional organs recover, particularly as many of them are poorly regenerative? Second, the lack of adequate biomarkers to indicate how, when, and to what degree to immunomodulate means that many patients are inappropriately treated and potentially harmed. The subset who may benefit are submerged within the considerable surrounding noise, leading to an overall intention-to-treat statistical analysis that is usually negative despite the promise held by preclinical and proof-of-principle trials. Finally, the impact of our therapies on the disease process, including the recovery phase, may be potentially deleterious, particularly as a reasoned argument could be made that much of what is currently perceived as pathologic may, in fact, be adaptive.

This article provides an overview of cellular dysfunction. The lack of definitive proof of the pathophysiology underlying organ failure necessitates the expounding of plausible hypotheses to explain the numerous conundrums surrounding multiple organ failure. Clearly, these hypotheses demand further scrutiny so that they can be verified, debunked, or further refined.

WHAT CAUSES ORGAN FAILURE?

In 2007, Professor Ed Abraham and I wrote the following summary,[6] which, I believe, neatly

Mervyn Singer received funding support through grants from the Medical Research Council and the Wellcome Trust.
University College London, Cruciform Building, Gower Street, London WC1E 6BT, UK
E-mail address: m.singer@ucl.ac.uk

Clin Chest Med 29 (2008) 655–660
doi:10.1016/j.ccm.2008.06.003

encapsulates a contemporary view of organ dysfunction:

> Current understanding of the pathophysiology underlying sepsis-induced multiple organ dysfunction highlights the multiple cell populations and cell-signaling pathways involved in interactions existing between different cells and organs affected by the septic process. The intricate cross-talk provided by temporal changes in mediators, hormones, metabolites, neural signaling, alterations in oxygen delivery and utilization, and by modifications in cell phenotypes underlines the adaptive and even coordinated processes beyond the dysregulated chaos in which sepsis was once perceived. Many pathologic processes previously considered to be detrimental are now viewed as potentially protective. Applying systems approaches to these complex processes will permit better appreciation of the effectiveness or harm of treatments, both present and future, and also will allow development not only of better directed, but also of more appropriately timed, strategies to improve outcomes from this still highly lethal condition.

The exaggerated inflammatory process that sepsis represents is associated with a complex interaction at one level among cytokines, mediators, and cell surface receptors. However, numerous other levels are also involved. These relate to, for example, genetic up- and down-regulation, hormonal-metabolic interactions, altered immune function, and perturbations of macro- and microcirculation. The net effect is cellular dysfunction. However, the precise manner by which organ function is affected has received scant attention. The traditional and rather simplistic view of circulatory defects is that they result from vasoconstriction, blood flow redistribution, and widespread microvascular occlusion from aggregated platelets and leukocytes, thus causing tissue hypoxia, cell death, and organ failure. A few straightforward observations demolish this view.

First, even with gross disseminated intravascular coagulation, a phenomenon infrequently seen in septic patients, there is relatively minimal evidence of cell death. In a postmortem study of patients dying of multiorgan failure,[7] Hotchkiss and colleagues took biopsy samples from numerous organs, including heart, lung, liver and kidney, and reported little or no cell death in most of them. An increase in the percentage of apoptotic cells was noted in tissues associated with immunity, such as the spleen, lymphocytes, and gut epithelium. Yet, even in these organs, the general architecture was preserved.

Second, organs affected by the septic process often have poor regenerative capacity. Yet, if the patient recovers, it is commonplace for these organs to recover without the need for lifelong support. For example, in one large audit of survivors of critical illness requiring renal replacement therapy, only 1.6% remained on long-term dialysis.[8]

Third, a lack of sufficient tissue oxygen delivery should compromise local tissue oxygenation. Yet studies in septic patients and animal models investigating organs as diverse as muscle, gut, and bladder showed elevations in tissue oxygen tension.[9–11] This value represents the balance between local oxygen supply and demand and thus implies that oxygen is available at the cellular level but is not being used.

There is clear evidence of microvascular abnormality in many organs during sepsis.[12] Assuming these measurements, any hypothesis must therefore reconcile the fact that tissue oxygen is available despite the presence of an abnormal microcirculation. The obvious corollary is that there is a failure of oxygen use by the cells. More than 90% of total body oxygen consumption is used by mitochondria toward generation of ATP and, to a lesser extent, heat and reactive oxygen species. As mitochondrial ATP generation is the major energy source for most cell types, this implicates mitochondrial dysfunction as central to the pathogenesis of organ dysfunction.

BIOENERGETIC-METABOLIC FUNCTION

ATP is generated by glycolysis (anaerobic respiration) and oxidative phosphorylation. As shown in **Fig. 1**, glucose is metabolized to pyruvate by glycolysis with a net gain of two ATP molecules per mole of glucose. Pyruvate enters the mitochondrion via the pyruvate dehydrogenase complex, which converts it into acetyl coenzyme A. This feeds into the Krebs' (tricarboxylic acid) cycle, which serves to donate electrons, via NADH and flavin adenine dinucleotide, to complexes I and II of the electron transport chain, respectively. The electrons are transported to complexes III and IV of the chain via specialized carriers, such as cytochrome c. By receiving and donating electrons, the redox states of complexes I, II, III, and IV are altered. As electrons pass down the chain, a proton gradient is also generated across the inner mitochondrial membrane. The last component of the chain, complex IV (cytochrome c oxidase), is the only point on the pathway where oxygen is involved. Oxygen is the terminal electron acceptor and is reduced to water in the process. This protonmotive force produced by hydrogen ion

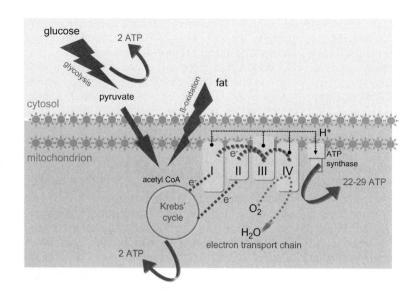

Fig. 1. Cellular energy production. CoA, coenzyme A.

movement drives ATP synthase to generate ATP from ADP. Approximately 24 to 31 molecules of ATP[13–20] are generated by the Krebs' cycle (2 ATP) and the electron transport chain from a molecule of glucose, thereby demonstrating the far greater efficiency of the mitochondrion relative to glycolysis. The cytosolic pyruvate not taken up by pyruvate dehydrogenase goes into equilibrium with lactate. Any substrate supply problem or blockade downstream, such as lack of oxygen or inhibition of mitochondrial complex, results in an increase in lactate levels. Apart from glucose, protein and fatty acid can also be used as substrates. Alanine can enter at the lower end of the glycolytic pathway while fatty acid can enter via acetyl coenzyme A, or through succinate at complex II.

The protonmotive force, which creates the membrane potential across the inner mitochondrial membrane, drives the rate of ATP synthesis. This force can be dissipated to some degree by protons recrossing the membrane ("proton leak"), either via specialized uncoupling proteins or a slippage at cytochrome c oxidase, rather than through ATP synthase. This uncoupling decreases the efficiency of aerobic respiration and generates heat. Uncoupling protein–1 in brown fat is the best clinical example of this phenomenon. Arguably, excessive uncoupling may be responsible for the pyrexia induced by sepsis and other inflammatory conditions.

Oxidative phosphorylation is tightly controlled by ATP consumption.[21] This factor is crucial for the cell as it has to respond promptly to any physiologic change in cellular energy demand. There is clearly some redundancy in the system to enable a rapid response, and this generally relies upon a modulation of the electron flux through each of the functional units of the electron transport chain. An increase in demand leads to a transient fall in ATP. At the same time, many extrinsic factors exert influence. A good example is thyroid hormone, which increases mitochondrial activity albeit at the expense of a decrease in efficiency as this hormone induces more uncoupling and heat production.[22] Longer-term adaptation to changes in ATP use is achieved by modifying the number of functional units. Thus, repeated exercise increases mitochondrial density in skeletal muscle whereas disuse leads to depletion.[23] As discussed later, this process of new mitochondrial protein turnover, mitochondrial biogenesis, may play a significant role in recovery following organ failure.

MITOCHONDRIAL DYSFUNCTION IN SEPSIS

For mitochondrial dysfunction in sepsis to occur, a number of possible mechanisms may be invoked: (1) direct inhibition or damage to mitochondria by inflammatory mediators, notably nitric oxide and its metabolites and other reactive species (this inhibition may be amplified by concurrent tissue hypoxia); (2) changes in hormonal activity that affect mitochondria directly and are known to occur during sepsis; and (3) genetic downregulation of mitochondrial protein turnover.

Direct Inhibition or Damage to Mitochondria by Inflammatory Mediators

The endogenously produced gases, nitric oxide, carbon monoxide, and hydrogen sulfide, are all inhibitors of cytochrome oxidase and most likely compete with oxygen for the same binding site.[24] All three gases are produced in excess during inflammation. Inhibition of complex IV allows a buildup of electrons and increased formation of the superoxide radical, which reacts to form peroxynitrite, a more potent reactive species that inhibits complex I either reversibly through nitrosylation or irreversibly by nitration.[25] Reduced glutathione, an important mitochondrial antioxidant, protects complex I from damage by reactive species. Once glutathione is depleted, inhibition of complex I occurs. Both human studies (using skeletal muscle biopsies from patients in septic shock) and laboratory models have demonstrated that complex I is one of the major targets of mitochondrial damage in sepsis.[26] The reduction in oxygen consumption measured ex vivo in skeletal muscle taken from septic rats 24 hours after induction of fecal peritonitis could be fully reversed by addition of succinate, which donates electrons to complex II and thus bypasses any block at complex I.[27] Direct damage to mitochondria (likely to be oxidant related) has been described in both long-term animal models and in patients.[26] These studies report minimal, if any, cell death.

Changes in Hormonal Activity

Mitochondria possess receptors for a variety of hormones, including thyroid hormone and glucocorticoids. They are also intimately involved in production of such hormones as, for example, cortisol. Mitochondrial activity, efficiency, and the rate of new protein turnover are influenced by, among others, triiodothyronine, cortisol, leptin, estrogen, and growth hormone.[13–15,28,29] In severe sepsis, some early changes in serum hormonal profiles are prognostic. Such early changes include, for example, a low triiodothyronine and thyroxine and an elevated reverse triiodothyronine.[16] Likewise, leptin and estrogen levels are elevated with systemic inflammation. However, while higher leptin levels are related to improved outcomes,[17] the opposite is true for estrogen.[15] Hyperglycemia also contributes to mitochondrial damage during sepsis, notably in the liver.[18] This may be related to increased oxidant damage and glycation of mitochondrial protein. The contribution of hormonal changes in sepsis to alterations in mitochondrial function needs to be further elucidated, but such changes appear to play an important role.

Down-Regulation of Mitochondrial Protein Turnover

In a small but tantalizing study of changes in neutrophil gene expression following injection of endotoxin into healthy volunteers, Calvano and colleagues[19] reported down-regulation of genes coding for mitochondrial proteins, notably components of the respiratory chain and pyruvate dehydrogenase. Temporal changes were not reported, but it does appear conceivable that a prolonged inflammatory insult may trigger a decrease in turnover of mitochondrial protein, leading to a further mechanism resulting in decreased energy production.

IS MULTIORGAN FAILURE AN ADAPTIVE, HIBERNATORYLIKE RESPONSE?

While direct damage to mitochondria may be viewed as a purely pathologic process, it is hard to reconcile genetic down-regulation of mitochondrial protein turnover and hormonal suppression of mitochondrial activity in a similar light, particularly as infection and inflammation have been constant companions through the evolutionary process. This opens the possibility that decreased energy production may be an adaptive response to a prolonged, severe inflammatory process.[20]

Sepsis is generally considered to be a hypermetabolic condition. This assumption is based upon extrapolation of the clinical features of pyrexia, tachycardia, and sweating, and an increase in oxygen delivery. However, multiple investigations in septic patients show that the degree of oxygen consumption is broadly comparable to that of normal people, and that resting energy expenditure (REE) actually *decreases* with increasing sepsis severity.[30–32] Moreover, every degree rise in temperature is associated with a 15% increase in REE,[33] implying a reduction in energy usage for normal physiologic functions. While many of these studies have not captured patients in the very early phase of sepsis, studies in volunteers given endotoxin do demonstrate an increase in REE.[34] During established sepsis, the REE falls toward normal levels but rebounds during the recovery phase.[30,32] This marked increase in energy use is likely due to both repair processes and restoration of normal cellular functioning.

The corollary of this progression of metabolic change over the course of sepsis is that metabolism initially increases to deal with the acute stress response of inflammation. If this first-line coping mechanism proves inadequate and severe inflammation persists, a new strategy of metabolic shutdown could be adopted whereby cells "retreat into their shell" and normal cellular functioning is discontinued until inflammation has abated.[20] Should the patient survive through this phase and inflammation settles, metabolism restarts and organ function is restored. An analogy can be made between metabolic shutdown and hibernation or estivation (the summer equivalent of hibernation) whereby a variety of organisms—including mammals, reptiles, snails, and even some species of fish and trees—go into a state of torpor until climactic conditions improve. This state is also recognized as dormancy in some types of bacteria, notably *Micrococcus luteus* and *Mycobacterium tuberculosis*.[35] Tellingly, mitochondria originate from probacteria and the human mitochondrial genome and bacteria share similar DNA. Thus, it is conceivable that sepsis may represent a form of hibernation. Indeed, Levy and colleagues[36] recently described histologic changes analogous to hibernation (glycogen deposition, up-regulation of glucose transporters) in the myocardium of septic rats. Indirect support for this hypothesis can be drawn from the lack of cell death in failed organs,[7] implying a functional rather than structural abnormality.

What triggers this metabolic shutdown in sepsis? This shutdown could be driven by a direct down-regulation of metabolic processes (possibly induced by the hormonal changes described earlier) and/or a progressive reduction in energy supply (again, induced by hormones), but also by decreased mitochondrial biogenesis, and by direct inhibition (eg, via nitric oxide and its congeners) or damage to the oxidative phosphorylation apparatus. This fall in energy should not be so abrupt as to cause ATP levels to plummet, thereby initiating cell death pathways. Rather, it should be more gradual, allowing the cell to achieve a new level of homeostasis and still maintain the possibility of long-term viability. Further investigation is required to determine the precise contribution of mitochondrial shutdown to organ dysfunction. Notably, we reported prognostic differences in skeletal muscle ATP levels taken on the day of intensive care unit admission in patients with septic shock, with levels being maintained (or even elevated) in survivors and significantly reduced in nonsurvivors, although their clinical severity was comparable.[37] A similar finding was reported in muscle and liver in a long-term rat model of fecal peritonitis.[38] As this level represents the balance between ATP generation and use, an ability to achieve adequate homeostasis, either in terms of reducing metabolic function or of maintaining sufficient energy production, could be a crucial determinant of survival.

RECOVERY PATHWAYS

As described earlier, three temporal phases to the septic response are apparent: (1) an early hypermetabolic response followed by (2) a period of metabolic down-regulation concurrent with clinical features of organ dysfunction, followed in the recovery phase by (3) an increase in metabolic activity as the organs recover. If mitochondria are inhibited or damaged, a restoration of normal or even elevated metabolism is contigent upon recovery of functioning mitochondria. New mitochondrial protein turnover (biogenesis) accelerates before and during the recovery process from sepsis.[39] Interestingly, nitric oxide is an important stimulator of this process.[40]

SUMMARY

Cellular dysfunction is a commonplace sequelum of sepsis and other systemic inflammatory conditions. Impaired energy production (related to mitochondrial inhibition, damage, and reduced protein turnover) appears to be a core mechanism underlying the development of organ dysfunction. The reduction in energy availability appears to trigger a metabolic shutdown that impairs normal functioning of the cell. This may well represent an adaptive mechanism analogous to hibernation that prevents massive degrees of cell death and thus enables eventual recovery in survivors.

REFERENCES

1. Martin GS, Mannino DM, Eaton S, et al. The epidemiology of sepsis in the United States from 1979 through 2000. N Engl J Med 2003;348:1546–54.
2. Available at: http://www.cdc.gov/nchs/products/pubs/pubd/hestats/finaldeaths03/finaldeaths03.htm. Accessed April 15 2008.
3. Available at: http://www.emea.europa.eu/human docs/Humans/EPAR/xigris/XigrisM2.htm. Accessed April 15 2008.
4. Singer M. The key advance in the treatment of sepsis in the last 10 years... doing less. Crit Care 2006; 10:122.
5. Singer M, Glynne P. Treating critical illness: the importance of first doing no harm. PLoS Med 2005; 2:108–13, e167.
6. Abraham EA, Singer M. Mechanisms of sepsis-induced organ dysfunction. Crit Care Med 2007; 35:2408–16.
7. Hotchkiss RS, Swanson PE, Freeman BD, et al. Apoptotic cell death in patients with sepsis, shock, and multiple organ dysfunction. Crit Care Med 1999;27:1230–48.
8. Noble JS, MacKirdy FN, Donaldson SI, et al. Renal and respiratory failure in Scottish ICUs. Anaesthesia 2001;56:124–9.
9. Boekstegers P, Weidenhofer S, Kapsner T, et al. Skeletal muscle partial pressure of oxygen in patients with sepsis. Crit Care Med 1994;22:640–50.
10. VanderMeer TJ, Wang H, Fink MP. Endotoxemia causes ileal mucosal acidosis in the absence of

mucosal hypoxia in a normodynamic porcine model of septic shock. Crit Care Med 1995;23:1217–26.

11. Rosser DM, Stidwill RP, Jacobson D, et al. Oxygen tension in the bladder epithelium rises in both high and low cardiac output endotoxemic sepsis. J Appl Physiol 1995;79:1878–82.

12. Boerma EC, van der Voort PH, Spronk PE, et al. Relationship between sublingual and intestinal microcirculatory perfusion in patients with abdominal sepsis. Crit Care Med 2007;35:1055–60.

13. Stark R, Roden M. Mitochondrial function and endocrine diseases. Eur J Clin Invest 2007;37:236–48.

14. Ritz P, Dumas JF, Ducluzeau PH, et al. Hormonal regulation of mitochondrial energy production. Curr Opin Clin Nutr Metab Care 2005;8:415–8.

15. Hsieh YC, Frink M, Choudhry MA, et al. Metabolic modulators following trauma and sepsis: sex hormones. Crit Care Med 2007;35(Suppl 9):S621–9.

16. Peeters RP, Wouters PJ, Kaptein E, et al. Reduced activation and increased inactivation of thyroid hormone in tissues of critically ill patients. J Clin Endocrinol Metab 2003;88:3202–11.

17. Arnalich F, López J, Codoceo R, et al. Relationship of plasma leptin to plasma cytokines and human survival in sepsis and septic shock. J Infect Dis 1999; 180:908–11.

18. Vanhorebeek I, De Vos R, Mesotten D, et al. Protection of hepatocyte mitochondrial ultrastructure and function by strict blood glucose control with insulin in critically ill patients. Lancet 2005;365:53–9.

19. Calvano SE, Xiao W, Richards DR, et al. A network-based analysis of systemic inflammation in humans. Nature 2005;437:1032–7.

20. Singer M, De Santis V, Vitale D, et al. Multiorgan failure is an adaptive, endocrine-mediated, metabolic response to overwhelming systemic inflammation. Lancet 2004;364:545–8.

21. Nogueira V, Rigoulet M, Piquet MA, et al. Mitochondrial respiratory chain adjustment to cellular energy demand. J Biol Chem 2001;276:46104–10.

22. Nogueira V, Walter L, Avéret N, et al. Thyroid status is a key regulator of both flux and efficiency of oxidative phosphorylation in rat hepatocytes. J Bioenerg Biomembr 2002;34:55–66.

23. Jubrias SA, Esselman PC, Price LB, et al. Large energetic adaptations of elderly muscle to resistance and endurance training. J Appl Physiol 2001;90:1663–70.

24. Szabó C. Hydrogen sulphide and its therapeutic potential. Nat Rev Drug Discov 2007;6:917–35.

25. Frost M, Wang Q, Moncada S, et al. Hypoxia accelerates nitric oxide–dependent inhibition of mitochondrial complex I in activated macrophages.

Am J Physiol Regul Integr Comp Physiol 2005;288: R394–400.

26. Brealey D, Singer M. Mitochondrial dysfunction in sepsis. Curr Infect Dis Rep 2003;5:365–71.

27. Protti A, Carré C, Frost MT, et al. Succinate recovers mitochondrial oxygen consumption in septic rat skeletal muscle. Crit Care Med 2007;35:2150–5.

28. Harper ME, Seifert EL. Thyroid hormone effects on mitochondrial energetics. Thyroid 2008;18:145–56.

29. Lee J, Sharma S, Kim J, et al. Mitochondrial nuclear receptors and transcription factors: who's minding the cell? J Neurosci Res 2008;86:961–71.

30. Uehara M, Plank LD, Hill GL. Components of energy expenditure in patients with severe sepsis and major trauma: a basis for clinical care. Crit Care Med 1999; 27:1295–302.

31. Zauner C, Schuster BI, Schneeweiss B. Similar metabolic responses to standardized total parenteral nutrition of septic and nonseptic critically ill patients. Am J Clin Nutr 2001;74:265–70.

32. Kreymann G, Grosser S, Buggisch P, et al. Oxygen consumption and resting metabolic rate in sepsis, sepsis syndrome, and septic shock. Crit Care Med 1993;21:1012–9.

33. Chioléro R, Revelly JP, Tappy L. Energy metabolism in sepsis and injury. Nutrition 1997;13(Suppl 9): 45S–51S.

34. Soop A, Albert J, Weitzberg E, et al. Complement activation, endothelin-1 and neuropeptide Y in relation to the cardiovascular response to endotoxin-induced systemic inflammation in healthy volunteers. Acta Anaesthesiol Scand 2004;48:74–81.

35. Mukamolova GV, Kaprelyants AS, Young DI, et al. A bacterial cytokine. Proc Natl Acad Sci U S A 1998; 95:8916–21.

36. Levy RJ, Piel DA, Acton PD, et al. Evidence of myocardial hibernation in the septic heart. Crit Care Med 2005;33:2752–6.

37. Brealey D, Brand M, Hargreaves I, et al. Association between mitochondrial dysfunction and severity and outcome of septic shock. Lancet 2002;360:219–23.

38. Brealey D, Karyampudi S, Jacques TS, et al. Mitochondrial dysfunction in a longterm rodent model of sepsis and organ failure. Am J Physiol Regul Integr Comp Physiol 2004;286:R491–7.

39. Haden DW, Suliman HB, Carraway MS, et al. Mitochondrial biogenesis restores oxidative metabolism during Staphylococcus aureus sepsis. Am J Respir Crit Care Med 2007;176:768–77.

40. Nisoli E, Falcone S, Tonello C, et al. Mitochondrial biogenesis by NO yields functionally active mitochondria in mammals. Proc Natl Acad Sci U S A 2004;101:16507–12.

The Right Ventricle in Sepsis

Chee M. Chan, MD[a],*, James R. Klinger, MD[b]

KEYWORDS

- Sepsis • Septic shock • Right ventricular function
- Critical care • Pulmonary circulation

The inflammatory response associated with sepsis typically results in increased vascular permeability and vasodilatation. These changes result in decreased intravascular volume and a fall in systemic vascular resistance that necessitates a robust increase in cardiac output. Numerous studies have described compensatory mechanisms for increased cardiac output despite a decrease in cardiac contractility. Most of these studies have been limited almost exclusively to left ventricular function, with little attention paid to right ventricular performance.[1–3] The lack of attention to the right ventricle (RV) in studies of cardiac output may seem reasonable considering its smaller muscle mass and its single organ responsibility, but its role as the second largest pump in the circulatory system connected in series to the left ventricle (LV) makes it a vital part of the mammalian circulation. Simply put, RV output must approximate LV output, provided that there are no significant shunts. Normally, the RV has little trouble keeping up with the LV; however, in the presence of decreased contractility, increased afterload, or insufficient filling, which are three conditions commonly associated with sepsis, RV output may be unable to keep pace with increased LV output. Under these conditions, the RV may fail to maintain adequate left atrial filling and can contribute to a fall in cardiac output from decreased LV preload. In addition to being connected to each other in series, the RV and LV also share a muscular wall, the interventricular septum. As a result, changes in intraventricular volume of one ventricle can affect the filling and contractility of the other via a process known as interventricular dependence.

For these reasons, a thorough understanding of RV performance and its potential derangements is essential to the proper hemodynamic management of patients who have sepsis. Over the past decade, growing interest focusing on the role of the RV in hemodynamic homeostasis has increased dramatically.[4–16] There is growing evidence that sepsis-associated cardiac dysfunction is not limited to the LV but often involves the RV as well.[17,18] Persistent RV dysfunction in sepsis has been associated with worse outcome.[19,20] In this article, we discuss the structural and functional differences between the RV and LV, the pathophysiology of RV depression caused by sepsis, methods of monitoring RV dysfunction, particularly in the intensive care unit, and potential strategies for managing RV dysfunction in patients who have sepsis.

THE NORMAL RIGHT VENTRICLE

Although the dual pump design of the human circulatory system has been known for centuries, hemodynamic differences between the systemic and pulmonary circulations were not well understood until recently. The first measurements of pulmonary arterial pressures were obtained in the 1940s.[21–24] Many investigators were surprised that pulmonary arterial pressures and resistance were only a fraction of systemic pressure and resistance. The pulmonary vascular resistance (PVR) was so low that some investigators hypothesized that RV contraction was not necessary to maintain cardiac output. Studies in dogs that obliterated the RV free wall by electrocautery demonstrated only a slight rise is central venous

[a] Division of Pulmonary and Critical Care Medicine, Washington Hospital Center, 110 Irving Street NW #2B-39, Washington, DC 20010, USA
[b] Division of Pulmonary Critical Care Medicine, Rhode Island Hospital, Brown University, Providence, RI, USA
* Corresponding author.
E-mail address: chee.m.chan@medstar.net (C.M. Chan).

Clin Chest Med 29 (2008) 661–676
doi:10.1016/j.ccm.2008.07.002
0272-5231/08/$ – see front matter © 2008 Elsevier Inc. All rights reserved.

pressure (CVP) and little change in cardiac output.[25–28] These studies were performed with the chest open and pericardium removed and likely underestimated the importance of RV systolic function under normal circumstances.

The cardiac output generated by the RV and LV is governed by the same three factors: preload, afterload, and myocardial contractility. The unique structural and functional characteristics of each ventricle results in different responses to these factors, however. During fetal life, PVR is higher in uninflated lungs than during adult life, and systemic vascular resistance (SVR) is lower. Increased PVR helps direct right-sided blood flow across the foramen ovale and into the left atrium. Hemodynamic loads are similar for both ventricles. Not surprisingly, the fetal ventricles are more similar in mass and shape, and the interventricular septum is flat and in a midline position. After birth, lung inflation dramatically drops PVR, and blood from the RV is redirected from the foramen ovale to the low-resistance pulmonary circulation. During normal development, LV demands increase considerably as systemic organs and skeletal muscle mass increase. By adult life, the ventricles develop distinct structural characteristics designed to compensate for the marked differences in afterload against which they work.

Systolic Function

Grossly, the LV is shaped like a thick-walled crucible (**Fig. 1**) and contains three distinct layers of myocytes: (1) the superficial muscle fibers with a longitudinal arrangement, (2) the more prominent middle layer, in which myocytes are oriented in the transverse axis, and (3) the deeper longitudinally oriented trabeculae and papillary muscles. High systolic pressures are achieved by circumferential contraction, which results in the lateral free wall and interventricular septum moving toward each other. The thick muscular walls of the LV make it capable of generating high systolic pressures and sustaining cardiac output, even when systemic vascular resistance is greatly elevated.

In contrast, the RV is a crescent-shaped chamber formed by a thinner, triangular-shaped piece of myocardial tissue wrapped around the interventricular septum (see **Fig. 1**). At end diastole, the normal RV wall is only 2 to 3 mm thick, compared with the thicker LV wall of 8 to 11 mm.[29] Microscopically, the RV free wall is comprised of only two layers of myocardiocytes: a superficial, transverse oriented muscle layer and a thicker deeper layer in which the fibers are longitudinally arranged from apex to base. Systolic

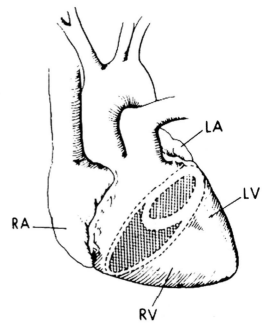

Fig. 1. Diagram of right and left ventricles shows partial cross section. Note the concentric shape of the left ventricle, thin right ventricular free wall, and the convex orientation of the interventricular septum away from the RV. (*From* Guyton AC. Textbook of medical physiology. 6th edition. Philadelphia: WB Saunders Company; 1981. p. 124; with permission.)

pressures in the RV are achieved more by longitudinal contraction, with the apex moving up toward the lateral leaflet of the tricuspid valve. The RV free wall moves inward at the same time as the interventricular septum is moving in the opposite direction toward the LV lateral free wall.

Blood flow through the RV can be divided into two parts. The initial stretch of the ventricular myocardium (end diastolic volume) begins as venous return from the right atrium enters the RV immediately after tricuspid valve opening. RV diastolic filling is completed by contraction of the right atrium. Contraction of the RV consists of a peristaltic pattern whereby the inflow region normally contracts approximately 25 to 50 msec before the outflow region, resulting in an intraventricular systolic pressure gradient of 15 to 25 mm Hg between the proximal and distal portions of the RV.[30] Dilatation of the outflow region occurs during contraction of the inflow region, which causes initial expansion of the pulmonary artery and primes the pulmonary artery for acceptance of a large volume of blood. Under normal circumstances, PVR remains low as long as the vascular bed can be recruited. Because the pulmonary circulation is highly compliant, ejection of blood from the RV is facilitated in part by the momentum of blood.

Some blood ejected from the RV during systole continues even during diastole.[31]

The different shape and function of the RV as compared with the LV result in different relationships between systolic pressure generated for any given volume. Its unique thin-walled crescent shape allows the RV to accommodate large increases in venous return without greatly increasing RV end diastolic pressure (RVEDP). As RV preload increases by volume expansion, stroke work increases only slightly (**Fig. 2**A). Cardiac output is well preserved over a range of volumes until dilatation of the ventricle is limited by the interventricular septum and pericardium.[32] As the RV begins to dilate and change its contour to mirror that of the LV, contribution of the Frank Starling mechanism becomes more apparent. Further increases in RV filling pressure overdistend myocardial fibers, which increases RV stroke work and decreases cardiac output.[33,34]

Afterload, defined as tension developed by muscle fibers to move a ventricular load during contraction, is affected by intraventricular pressure and chamber size. The same unique properties of RV construction that allow it to accommodate large increases in preload make it exquisitely sensitive to increases in afterload. Its inability to generate high pressures limits the ability of the RV to compensate for acute rises in PVR. As shown in **Fig. 2**B, stroke volume and cardiac output decline dramatically as resistance is increased by constricting the main pulmonary artery.

Diastole

The same property of the RV free wall that makes it intolerant of an abrupt rise in afterload, namely its highly compliant RV free wall, allows it to accommodate large increases in venous return without marked increases in end diastolic pressure.[35–37] At the same time, the high compliance and low inward elastic recoil of the RV permit greater transmission of negative intrathoracic pressures. Deep inhalation greatly increases RV transmural pressure and allows the diaphragm to facilitate RV loading by literally sucking blood into the chest.

The greater compliance of the RV is important because it is subject to substantially more variation in filling volumes than the LV. The lungs normally contain only approximately one tenth of the total intravascular volume or approximately 500 mL in an average sized adult,[38] and LV filling largely depends on blood flow through the lungs determined by RV output. In contrast, RV filling is determined not only by LV output but also by systemic venous tone. RV filling can be affected by fluid shifts from the extravascular to intravascular space. Changes in intrathoracic pressures also affect RV filling considerably more than they do the LV. As intrathoracic pressure falls during inspiration, pericardial pressure falls while CVP remains constant, which increases RV transmural pressures. In contrast, any change in pericardial pressure applied to the left heart is also applied to the lung and the major pulmonary veins that supply the LV, which keeps LV transmural pressure essentially unchanged.

Contractility and Perfusion

The contractility of the RV is also affected by its unique geometric shape. Although its smaller mass results in less maximal contractile force, the RV has a greater end diastolic volume than

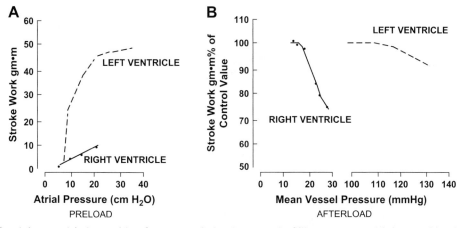

Fig. 2. The right ventricle is capable of accommodating increases in filling pressure with less workload than the left (*A*) but is unable to sustain systolic function in response to an acute increase in afterload as evidenced by a rapid decline in stroke volume (*B*). Atrial filling pressure was elevated by volume loading. Afterload was increased by constricting the main pulmonary artery or aorta. (*From* Braunwald E. Textbook of cardiovascular medicine. 1st edition. Philadelphia: WB Saunders Company; 1980. p. 532; with permission.)

the LV and a greater surface area per volume of blood. Flattening of the RV during systole allows large changes in volume without much change in RV free wall area (**Fig. 3**), which allows the RV to achieve a similar stroke volume as the LV with lower energy expenditure.[39]

The interventricular septum is generally supplied by the right coronary artery and left anterior descending artery, whereas the free wall of the RV is supplied primarily by the right coronary artery. Oxygen extraction and blood flow to the RV are comparatively less than the LV, given its smaller muscle mass. In the absence of significant coronary artery disease, perfusion of the RV free wall is determined primarily by the difference in RV free wall tension and aortic pressure that supplies the right coronary artery.[40] The combination of increased RV free wall tension and decreased systemic arterial pressure—two conditions that often occur in sepsis—may result in profound hypoperfusion of the RV and depressed cardiac output. When coronary artery perfusion reduces below a critical threshold, acute myocardial ischemia ensues along with rapid cardiovascular collapse.[40]

Ventricular Interdependance

As two pumps connected in series, each ventricle is capable of affecting the performance of the other via the amount of blood pumped forward. LV dysfunction impairs RV performance by increasing RV afterload, and RV dysfunction can impede LV performance by failing to provide adequate preload. The ventricles are also physically connected to each other via the interventricular septum. Changes in intraventricular pressures of one ventricle can be transmitted across the septum and affect transmural pressures and compliance of the other ventricle. When the RV is subjected to increases in filling pressure or afterload, it begins to dilate and compensates by increasing intraventricular volume and end diastolic pressure. The result is a larger, rounder RV pushing the interventricular septum toward the LV. Normally, LV end diastolic pressure is greater than RVEDP, which allows the interventricular septum to move toward the RV during diastole. This motion, coupled with the lateral movement of the LV free wall, allows for maximal chamber enlargement in the concentric LV. If RVEDP begins to equal or exceed LV end diastolic pressure, the interventricular septum can move paradoxically toward the LV free wall during diastole. This is best seen on two-dimensional echocardiography as a flattening of the normal concave shape of the septum relative to the LV or a bowing of the septum away from the RV (**Fig. 4**). Compression of the septum toward the LV free wall also impairs LV systolic function.

The degree of ventricular interdependence is greatly affected by the pericardium. As pericardial compliance decreases, more of the increase in intraventricular pressure from one ventricle is transmitted through the septum to the other

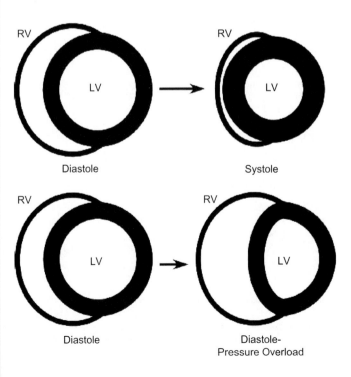

Diastole   Systole

Diastole   Diastole-
                  Pressure Overload

Fig. 3. The crescent shape of the right ventricle (RV) allows it to accommodate a large increase in interventricular volume during diastole with only a slight increase in RV free wall area. (*From* Greyson CR. Pathophysiology of right ventricular failure. Crit Care Med 2008;36(1):S57–65; with permission.)

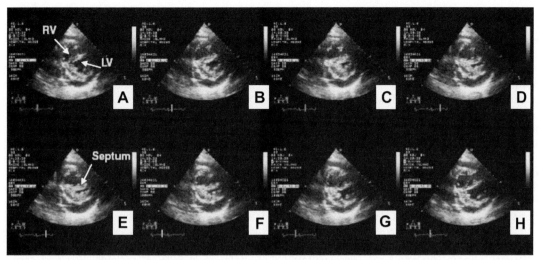

Fig. 4. Echocardiographic images of a heart from a patient with right ventricular overload caused by pulmonary arterial hypertension during systole (*A–D*) and diastole (*E–H*). Note the enlarged right ventricle (RV) and bowing of the interventricular septum toward the left ventricle (LV) during diastole preventing normal LV filling. (*From* Stone A, Klinger JR. The right ventricle in pulmonary hypertension, contemporary cardiology pulmonary hypertension. In: Hill NS, Farber HW, editors. Humana Press; 2008. p. 93–126; with permission.)

ventricle. RV dilatation in the presence of pericardial disease or even increased intrathoracic pressure may have more salient effects on LV filling than under normal conditions.[41]

RIGHT VENTRICULAR FUNCTION AND THE PULMONARY CIRCULATION IN SEPSIS

Early circulatory response to sepsis and septic shock is characterized by vasodilation and increased vascular permeability, which leads to a marked reduction in intravascular filling pressures.[42] A concomitant imbalance in oxygen supply and demand may lead to myocardial depression.[43] Circulating cytokines, such as tumor necrosis factor–α, may further worsen contractility.[44–47] As a result, LV ejection fraction (LVEF) often decreases during sepsis. A fall in LVEF may decrease stroke volume initially, but in response to fluid resuscitation, LV end diastolic volume rises and stroke volume begins to normalize. Cardiac output is elevated primarily by increased heart rate. A reduction in LV afterload also helps to achieve elevated cardiac output in the face of depressed LV contractility.[48,49]

Unlike the systemic circulation, resistance in the pulmonary vasculature is often increased in sepsis, especially in the presence of acute lung injury. Decreased production of nitric oxide, an endogenous vasodilator, likely contributes to increased PVR and pulmonary hypertension in sepsis.[50,51] Increases in circulating levels of other vasoactive substances, such as thromboxane, endothelin,

and serotonin release from platelets also may contribute.[52–55] Acute lung injury leads to hypoxic pulmonary vasoconstriction, and this pulmonary pressor response is enhanced by hypercarbia or acidosis. Coagulation abnormalities are also common in the pulmonary vascular bed during sepsis and acute lung injury and may lead to pulmonary arterial thrombosis that further raises PVR.[56] During sepsis, the RV faces substantial increases in PVR during a time when the LV needs to increase cardiac output considerably to compensate for a fall in systemic vascular resistance.

The RV is poorly prepared to compensate for acute elevations in afterload. Its inability to acutely raise pulmonary pressure partly explains development of cardiogenic shock in large pulmonary embolism. In sepsis, the RV is even less tolerant of increases in afterload because of the imbalance in oxygen supply and demand and systemic hypotension that reduce RV perfusion.[57,58] One of the few mechanisms that the RV has to elevate pulmonary artery pressure (PAP) and maintain systolic function is to increase end diastolic pressure. As shown in **Fig. 2**A, RV systolic function is maintained over a wide range of increasing filling pressures. Increasing RV transmural filling pressures is a vital part of hemodynamic resuscitation; however, expansion of intravascular volume in the patient who has sepsis may be difficult because of decreased venous tone and increased vascular permeability. Positive airway pressure from mechanical ventilation may further decrease transmural filling pressures. As a consequence, aggressive fluid resuscitation and frequent CVP monitoring are often necessary to ensure adequate right-sided filling pressures. Much of the success of early goal-directed therapy in septic shock may be caused by targeting an elevated CVP.[59] Excessive fluid resuscitation eventually may impair LV filling via ventricular interdependence, however.[60] This effect is most pronounced when dilation of one or both ventricles has stretched the pericardium to its limit. Further expansion of the RV under these conditions encroaches upon the LV cavity, especially during diastole and impairs LV filling.[61] In dog models in which PVR was raised by artificially inducing pulmonary embolism, cardiac output dropped significantly when RV filling pressures were elevated enough to impede LV filling.[62]

Several clinical studies have demonstrated reduced RV systolic function in sepsis (**Table 1**). Before volume expansion, RV ejection fraction (EF) is usually reduced in sepsis with a high RV end diastolic volume index (RVEDVI). In survivors of sepsis, fluid resuscitation is associated with an increase in cardiac index, CVP, pulmonary capillary wedge pressure, mean PAP (mPAP), and stroke volume index. RV stroke work index, RVEDVI, and RV end systolic volume index increase, whereas RVEF continues to decrease.[63] An increase in filling pressures from volume replacement produces a concomitant rise in RVEDVI. Further reduction in RVEF after fluid resuscitation may be caused by the increase in preload or an increase in PAP and PVR. These findings suggest that initial RV function is depressed at the onset of sepsis and that increasing cardiac output depends on increasing RV filling volumes.

Decreased RVEF persists in patients who have sepsis even after fluid resuscitation. Hoffman and colleagues[17] noted significant RV systolic dysfunction in patients who received fluid resuscitation for sepsis compared with patients undergoing elective surgery who received at least 6 L of fluid replacement. The average RVEF was 35% ± 16% for septic patients versus 52% ± 7% in patients undergoing elective surgery. At the same time, RVEDVI was nearly threefold higher (143 ± 28 and 55.8 ± 7.4 mL/m^2). Similarly, Mitsuo and colleagues[18] reported an RVEF of 36% ± 9.7% in patients who had sepsis compared with 47% ± 7% in trauma patients ($P < .005$), along with greater RVEDVI (122 ± 40 versus 101 ± 34, respectively; $P < .01$). In contrast to other studies, patients in this study did not have circulatory shock.

How much of the decrease in RV systolic function in sepsis is caused by LV dysfunction is uncertain. Concordant depression of RVEF and LVEF was found in 82% of patients who had sepsis with unidirectional changes in RVEDVI and LV end diastolic volume index (LVEDVI) in 76%.[64] RVEF often improves in concert with LVEF. In one study,[63] RVEF and LVEF were both substantially depressed to 35% and 31%, respectively, and recovered subsequently to 51% and 47%, respectively, in survivors. Similar to RVEDVI, LVEDVI was elevated and decreased to normal values with recovery. During fluid resuscitation, LVEDVI and LVEDSI increased similarly to RVEDVI and RVEDSI. Improved LV systolic function may improve RV performance by decreasing pulmonary venous pressure and lowering PAP. It is also possible, however, that resolving sepsis simply improves right and left myocardial contractility as chemokine levels fall and coronary perfusion increases.

Regardless of the cause, decreased RV systolic function in sepsis has been associated with increased mortality. Dhainaut and colleagues[19] found that nonsurvivors had lower RVEF (29% ± 11%) than survivors (32% ± 13%). Although the

Table 1
Effect of initial and subsequent right ventricular ejection fraction on survival in patients with sepsis

	n	Survivors Initial RVEF	Nonsurvivors Initial RVEF	Survivors Follow-up RVEF	Nonsurvivors Follow-up RVEF
Hoffman et al, 1983	9	0.29 ± 0.06	0.36 ± 0.15	0.35 ± 0.10	0.34 ± 0.07
Vincent et al, 1988	56	0.28 ± 0.09	0.21 ± 0.07	—	—
Dhainaut et al, 1988	23	0.32 ± 0.13	0.29 ± 0.11	0.31 ± 0.12	0.22 ± 0.11
Parker et al, 1990	39	0.35	0.41	0.51	0.39

Abbreviation: RVEF, right ventricular ejection fraction.

difference in RVEF was small, their findings were confirmed the following year in a similar study by Vincent and colleagues,[65] who found nonsurvivors to have an RVEF of only 20.9% ± 6.7% compared with 27.8% ± 8.6% in survivors. Other hemodynamic parameters in this study, such as mPAP, mean arterial pressure, and cardiac index of the RV, were not predictive of survival. In another study,[20] preserved RV function, defined as RVEF more than 45% at time of diagnosis, predicted better response to fluid alone and less need for inotropes or vasoactive agents. Parker and colleagues[64] found that nonsurvivors had only mild reductions in RVEF and LVEF (41% and 40%, respectively) despite fluid resuscitation to a pulmonary capillary wedge pressure between 15 and 18 mm Hg, suggesting that lack of ventricular depression may be a maladaptive response to sepsis.

As with LV function, patients who survive sepsis eventually develop improvement in RV function. In one study,[17] RVEF improved in survivors with a significant decrease in RVEDVI, whereas RVEDVI, stroke volume index, and RV stroke work index all increased in patients whose condition deteriorated. Although an initial negative linear regression was noted between RVEF and mPAP in survivors and nonsurvivors, this relationship failed to be significant in nonsurvivors within 48 hours but was still significant in survivors. RVEDP and RVEDV had an initial positive linear relationship that persisted in survivors but not in nonsurvivors.[64] The lack of persistent correlation in these variables may be the result of progressive deterioration of ventricular function. Ultimately, survivors had resolution of these changes within 7 to 14 days.[64]

PVR is persistently elevated in fluid resuscitated patients with sepsis; however, evidence that RV dysfunction in sepsis is caused by increased afterload alone is lacking. Most studies have not found any correlation between the degree of PVR elevation and RVEF or RVEDVI.[64] Patients without sepsis (patients who have hypovolemia, postoperative patients, trauma patients) but with similar elevations in PVR do not develop RV dysfunction.[17] Although elevated PVR likely contributes to RV dysfunction in sepsis, the cause of depressed RV function is probably multifactorial and likely includes decreased contractility and LV dysfunction.

Decreased myocardial perfusion could have a profound negative impact on contractility. Ventricular enlargement during fluid resuscitation acutely increases RV free wall tension and makes the RV particularly vulnerable to reduced coronary blood flow from hypotension.[66] As a consequence, subendocardial ischemia can be exacerbated by increasing oxygen demand on the RV

myocardium.[67] The contribution of decreased coronary blood flow to RV dysfunction in sepsis seems to be insignificant, however. Using thermodilution coronary sinus catheters, recent studies found that coronary blood flow is either preserved or elevated in sepsis (**Fig. 5**).[68,69] There was no difference in coronary blood flow in patients with myocardial depression compared with those without. Another mechanism explaining decreased contractility, such as impaired perfusion of the myocardial microcirculation or the presence of a humoral mediator, must exist. Circulating tumor necrosis factor–α, in particular, has been found to be a major contributor to depressed myocardial contractility in septic shock.[44–47,70–72] Along with its inflammatory and immune function, tumor necrosis factor–α depresses myocardial function through alterations of several pathways, including impaired nitric oxide signaling, the sphingomyelinase pathway,[73,74] and calcium flow.[75,76]

Thus, there are many mechanisms that contribute to RV dysfunction in sepsis. If stress on the RV is severe, a vicious cycle begins in which rapid circulatory collapse occurs (**Fig. 6**).

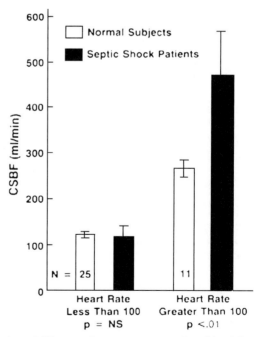

Fig. 5. Differences in mean coronary sinus blood flow (CSBF) in patients with (*n* = 7) and without (*n* = 25) septic shock. CSBF was similar in patients without tachycardia and greater in septic patients when heart rate exceeded 100 beats/min. (*From* Cunnion RE, Schaer GL, Parker MM, et al. The coronary circulation in human septic shock. Circulation 1986;73:637–44; with permission.)

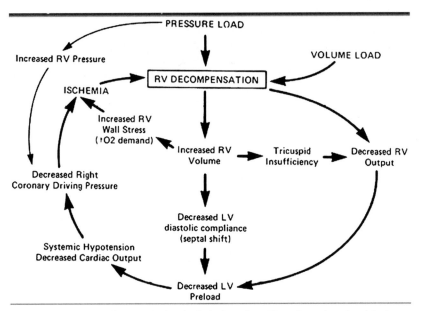

Fig. 6. Factors that contribute to right ventricular (RV) dysfunction. Elevation of preload (volume overload) and afterload (pressure overload) lead to increased RV volume increasing myocardial O$_2$ demands, whereas decreasing RV perfusion pressure leads to decreased RV contractility. At the same time, increased RV pressure is transmitted to the left ventricle (LV) via the interventricular septum and impedes LV filling, which results in decreased LV output that worsens RV coronary perfusion pressure and further decreases RV output. (*From* Wiedemann HP, Matthay RA. Acute right heart failure. Crit Care Clin 1985;1(3):631–61; with permission.)

RIGHT VENTRICULAR MONITORING IN CRITICALLY ILL PATIENTS WHO HAVE SEPSIS

Several techniques can be used to assess or monitor RV function. Contrast ventriculography is the traditional method for estimating RV wall motion, volume, and EF.[77–79] Using this technique, reports of normal RVEF have ranged from 45% to 75%.[80] The wide variation may be caused by the complex shape and contraction of the RV, which make it difficult to calculate accurate end diastolic and end systolic volumes using a two-dimensional technique. The need for special equipment and invasive nature of this test also makes it impractical for critically ill patients,[27] not to mention the risk of contrast-induced nephropathy in patients who already have tenuous renal function from septic shock.

Radionuclide angiography can provide an accurate and reproducible measurement of RVEF, size, and regional wall motion. The normal RVEF reported with this technique has ranged from 45% to 65%.[81,82] The first-pass and equilibrium gated blood pool techniques can determine RVEF using autologous erythrocytes labeled with [99m]Technetium pyrophosphate.[83–87] In the first-pass technique, repeated images are obtained as the radionuclide mixes and circulates through the heart. EF is estimated from computer-generated time curves. This technique requires a large quantity of radioactive injection. The equilibrium gated blood pool technique acquires repeated images in line with the R wave of the electrocardiogram. Time curves are used to estimate EF. Determination of RVEF correlates well between the two techniques.[87] The limiting factor is potential underestimation of RVEF because it is often difficult to account for radioactivity within the right atrium.[84] The ability to perform the equilibrium gated blood pool technique at bedside with a mobile gamma camera makes it appealing, but equipment is often bulky and radiologists must be skilled at interpretation.[32]

A pulmonary artery catheter (PAC) capable of measuring cardiac output by thermodilution is a bedside technique that produces reliable data with little equipment and can be used to assess and monitor ventricular function in critically ill patients. Although this is an invasive technique, it allows for direct measurement of right atrial pressure, RV systolic and diastolic pressures, PAP, pulmonary capillary wedge pressure, and measurement of cardiac output. Thermodilution techniques also have been used to measure RVEF and RV volumes and have been found to correlate closely with measurements made by radionuclide angiography.[88,89] Using this technique, cardiac output and RVEF can be serially measured throughout the day to determine hemodynamic effects of various therapeutic strategies in the intensive care unit.[32] Insertion of a PAC is not without inherent risks, and a growing body of evidence suggests that there is no mortality benefit in using PACs in managing critically ill patients who have sepsis.[90–93] Regardless of whether PACs can improve outcome in patients who have sepsis with acute RV failure remains to be determined.

Transthoracic two-dimensional echocardiography is a noninvasive technique with minimal risks that provides reproducible estimates of LV and RV size, contractility, and EF. It can be performed at the patient's bedside, obviating the need for transport, and can be repeated frequently in the same patient. Echocardiography also can assess the position and movement of the interventricular septum.[80] Septal flattening and paradoxical movement of the septum toward the LV free wall during diastole suggests RV pressure or volume overload.[94] Jardin and colleagues[95] showed that echocardiographic estimates of RVEF, RV area, and volumes were similar to measurements made by catheter-based thermodilution techniques, suggesting that transthoracic echocardiography is capable of providing assessments of RV function that are similar to PAC. Its ready availability in most institutions and ease of use have made it one of the most valuable tools for initial evaluation and subsequent monitoring of RV function in the intensive care unit.

APPROACH TO RIGHT VENTRICULAR FAILURE IN THE PATIENT WHO HAS SEPSIS

Medical management of the patient who has sepsis has progressed rapidly over the last decade. Current recommendations for antibiotic treatment, volume resuscitation, adjunctive steroid therapy, glucose control, and administration of activated protein C have been summarized by professional societies and recently organized into care bundles.[96] When treating patients who have chronic pulmonary disease and sepsis, there is often concern that rigorous fluid resuscitation and high-dose pressors may worsen right heart function, but the overriding concern always should be systemic tissue perfusion. As such, the initial approach to patients who have sepsis and RV failure should not be much different than for any other patient. Adequate ventilation, oxygenation, and stabilization of systemic hemodynamics are the greatest priorities. Rapid identification of the source of infection, treatment with appropriate antibiotics, and source control are imperative to improving outcome. Once these measures have

been initiated, RV function should be considered, particularly in patients who demonstrate depressed cardiac output. When RV failure is found, management should be directed toward optimizing RV preload, reducing afterload, and improving contractility.

Aggressive fluid hydration and volume expansion are critical to maintaining adequate preload to the RV and improving cardiac output.[97] There is, however, a point at which systolic function begins to decline as RV myocytes are stretched beyond their mechanical advantage point. High right-sided filling pressure also begins to impede LV diastolic filling if RVEDP approaches or exceeds LV end diastolic pressure. Increased wall tension from an excessively dilated RV increases oxygen demand while reducing coronary perfusion, and if not accompanied by adequate systemic blood pressure, it can precipitate myocardial ischemia.[98–100] RV failure and cardiovascular collapse have been demonstrated with continued volume expansion in anesthetized dogs facing elevated PVR.[101–103] Although volume expansion should be the initial treatment for RV dysfunction in septic shock, a threshold exists beyond which further fluid resuscitation is detrimental.

Upper limits for LV filling have been well established in clinical practice and can be monitored hemodynamically or by the clinical development of pulmonary edema. Similar hemodynamic and clinical endpoints have not been established for the RV. The presence of peripheral edema or jugular venous distension may indicate elevated right-sided pressures but may not necessarily indicate RV failure or even adequate RV filling. A prudent approach is to assess RV function in patients who continue to show signs of inadequate cardiac output after initial volume resuscitation. If echocardiography reveals decreased RV contractility, measurement of CVP should be obtained and monitored during further attempts at volume expansion. Placement of a PAC may be necessary to monitor cardiac output. Increases in CVP that increase RV diameter to the point of impeding LV filling or cause RV ischemia on ECG strongly suggest that further elevation of right-sided pressures is detrimental. On the other hand, if cardiac output increases with further elevation of CVP, maintenance of higher right-sided filling pressures may be indicated.

Another goal of volume expansion is to raise aortic blood pressure to preserve right coronary perfusion. When systemic pressure does not correct with fluid resuscitation, initiation of vasopressor agents is needed to increase systemic pressures and maintain adequate coronary perfusion. Norepinephrine, an α_1- and β_1-adrenergic stimulant, has been shown to increase mPAP and PVR without affecting RVEF or RVEDVI.[104,105] Increased oxygen extraction is also noted. Despite worsening PVR, RVEF is maintained with improvement in oxygen extraction using this agent. Dopamine is an adrenergic and dopaminergic agonist that improves mean systemic arterial pressure, cardiac index, and mPAP but does not affect PVRI, RVEF, or RVEDVI. In one study,[106] oxygen delivery and consumption increased by approximately 20% in patients who had sepsis with mildly depressed RVEF of less than 50%. Similarly, epinephrine, a potent α- and β-adrenergic agent, increases mPAP but not RVEDVI while it increases RVEF by approximately 25%.[107]

Dobutamine is a β_1-adrenergic inotrope that augments contractility and reduces LV afterload.[108] Low doses of dobutamine, in the range of 1 to 5 μg/kg/min, decrease PVR and increase cardiac output. At higher dosages, however, dobutamine causes significant tachycardia without further reduction in PVR.[105] Its use in sepsis is limited because it may cause systemic hypotension. Dobutamine has been advocated to increase RV contractility and augment cardiac output in chronic RV failure or acute RV failure in patients with chronic pulmonary vascular disease,[97] but its effect on RV function during sepsis has not been well studied. Similarly, milrinone is a selective phosphodiesterase-3 inhibitor with inotropic and vasodilatory effects. Milrinone significantly improves RV function and reduces PVR in acute and chronic pulmonary hypertension in animal models.[109,110] Used in conjunction with nitric oxide in the pediatric population, it produced selective pulmonary vasodilation after cardiac surgery for congenital heart defects.[111] Its systemic vasodilatory effects limit its use, however, because it may worsen hypotension.

The effects of phenylephrine, isoproterenol, and vasopressin on RV function are also not well known in sepsis or septic shock. Phenylephrine is an α_1-adrenergic agent. Its potent arteriolar vasoconstriction promotes right coronary perfusion but has been shown to increase mPAP and PVR while reducing cardiac output in patients with chronic pulmonary hypertension.[112,113] Isoproterenol, a β_1- and β_2-adrenergic agent, improves PVR and cardiac output for surgical patients with pulmonary hypertension.[114,115] Vasopressin is a nonadrenergic agent that causes systemic vasoconstriction and selective pulmonary vasodilation.[116] Higher doses of vasopressin than those used for septic shock have been shown to increase mPAP and PVR and decrease cardiac output.[117]

The use of digoxin as an inotrope in acute RV dysfunction is controversial. Although digoxin increases RV myocardial contractility, the effect is generally mild and it has been shown to increase pulmonary vasoconstriction.[118,119] Increasing contractility is offset by an increase in afterload. Several studies have suggested that use of digoxin improves RV function only in the setting of concomitant left heart dysfunction.[120–122] Otherwise, the role of digoxin is nominal in the setting of right heart failure.

Pulmonary vasoconstriction from hypoxemia and decreased production of nitric oxide can worsen pulmonary hypertension in sepsis.[97] Hypercapnea and acidemia potentiate hypoxic vasoconstriction, and every effort should be made to control these complications of sepsis as much as possible. Selective pulmonary vasodilators have become the mainstay of treating right heart failure in pulmonary hypertension, but their use in sepsis is complicated by their ability to lower systemic vascular resistance and worsen V/Q matching by inhibiting hypoxic pulmonary vasoconstriction. Prostacyclin analogs, such as epoprostenol and treprostinil, exert their pulmonary vasodilator effects by increasing intracellular cAMP levels and have some inotropic effect, but most of the increase in cardiac output is attributed to their ability to decrease SVR. The systemic vasodilator effect of prostacyclin can be mostly eliminated by administration via the inhaled route. Continuous inhalation of nebulized epoprostenol has been used successfully to manage patients with pulmonary hypertension and RV failure after cardiac surgery[123] and has been shown to improve gastric mucosal pH in patients who have sepsis and pulmonary hypertension.[124] When given orally, sildenafil is a less selective pulmonary vasodilator than inhaled epoprostenol or nitric oxide. It has been shown to maintain ventilation-perfusion matching[125] but causes systemic hypotension.[126] Its use should be reserved for patients who show significant hemodynamic improvement with inhaled prostacyclins or nitric oxide.

Inhaled nitric oxide is a potent and selective pulmonary vasodilator.[127] Rapid inactivation by hemoglobin in the pulmonary circulation prevents its systemic effects.[128,129] Its limited effect to ventilated areas of the lung usually results in improved oxygenation by stealing pulmonary blood flow from intrapulmonary shunts.[130] When used in combination with dobutamine for acute and chronic pulmonary hypertension, there is a rise in cardiac index, drop in PVR, and improvement in Pao_2/Fio_2.[131,132] Although its use in mechanically ventilated patients with acute respiratory distress syndrome has not been shown to improve patient outcome,[133] it has been shown to improve RVEF and RVEDV in patients with acute respiratory distress syndrome.[134] Rarely, nitric oxide can cause methemoglobinemia or nitrogen dioxide formation, a significant oxidant, when combined with high concentrations of oxygen.[135,136] Overall, nitric oxide is a safe medication to improve PVR and decrease RV afterload and may be useful therapy in bridging patients with acute RV failure in septic shock.

Finally, positive pressure mechanical ventilation is often used in patients who have sepsis and acute lung injury. Increasing intrathoracic pressure not only decreases RV preload but also can increase PVR and RV afterload by overdistending normal lung. Positive end expiratory pressure has been shown to increase PAP and hinder RV outflow.[137] Avoiding overdistention of the lung may preserve RV function in the setting of sepsis with acute lung injury. Some investigators feel that some of the improvement in survival observed with low volume lung protection strategy in patients who have acute respiratory distress syndrome may be attributable to a decrease in the incidence of right heart failure caused by lung hyperinflation.[138–140] At the same time, careful consideration must be given to avoiding acute hypercapnia and acidosis, because both have been shown to exacerbate hypoxic pulmonary hypertension and increase PVR after cardiac surgery.[141]

SUMMARY

Right ventricular dysfunction is common in sepsis and septic shock because of decreased myocardial contractility and elevated PVR despite a concomitant decrease in systemic vascular resistance. Aggressive volume replacement may be vital to maintaining RV function, but excess hydration can cause RV dilation, decreased LV diastolic filling, and reduced cardiac output. Myocardial depression from decreased myocardial perfusion and circulating cytokines lower RVEF. The mainstay of treatment for acute right heart failure includes treating the underlying cause of sepsis, reversing circulatory shock to maintain tissue perfusion and oxygen delivery. Vasoconstrictor agents have been shown to improve RV cardiac function by augmenting coronary perfusion. Decreasing PVR with selective pulmonary vasodilators, such as inhaled nitric oxide and prostacyclins, is a reasonable approach to improving cardiac output in patients who have sepsis and RV dysfunction, as is the addition of inotropic agents, such as dobutamine and milrinone. Clinical data to support this strategy are lacking, however. Currently, treatment for RV dysfunction in the setting of sepsis should concentrate on fluid repletion, monitoring for signs of RV overload, and correcting reversible causes of elevated PVR, such as hypoxia, acidosis, and lung hyperinflation.

REFERENCES

1. Rackow EC, Kaufman BS, Falk JL, et al. Hemodynamic response to fluid repletion in patients with septic shock: evidence for early depression of cardiac performance. Circ Shock 1987;22:11–22.
2. Weisel RD, Vito L, Dennis RC, et al. Myocardial depression during sepsis. Am J Surg 1977;133: 512–21.
3. Kumar A, Haery C, Parrillo JE. Myocardial dysfunction in septic shock. Crit Care Clin 2000;16(2): 251–87.
4. Stein PD, Beemath A, Matta F, et al. Enlarged right ventricle without shock in acute pulmonary embolism: prognosis. Am J Med 2008;121(1):34–42.
5. Grifoni S, Olivotto I, Cecchini P, et al. Short-term clinical outcome of patients with acute pulmonary embolism, normal blood pressure, and echocardiographic right ventricular dysfunction. Circulation 2000;101(24):2817–22.
6. Vieillard-Baron A, Page B, Augarde R, et al. Acute cor pulmonale in massive pulmonary embolism: incidence, echocardiographic pattern, clinical implications and recovery rate. Intensive Care Med 2001;27(9):1481–6.
7. Vonk-Noordegraaf A, Marcus JT, Holverda S, et al. Early changes of cardiac structure and function in COPD patients with mild hypoxemia. Chest 2005; 127(6):1898–903.
8. Brent BN, Berger HJ, Matthay RA, et al. Physiologic correlates of right ventricular ejection fraction in chronic obstructive pulmonary disease: a combined radionuclide and hemodynamic study. Am J Cardiol 1982;50:255–62.
9. Han MK, McLaughlin VV, Criner GJ, et al. Pulmonary disease and the heart. Circulation 2007; 116(25):2992–3005.
10. Vieillard-Baron A, Schmitt JM, Augarde R, et al. Acute cor pulmonale in acute respiratory distress syndrome submitted to protective ventilation: incidence, clinical implications, and prognosis. Crit Care Med 2001;29(8):1641–2.
11. Moloney ED, Evans TW. Pathophysiology and pharmacologic treatment of pulmonary hypertension in acute respiratory distress syndrome. Eur Respir J 2003;21(4):720–7.
12. Yu CM, Sanderson JE, Chan S, et al. Right ventricular diastolic dysfunction in heart failure. Circulation 1996;93(8):1509–14.
13. Bowers TR, O'Neill WW, Pica M, et al. Patterns of coronary compromise resulting in acute right

ventricular ischemic dysfunction. Circulation 2002; 106(9):1104–9.

14. La Vecchia L, Luca Spadaro G, Paccanaro M, et al. Predictors of right ventricular dysfunction in patients with coronary artery disease and reduced left ventricular ejection fraction. Coron Artery Dis 2002;13(6):319–22.

15. Klinger JR, Hill NS. Pulmonary hypertension in the intensive care unit: critical role of the right ventricle. Crit Care Med 2007;35(9):2210–1.

16. Stone A, Klinger JR. The right ventricle in pulmonary hypertension. In: Hill NS, Farber HW, editors. Contemporary cardiology pulmonary hypertension. Totowa (NJ): Humana Press; 2008. p. 93–126.

17. Hoffman MJ, Lazar JG, Sugerman HF, et al. Unsuspected right ventricular dysfunction in shock and sepsis. Ann Surg 1983;198(3):307–18.

18. Mitsuo T, Shimazaki S, Matsuda H. Right ventricular dysfunction in septic patients. Crit Care Med 1992; 20(5):630–4.

19. Dhainaut JF, Lanore JJ, de Gournay JM, et al. Right ventricular dysfunction in patients with septic shock. Intensive Care Med 1988;14:488–91.

20. Redl G, Germann P, Plattner H, et al. Right ventricular function in early septic shock states. Intensive Care med 1993;19:3–7.

21. Hellems HK, Haynes FW, Dexter L, et al. Pulmonary capillary pressure in animals estimated by venous and arterial catheterization. Am J Physiol 1948; 155(1):98–105.

22. Haddy FJ, Campbell GS, Adams WL, et al. A study of pulmonary venous and arterial pressures and other variables in the anesthetized dog by flexible catheter techniques. Am J Physiol 1949;158(1): 89–95.

23. Werko L, Lagerlof H. Studies on the circulation in man: cardiac output and blood pressure in the right auricle, right ventricle and pulmonary artery in patients with hypertensive cardiovascular disease. Acta Med Scand 1949;133(6):427–36.

24. Warren JV, Wilson JS, Doyle JT. Induced variations in pulmonary arterial and pulmonary capillary pressures in man. J Clin Invest 1950;29(6):850–1.

25. Bakos ACP. The question of the function of the right ventricular myocardium: an experimental study. Circulation 1950;1:724–32.

26. Kagan A. Dynamic responses of the right ventricle following extensive damage by cauterization. Circulation 1952;5:816–23.

27. Wiedemann HP, Matthay RA. Acute right heart failure. Crit Care Clin 1985;1(3):631–61.

28. Starr I, Jeffers WA, Meade RH. The absence of conspicuous increments of venous pressure after severe damage to the RV of the dog, with discussion of the relation between clinical congestive heart failure and heart disease. Am Heart J 1943; 26:291–301.

29. Dell'Italia LJ. The right ventricle: anatomy, physiology, and clinical importance. Curr Probl Cardiol 1991;16:653–720.

30. James TN. Anatomy of the crista supraventricularis: its importance for understanding the right ventricular function, right ventricular infarction and related conditions. J Am Coll Cardiol 1985;6:1083–95.

31. Pouleur H, Lefevre J, Van Mechelen H, et al. Free wall shortening and relaxation during ejection in the canine right ventricle. Am J Physiol 1980;239: H601–13.

32. Janicki JS, Weber KT. The pericardium and ventricular interaction, distensibility, and function. Am J Phys 1980;238(4):H494–503.

33. Szabo G, Soos P, Bahrle S, et al. Adaptation of the right ventricle to an increased afterload in the chronically volume overloaded heart. Ann Thorac Surg 2006;82:989–95.

34. De Vroomen M, Cardozo RH, Steendijk P, et al. Improved contractile performance of right ventricle in response to increased RV afterload in newborn lamb. Am J Physiol Heart Circ Physiol 2000;278: H100–5.

35. Maughan WL, Shoukas AA, Sagawa K, et al. Instantaneous pressure-volume relationship of the canine right ventricle. Circ Res 1979;44(3): 309–15.

36. Hurtford WE, Barlai-Kovach M, Strauss HW, et al. Canine biventricular performance during acute progressive pulmonary microembolization: regional myocardial perfusion and fatty acid uptake. J Crit Care 1987;2(4):270–81.

37. Hurtford WE, Zapol WM. The right ventricle and critical illness: a review of anatomy, physiology, and clinical evaluation of its function. Intensive Care Med 1988;14:448–57.

38. De Freitas FM, Faraco EZ, De Azevedo DF, et al. Behavior of normal pulmonary circulation during changes of total blood volume in man. J Clin Invest 1965;44:366–78.

39. Greyson CR. Pathophysiology of right ventricular failure. Crit Care Med 2008;36(1):S57–65.

40. Urabe Y, Tomoike H, Ohzono K, et al. Role of afterload in determining regional right ventricular performance during coronary underperfusion in dogs. Circ Res 1985;57:96–104.

41. Bove AA, Santamore WP. Ventricular interdependence. Prog Cardiovasc Dis 1981;23:365–88.

42. Rudiger A, Singer M. Mechanisms of sepsis induced cardiac dysfunction. Crit Care Med 2007; 35(6):1599–608.

43. Hotchkiss RS, Karl IE. Reevaluation of the role of cellular hypoxia and bioenergetic failure in sepsis. JAMA 1992;267:1503–10.

44. Kadokami T, McTiernan CF, Kubota T, et al. Effects of soluble TNF receptor treatment on lipopolysaccharide-induced myocardial cytokine expression.

Am J Physiol Heart Circ Physiol 2001;280: H2281–91.

45. Meldrum D. Tumor necrosis factor in the heart. Am J Physiol 1998;274:R577–95.

46. Kapadia S, Lee J, Torre-Amione G, et al. Tumor necrosis factor-α gene and protein expression in adult feline myocardium after endotoxin administration. J Clin Invest 1995;96:1042–52.

47. Carlson DL, Willis MS, White J, et al. Tumor necrosis factor-α induced caspase activation mediates endotoxin related cardiac dysfunction. Crit Care Med 2005;33:1021–8.

48. Parker MM, Shelhamer JH, Bacharach SL, et al. Profound but reversible myocardial depression I patients with septic shock. Ann Intern Med 1984; 100:483–90.

49. Ellrodt AG, Riedinger MS, Kimchi A, et al. Left ventricular performance in septic shock: reversible segmental and global abnormalities. Am Heart J 1985;110:402–9.

50. Ogata M, Ohe M, Katayose D, et al. Modulatory role of EDRF in hypoxic contraction of isolated porcine pulmonary arteries. Am J Physiol 1992;262:H691–7.

51. Myers PR, Wright TF, Tanner MA, et al. EDRF and nitric oxide production in cultured endothelial cells: direct inhibition by E. coli endotoxin. Am J Physiol 1992;262:H710–8.

52. Stewart DJ, Levy RD, Cernacek P, et al. Increased plasma endothelin-1 in pulmonary hypertension: marker or mediator of disease? Ann Intern Med 1991;114:464–9.

53. Pittet JF, Morel DR, Hemsen A, et al. Elevated plasma endothelin-1 concentrations are associated with the severity of illness in patients with sepsis. Ann Surg 1991;213(3):261–4.

54. Herve P, Launay JM, Scrobohaci ML, et al. Increased plasma serotonin in primary pulmonary hypertension. Am J Med 1995;99:249–54.

55. Sibbald W, Peters S, Lindsay RM. Serotonin and pulmonary hypertension in human septic ARDS. Crit Care Med 1980;8(9):490–4.

56. Aihara M, Nakazawa T, Dobashi K, et al. A selective pulmonary thrombosis associated with sepsis-induced disseminated intravascular coagulation. Intern Med 1997;36(2):97–101.

57. Calvin JE. Acute right heart failure: pathophysiology, recognition, and pharmacological management. J Cardiothorac Vasc Anesth 1991;5:507–13.

58. Vlahakes GJ, Turley K, Hoffman JI. The pathophysiology of failure in right ventricular hypertension: hemodynamic and biochemical correlates. Circulation 1981;63:87–95.

59. Rivers E, Nguyen B, Havstad S, et al. Early goal directed therapy in the treatment of severe sepsis and septic shock. N Engl J Med 2001;345(19): 1368–77.

60. Ama R, Leather HA, Sege rs P, et al. Acute pulmonary hypertension causes depression of left ventricular contractility and relaxation. Eur J Anaesthesiol 2006;23:824–31.

61. Pinsky MR. The role of the right ventricle in determining cardiac output in the critically ill. Intensive Care Med 1993;19:1–2.

62. Belenkie I, Dani R, Smith ER, et al. Effects of volume loading during experimental acute pulmonary embolism. Circulation 1989;80:178–88.

63. Schneider AJ, Teule GJ, Groeneveld ABJ, et al. Biventricular performance during volume loading in patients with early septic shock, with emphasis on the right ventricle: a combined hemodynamic and radionuclide study. Am Heart J 1988;116: 103–12.

64. Parker MM, McCarthy KE, Ognibene FP, et al. Right ventricular dysfunction and dilatation, similar to left ventricular changes, characterize the cardiac depression of septic shock in humans. Chest 1990; 97:126–31.

65. Vincent JL, Reuse C, Frank N, et al. Right ventricular dysfunction in septic shock: assessment by measurements using the thermodilution technique. Acta Anaesthesiol Scand 1989;33:34–8.

66. Kleinman WM, Krause SM, Hess ML. Differential subendocardial perfusion and injury during the course of gram negative endotoxemia. Adv Shock Res 1980;4:139–52.

67. Gold FL, Bache RJ. Transmural right ventricular blood flow during acute pulmonary artery hypertension in the sedated dog: evidence for subendocardial ischemia despite residual vasodilator reserve. Circ Res 1982;51:196–204.

68. Dhainaut JH, Huyghenbaert MF, Monsallier JH, et al. Coronary hemodynamics and myocardial metabolism of lactate, free fatty acids, glucose and ketones in patients with septic shock. Circulation 1987;75:533–41.

69. Cunnion RE, Schaer GL, Parker MM, et al. The coronary circulation in human septic shock. Circulation 1986;73:637–44.

70. Parrillo JE, Burch C, Shelhamer JH, et al. A circulating myocardial depressant substance in humans with septic shock. J Clin Invest 1985;76: 1539–53.

71. Maksad AK, Cha CJ, Stuart RC, et al. Myocardial depression in septic shock: physiologic and metabolic effects of a plasma factor on an isolated heart. Circ Shock 1979;1(Suppl):1–8.

72. Reilly JM, Cunnion RE, Burch-Whitman C, et al. A circulating myocardial depressant substance is associated with cardiac dysfunction and peripheral hypoperfusion (lactic acidemia) in patients with septic shock. Chest 1989;95:1072–80.

73. Krown KA, Page MT, Nguyen C, et al. Tumor necrosis factor-α induced apoptosis in cardiac

myocytes. Involvement of the sphingolipid signaling cascade in cardiac cell death. J Clin Invest 1996;98:2854–65.

74. Oral H, Dorn GW, Mann DL. Sphingosine mediates the immediate negative inotropic effects of tumor necrosis factor-α in the adult mammalian cardiac myocyte. J Biol Chem 1997;272:4836–42.

75. Muller-Werdan U, Engelmann H, Werdan K. Cardiodepression by tumor necrosis factor-α. Eur Cytokine Netw 1998;9:689–91.

76. Yokoyama T, Vaca L, Rossen RD, et al. Cellular basis for the negative inotropic effects of tumor necrosis factor-α in the adult mammalian heart. J Clin Invest 1993;92:2303–12.

77. Matthay RA, Berger HJ. Cardiovascular function in cor pulmonale. Clin Chest Med 1983;4:269–95.

78. Banka VS, Agarwal JB, Bodenheimer MM, et al. Interventricular septal motion: biventricular angiographic assessment of its relative contribution to left and right ventricular contraction. Circulation 1981;64:992–6.

79. Manno BV, Iskandrian AS, Hakki AH. Right ventricular function: methodologic and clinical considerations in noninvasive scintigraphic assessment. J Am Coll Cardiol 1984;3:1072–81.

80. Ferlinz J. Right ventricular function in adult cardiovascular disease. Prog Cardiovasc Dis 1982;25: 225–67.

81. Berger HJ, Zaret BL. Noninvasive radionuclide assessment of right ventricular performance in man. Cardiovasc Clin 1979;10:91–104.

82. Morrison D, Goldman S, Wright AL, et al. The effect of pulmonary hypertension on systolic function of the right ventricle. Chest 1983;84:250–7.

83. Berger HJ, Matthay RA. Noninvasive radiographic assessment of cardiovascular function in acute and chronic respiratory failure. Am J Cardiol 1981;47:950–62.

84. Berger HJ, Matthay RA. Radionuclide right ventricular ejection fraction: applications in valvular heart disease. Chest 1981;79:497–8.

85. Matthay RA, Berger HJ. Noninvasive assessment of right and left ventricular function in acute and chronic respiratory failure. Crit Care Med 1983;11: 329–38.

86. Morrison DA, Turgeon J, Ovitt T. Right ventricular ejection fraction measurement: contrast ventriculography versus gated blood pool and gated first pass radionuclide methods. Am J Cardiol 1984; 54:651–3.

87. Maddahi J, Berman DS, Matsuoka DT, et al. A new technique for assessing right ventricular ejection fraction using rapid multiple gated equilibrium cardiac blood pool scintigraphy. Circulation 1979;60: 581–9.

88. Dhainaut JF, Brunet F, Mansallier JF, et al. Bedside evaluation of right ventricular performance using a rapid computerized thermodilution method. Crit Care Med 1987;15:148–52.

89. Kay HR, Afshari M, Barash P, et al. Measurement of ejection fraction by thermal dilution techniques. J Surg Res 1983;34:337–46.

90. Connors AF Jr, Speroff T, Dawson NV, et al. The effectiveness of right heart catheterization in the initial care of critically ill patients: SUPPORT investigators. JAMA 1996;276(11):889–97.

91. Harvey S, Harrison DA, Singer M, et al. Assessment of the clinical effectiveness of pulmonary artery catheters in management of patients in intensive care (PAC-Man): a randomized controlled trial. Lancet 2005;366(9484):472–7.

92. Wheeler AP, Bernard GR, Thompson BT, et al. National Heart, Lung, and Blood Institute Acute Respiratory Distress Syndrome (ARDS) Clinical Trials Network. Pulmonary artery versus central venous catheter to guide treatment of acute lung injury. N Engl J Med 2006;354(21):2213–24.

93. Richard C, Warszawski J, Anquel N, et al. Early use of the pulmonary artery catheter and outcomes in patients with shock and acute respiratory distress syndrome: a randomized controlled trial. JAMA 2003;290(20):2713–20.

94. Weyman AE, Wann S, Feigenbaum H, et al. Mechanism of abnormal septal motion in patients with right ventricular volume overload: a cross sectional echocardiographic study. Circulation 1976;54:179–86.

95. Jardin F, Farcot JC, Boisante L, et al. Influence of positive end expiratory pressure on left ventricular performance. N Engl J Med 1981;304:387–92.

96. Dellinger RP, Levy MM, Carlet JM, et al. Surviving sepsis campaign: international guidelines for management of severe sepsis and septic shock. Crit Care Med 2008;36(1):296–327.

97. Zamanian RT, Haddad F, Doyle RL, et al. Management strategies for patients with pulmonary hypertension in the intensive care unit. Crit Care Med 2007;35(9):2037–50.

98. Schneider AJ, Groeneveld ABJ, Nauta J, et al. Volume loading, dobutamine and noradrenaline for treatment of right ventricular dysfunction in porcine septic shock. Circ Shock 1987;23:93–106.

99. Schneider AJ, Teule GJJ, Kester ADM, et al. Biventricular function during volume loading in porcine E coli septic shock, with emphasis on right ventricular function. Circ Shock 1986;18:53–63.

100. Via G, Braschi A. Pathophysiology of severe pulmonary hypertension in the critically ill patient. Minerva Anestesiol 2004;70:233–7.

101. Paetkau D, Kettner J, Girling L, et al. What is the appropriate therapy to maintain cardiac output as pulmonary vascular resistance increases? Anesthesiology 1982;5:A56.

102. Ghignone M, Girling L, Prewitt RM. Effects of vasodilators on canine cardiopulmonary function when

a decrease in cardiac output complicates an increase in right ventricular afterload. Am Rev Respir Dis 1985;131:527–30.

103. Prewitt RM, Ghignone M. Treatment of right ventricular dysfunction in acute respiratory failure. Crit Care Med 1983;11:346–52.

104. Martin C, Perrin G, Saux P, et al. Effects of norepinephrine on right ventricular function in septic shock patients. Intensive Care Med 1994;20:444–7.

105. Kerbaul F, Rondelet B, Motte S, et al. Effects of norepinephrine and dobutamine on pressure load induced right ventricular failure. Crit Care Med 2004;32:1035–40.

106. Schreuder WO, Schneider AJ, Groeneveld ABJ, et al. Effect of dopamine vs norepinephrine on hemodynamics in septic shock: emphasis on right ventricular performance. Chest 1989;95:1282–8.

107. Le Tulzo Y, Seguin P, Gacouin A, et al. Effects of epinephrine on right ventricular function in patients with severe septic shock and right ventricular failure: a preliminary descriptive study. Intensive Care Med 1997;23:664–70.

108. Leier CV, Webel J, Bush CA. The cardiovascular effects of the continuous infusion of dobutamine in patients with severe cardiac failure. Circulation 1977;56:468–72.

109. Deb B, Bradford K, Pearl RG. Additive effects of inhaled nitric oxide and intravenous milrinone in experimental pulmonary hypertension. Crit Care Med 2000;28:795–9.

110. Chen EP, Bittner HB, Davis RD Jr, et al. Milrinone improves pulmonary hemodynamics and right ventricular function in chronic pulmonary hypertension. Ann Thorac Surg 1997;63:814–21.

111. Khazin V, Kaufman Y, Zabeeda D, et al. Milrinone and nitric oxide: combined effect on pulmonary artery pressures after cardiopulmonary bypass in children. J Cardiothorac Vasc Anesth 2004;18:156–9.

112. Kwak YL, Lee CS, Park YH, et al. The effect of phenylephrine and norepinephrine in patients with chronic pulmonary hypertension. Anaesthesia 2002;57:9–14.

113. Rich S, Gubin S, Hart K. The effects of phenylephrine on right ventricular performance in patients with pulmonary hypertension. Chest 1990;98:1102–6.

114. Ducas J, Duval D, Dasilva H, et al. Treatment of canine pulmonary hypertension: effects of norepinephrine and isoproterenol on pulmonary vascular pressure flow characteristics. Circulation 1987;75: 235–42.

115. Prielipp RC, McLean R, Rosenthal MH, et al. Hemodynamic profiles of prostaglandin E1, isoproterenol, prostacyclin, and nifedipine in experimental porcine pulmonary hypertension. Crit Care Med 1991;19:60–7.

116. Garcia-Villalon AL, Garcia JL, Fernandez N, et al. Regional differences in the arterial response to vasopressin: role of endothelial nitric oxide. Br J Pharmacol 1996;118:1848–54.

117. Leather HA, Segers P, Berends N, et al. Effects of vasopressin on right ventricular function in an experimental model of acute pulmonary hypertension. Crit Care Med 2002;30:2548–52.

118. Smith DE, Bissett JK, Phillips JR, et al. Improved right ventricular systolic time intervals after digitalis in patients with cor pulmonale and chronic obstructive pulmonary disease. Am J Cardiol 1978;41: 1299–304.

119. Green LH, Smith TW. The use of digitalis in patients with pulmonary disease. Ann Intern Med 1977;87: 459–65.

120. Coates AL, Desmond K, Asher MI, et al. The effect of digoxin on exercise capacity and exercising cardiac function in cystic fibrosis. Chest 1982;82:543–7.

121. Mathur PN, Powles P, Pugsley SO, et al. Effect of digoxin on right ventricular function in severe chronic airflow obstruction. Ann Intern Med 1981; 95:283–8.

122. Hirschfeld SS. Ventricular interdependence during exercise in cystic fibrosis. Chest 1982;82:524–5.

123. Muzaffar S, Shukla N, Angelini GD, et al. Inhaled prostacyclin is safe, effective, and affordable in patients with pulmonary hypertension, right-heart dysfunction, and refractory hypoxemia after cardiothoracic surgery. J Thorac Cardiovasc Surg 2004; 128(6):949–50.

124. Eichelbrönner O, Reinelt H, Wiedeck H, et al. Aerosolized prostacyclin and inhaled nitric oxide in septic shock: different effects on splanchnic oxygenation? Intensive Care Med 1996;22(9):880–7.

125. Ghofrani HA, Wiedemann R, Schermuly RT, et al. Sildenafil for treatment of lung fibrosis and pulmonary hypertension: a randomised controlled trial. Lancet 2002;360(9337):895–900.

126. Arruda-Olson AM, Mahoney DW, Nehra A, et al. Cardiovascular effects of sildenafil during exercise in men with known or probable coronary artery disease: a randomized crossover trial. JAMA 2002; 287(6):719–25.

127. Offner PJ, Ogura H, Jordan BS, et al. Effects of inhaled nitric oxide on right ventricular function in endotoxin shock. J Trauma 1995;39(2):179–86.

128. Rimar S, Gillis CN. Pulmonary vasodilation by inhaled nitric oxide after endothelial injury. J Appl Physiol 1992;73:2179–83.

129. Rich GF, Roos CM, Anderson SM, et al. Inhaled nitric oxide: dose response and the effects of blood in the isolated rat lung. J Appl Physiol 1993;75: 1278–84.

130. Dembinski R, Max M, Lopez F, et al. Effect of inhaled nitric oxide in combination with almitrine on ventilation-perfusion distributions in experimental lung injury. Intensive Care Med 2000;26(2): 221–8.

131. Bradford KK, Deb B, Pearl RG. Combination therapy with inhaled nitric oxide and intravenous dobutamine during pulmonary hypertension in the rabbit. J Cardiovasc Pharmacol 2000;36:146–51.

132. Vizza CD, Rocca GD, Roma AD, et al. Acute hemodynamic effects of inhaled nitric oxide, dobutamine, and a combination of the two in patients with mild to moderate secondary pulmonary hypertension. Crit Care 2001;5:355–61.

133. Taylor RW, Zimmerman JL, Dellinger RP, et al. Low dose inhaled nitric oxide in patients with acute lung injury: a randomized controlled trial. JAMA 2004; 291:1603–9.

134. Rossaint R, Slama K, Steudel W, et al. Effects of inhaled nitric oxide on right ventricular function in severe acute respiratory distress syndrome. Intensive Care Med 1995;21(3):197–203.

135. Weinberger B, Laskin DL, Heck DE, et al. The toxicology of inhaled nitric oxide. Toxicol Sci 2001;59:5–16.

136. Wang T, El Kebir D, Blaise G. Inhaled nitric oxide in 2003: a review of its mechanisms of action. Can J Anaesth 2003;50:839–46.

137. Artucio H, Hurtado J, Zimet L, et al. PEEP induced tricuspid regurgitation. Intensive Care Med 1997; 23:836–40.

138. Jardin F, Vieillard-Baron A. Is there a safe plateau pressure in ARDS? The right heart only knows. Intensive Care Med 2007;33(3):444–7.

139. Vieillard-Baron A, Jardin F. Why protect the right ventricle in patients with acute respiratory distress syndrome? Curr Opin Crit Care 2003;9(1):15–21.

140. Jardin F, Vieillard-Baron A. Right ventricular function and positive pressure ventilation in clinical practice: from hemodynamic subsets to respirator settings. Intensive Care Med 2003;29:1426–34.

141. Viitanen A, Salmenpera M, Heinonen J. Right ventricular response to hypercarbia after cardiac surgery. Anesthesiology 1990;73:393–400.

Antimicrobial Management of Sepsis and Septic Shock

Sat Sharma, MD, FRCPC, FCCP[a], Anand Kumar, MD, FCCM[b,c],*

KEYWORDS

• Infections • Antibiotics • Sepsis • Septic shock

Sepsis affects millions of patients worldwide each year, including approximately 800,000 people in the United States.[1,2] Of those, approximately half develop septic shock and half of those afflicted with septic shock die.[1,2] Sepsis mortality, estimated at 9.3% of all deaths in the United States, is numerically equivalent to mortality from acute myocardial infarction and far exceeds mortality related to either AIDS or breast cancer.[1] The rate of severe sepsis (sepsis with organ failure) hospitalization (132 per 100,000) almost doubled during the 21-year period from 1979 to 2000 and is considerably greater than has been previously predicted.[3] Along with the incidence, the associated total mortality has been steadily increasing over the past several decades.[4] The cost of treatment of this condition is staggering, estimated to be up to $20 billion annually in the United States alone.[2,4] An understanding of basic pharmacologic principles of antimicrobial therapy is crucial for its appropriate use in critically ill patients with sepsis and septic shock. This article reviews sepsis pathophysiology and the rational use of antibiotics in sepsis and presents evidence-based recommendations for optimal antibiotic therapy.

SEPSIS PATHOPHYSIOLOGY

Our understanding of the pathophysiologic processes involved in sepsis has significantly advanced in recent years. Current thinking envisions activation of inflammatory cytokine and coagulation cascades as central to the pathogenesis of sepsis. Bacterial products and toxins activate cells of the innate immune system (macrophages and neutrophils) to synthesize proinflammatory mediators (tumor necrosis factor, IL-1) and regulatory cytokines (IL-6).[5] Consequently, feedback activation of host cells releases counter-inflammatory mediators (IL-10 and transforming growth factor–β) that may inhibit the inflammatory processes.[6] The inflammatory cascade results in neutrophil-endothelial-cell adhesion, activation of clotting, and generation of secondary inflammatory mediators (other cytokines, prostaglandins, leukotrienes, and proteases).[6] Tissue factors and activated monocytes/macrophages play a key role in triggering a coagulant response that stimulates multiple inflammatory pathways.[7] The release of plasminogen-activator inhibitor–1 suppresses endogenous fibrinolysis and activates thrombin-activateable fibrinolysis inhibitor.[8] The sepsis pathophysiology comprises diffuse endothelial injury, increased capillary permeability, distributive hemodynamics, microvascular thrombosis, tissue ischemia, and multiorgan failure and apoptosis.

Except for antimicrobial and activated protein C therapy, all other therapies for severe sepsis, septic shock, and sepsis-associated multiple-organ failure are substantially supportive in nature. These include hemodynamic support with fluid

[a] Sections of Pulmonary and Critical Care Medicine, Department of Internal Medicine, University of Manitoba, 700 William Avenue, Winnipeg, Manitoba, Canada R3E-0Z3

[b] Sections of Pulmonary and Critical Care Medicine and Infectious Diseases, Department of Medicine, University of Manitoba, 700 William Avenue, Winnipeg, Manitoba, Canada R3E-0Z3

[c] Department of Medicine, University of Medicine and Dentistry of New Jersey, Camden, NJ, USA

* Corresponding author. Section of Critical Care Medicine, Section of Infectious Diseases, Health Sciences Centre, JJ 399, University of Manitoba, 700 William Avenue, Winnipeg, Manitoba, Canada R3E-0Z3.

E-mail address: akumar61@yahoo.com (A. Kumar).

Clin Chest Med 29 (2008) 677–687
doi:10.1016/j.ccm.2008.06.004

administration, inotropic/vasopressor therapy, metabolic support, adrenal replacement therapy, and nutritional support. This article reviews the basic principles of antimicrobial therapy that continue to hold an important place in the therapeutic armamentarium of sepsis and septic shock therapy. To properly understand antimicrobial therapy, clinicians need especially to understand the importance of (1) ensuring that empiric therapy is effective against the pathogen, (2) initiating therapy as quickly as possible, and (3) achieving optimum target levels of antibiotics as rapidly as possible.[9]

RATIONAL USE OF ANTIBIOTICS IN SEPSIS

Along with appropriate resuscitation, optimal use of antibiotic therapy is the critical determinant of survival in sepsis and septic shock (**Figs. 1** and **2**).[10-12] A judicious and thoughtful approach to antibiotic therapy is mandatory given that ineffective initial therapy worsens the outcome in sepsis. Beyond the issues related to the infecting organisms and their sensitivity profile, optimal antimicrobial therapy includes assessment of host factors (eg, immune status, organ function, site of infection), pharmacokinetics (eg, drug absorption, distribution, elimination), and pharmacodynamics (eg, mode of action, bacteriocidal versus bacteriostatic activity, rate of killing).[12,13] In many circumstances in the critically ill, standard antimicrobial regimens require modification (**Table 1**). Because the infecting organism is not known at the time of antibiotic initiation, empiric

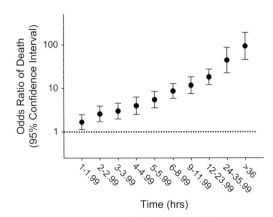

Fig. 2. Effect of septic shock-associated hypotension and appropriate antibiotic administration. The Y axis represents the odds ratio of death. The X axis represents time (hours) following recognition of septic shock–associated hypotension. (*From* Kumar A, Roberts D, Wood KE, et al. Duration of hypotension before initiation of effective anti-microbial therapy is the critical determinant of survival in human septic shock. Crit Care Med 2006;34(6):1593; with permission.)

antibiotic therapy is based on clinical presentation and epidemiologic factors, including local flora, resistance patterns, and resistance patterns and previous antibiotic exposure. Other patient factors that may affect antibiotic choice and dose include specific susceptibilities (eg, encapsulated organisms in splenectomized patients, *Pseudomonas* in neutropenics), antibiotic toxicity (anaphylaxis, angioneurotic edema, Stevens-Johnson syndrome, allergic interstitial nephritis), and organ dysfunction (impaired clearance of antibiotics). The metabolic and immunologic derangements in critically ill patients and simultaneous use of many other pharmacologic agents can substantially affect the pharmacokinetics and pharmacodynamics of antimicrobial therapy. An inappropriate antibiotic prescription in critically ill septic patients can markedly increase mortality (septic shock, nosocomial pneumonia) and morbidity (seeding of prosthetic valves, vascular grafts, artificial joints).[10,11]

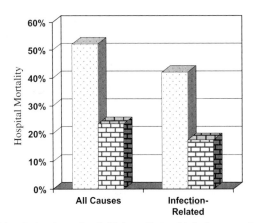

Fig. 1. Inadequate initial antimicrobial therapy is associated with marked increases of all-cause and infection-related mortality in patients admitted to intensive care units with life-threatening infections. (*Data from* Kollef MH, Sherman G, Ward S, et al. Inadequate antimicrobial treatment of infections. A risk factor for hospital mortality among critically ill patients. Chest 1999;115:469.)

CLINICAL PHARMACOLOGY OF ANTIBIOTICS

Effective treatment of an established infection requires delivery of a sufficient amount of drugs to the local site of infection for an adequate time to bring about a cure.[10-13] Since this cannot be directly measured, substitute in vitro parameters reflecting probability of success of antimicrobial therapy have been established. These are antibiotic susceptibility tests.

Table 1
Indications for extended empiric antibiotic therapy of severe sepsis/septic shock

Therapy	Indications
Gram-negative coverage	Nosocomial infection Patient neutropenic or immunosuppressed Patient immunocompromised due to chronic organ failure (eg, liver, renal, lung, heart,)
↑ Gram-positive coverage (vancomycin or alternate novel gram-positive agent)	High level endemic MRSA (community or nosocomial) Neutropenic patient Intravascular catheter infection Nosocomial pneumonia
↑ Fungal/yeast coverage (triazole, echinocandin, amphotericin B)	Neutropenic fever or other immunosuppressed patient Unresponsive to standard antibiotic therapy Cases requiring prolonged broad-spectrum antibiotic therapy Positive relevant fungal cultures Consider empiric therapy if high-risk patient with severe shock

Abbreviation: MRSA, methicillin-resistant Staphylococcus aureus.

Susceptibility testing involves serially diluting antibiotic solutions overnight until the growth of the specific pathogen occurs. An organism is deemed susceptible to the antibiotic if the minimum inhibitory concentration (MIC) is one sixteenth to one fourth of the peak achievable serum concentration (or urine concentration if a urinary pathogen). Despite a satisfactory MIC, failure of antibiotic therapy may occur if the antibiotic concentrations at the target site (cerebrospinal fluid, bile, prostatic tissue, pancreas, necrotic avascular tissue) are not well equilibrated with serum. Another cause of antibiotic failure is failure of the drug to penetrate the bacterial cell wall (β-lactam therapy in *Legionella*). Conversely, an antibiotic considered modestly effective through in vitro susceptibility testing may be highly effective clinically if concentrated well at the target site (aminoglycosides for some urosepsis, macrolides for *Legionella*).[10]

The use of the MIC as the sole factor while deciding antibiotic therapy is problematic. With certain antibiotics (aminoglycosides, fluoroquinolones), a substantial proportion of the bacteria may be inhibited or killed when the MIC is subtherapeutic (postantibiotic effect). A similar effect occurs because of the impaired resistance to phagocytosis by the pathogens recently exposed to therapeutic antibiotic concentrations. Another reason that MIC testing has a limited association with clinical response is that the test evaluates a pathogen's response to a constant concentration of antibiotic, whereas the standard dosing actually is intermittent, resulting in varying concentrations at the target site. Furthermore, it is important to note that MIC does not distinguish between bacterial killing and inhibition of bacterial growth.[11]

Pharmacokinetics

The goal of antibiotic therapy is to deliver an appropriate drug at a high enough concentration to the infectious site to kill the pathogenic organism. In serious infections, the local drug concentration must exceed the MIC for the best cure rates. Several pharmacokinetics factors can affect the local drug concentration. These include factors related to drug absorption, distribution, and elimination.[14] Because of poor absorption from the gastrointestinal tract in critically ill patients who develop poor gut perfusion, bowel edema, and ileus, only intravenous administration results in consistently predictable peak levels crucial for the efficacy of many antimicrobial agents.[15,16]

Overall, antimicrobial distribution is affected by the patient's size, percentage of body fat, and degree of edema. Each has a significant impact on drug concentration at the target site. Drug volume of distribution, which equals the amount of drug administered divided by the plasma drug concentration, describes the relative distribution of the drug within the body compartments. Extracellular volume is markedly increased in states of total body fluid overload (cirrhosis, renal failure, congestive heart failure, sepsis with fluid resuscitation, trauma, and anasarca) commonly seen in the intensive care unit (ICU). In these circumstances, the serum level of drugs that primarily distribute to the extracellular fluid can be markedly low (eg, aminoglycosides).[17] Decreased serum proteins and albumin can substantially increase free drug levels and should be factored in when performing dosage calculations.

Local factors determining antibiotic concentration at the site of infection are also important. The vascularity index of a site (vascular endothelial area divided by the tissue volume) can be important in infections of bone or limbs with impaired blood flow, thus requiring debridement of necrotic tissue or vascular repair for antibiotics to be effective. Because of the high vascularity index, adequate drug levels are easily achieved in joint, pleural, and peritoneal space infections. Nonfenestrated capillaries that limit the movement of larger molecules, including antibiotics, often perfuse organs, such as the brain, the eyes, and the prostate. The antibiotic must diffuse through the endothelial membrane (depending on its lipid solubility, the pharmacokinetics of the drug, and the fluid pH) or be instilled directly.[18] Abscesses present a series of barriers to effective therapy because antimicrobials cannot be effectively delivered into the avascular core of abscesses or other necrotic tissue (depending on size). Also, aminoglycosides and erythromycin show decreased activity at the acid pHs that exist in abscesses. Furthermore, aminoglycosides and vancomycin are bound to and inactivated by DNA that exists in abundance in pus. Finally, because β-lactams work best on rapidly growing cell populations, longer duration of therapy is required for the slow-growing organisms in abscesses.

In ICU patients, an abnormal clearance rate of the drug will usually prolong the half-life of antibiotics; in some cases, elimination may be more rapid. In either case, close attention must be paid to dosage adjustments and dosing intervals.[10,11] Many antibiotics (aminoglycosides, quinolones, tetracyclines, vancomycin, sulfonamides, and amphotericin) are primarily eliminated through glomerular filtration. Shock states will substantially lower the glomerular filtration rate, whereas the hyperdynamic phase of burn injury and sepsis (without shock) can be associated with increased glomerular filtration rate. Although renal injury will impair drug clearance, dosage adjustment is generally not required for most drugs until the creatinine clearance falls under 30% of normal. Drug dosing in septic shock must anticipate that serum creatinine may inaccurately reflect true renal function as reflected by creatinine clearance, and is better reflected by the urine output. No good measure exists for estimation of altered liver clearance. No substantial dosage adjustments are required until serum conjugated bilirubin exceeds 5 mg/dL. Antibiotics that may require dosage adjustment with liver failure include erythromycin, nafcillin, mezlocillin, rifampin, tetracycline, isoniazid, clindamycin, chloramphenicol, and metronidazole.[10]

Pharmacodynamics

The goal of antibiotic therapy is to maximize efficacy while minimizing toxicity. Pharmacodynamics includes microbiologic activity, pharmacokinetic properties, and interactions among the drug, the host, and the organism.[19] Whether a drug is bacteriostatic or bacteriocidal basically depends on the pharmacodynamic properties of the drug. Bacteriostatic antibiotics inhibit growth of organisms, whereas bacteriocidal antibiotics kill the organisms. A bacteriocidal drug has a maximal bactericidal concentration that is only two to four times the MIC, as opposed to a bacteriostatic drug that has an maximal bactericidal concentration more than 16 times higher MIC. An alternative approach defines a bacteriocidal antimicrobial as one that yields 3-log bacterial kill (1000-fold reduction in organisms) over 24 hours. Some drugs can be bacteriostatic for one group of organisms but bacteriocidal for another. Because host immune defenses augment antibiotic efficacy in vivo, bacteriocidal activity of antibiotic regimens is only definitively required for clinical cure in limited circumstances. These include endovascular infections, particularly endocarditis, meningitis, and cerebral abscess; infections in neutropenics; and osteomyelitis (particularly *Staphylococcus aureus* osteomyelitis). For other infections, exceeding the MIC of the target organism by several factors is sufficient to bring about cure.[10,11]

The use of multiple antibiotics is common in the ICU for many reasons. Treatment of life-threatening infections is commenced on an empiric basis. Therefore, missing a causative organism can worsen probability of its survival. Although broad-spectrum agents have become available, only rarely can one be certain that all likely pathogens are effectively covered with a single agent. Multicenter trials suggest that clinical outcome is greatly improved if patients are started on empiric broad-spectrum therapy on presentation rather than waiting until an infection is identified.[20,21] Outcome in such patients is clearly improved if the causative organism is included in the initial empiric regimen and is substantially degraded if it is not. In neutropenic patients, a successful empiric regimen should be continued until resolution of neutropenia, whereas narrowing the regimen to a single agent following identification of the organism is reasonable in other cases.

Use of multiple antimicrobial agents remains contentious in nonneutropenic patients because many of the newer compounds (cefoxitin, cefotetan, meropenem, imipenem-cilastatin, piperacillin-tazobactam, gatifloxacin, moxifloxacin) achieve similar breadth of coverage with single drugs and it may be unnecessary to cover every organism present in an infection.[22] Another reason for multiantibiotic therapy may be to prevent the emergence of resistance. This phenomenon has only been demonstrated for treatment of tuberculosis and is speculative otherwise. Many clinical and animal studies demonstrate that *Pseudomonas aeruginosa* can develop resistance to β-lactam antibiotics during therapy. Although not proven, the addition of aminoglycosides to prevent resistance is one basis of recommendations for double therapy in serious *Pseudomonas* infections.

With rare exceptions (amphotericin plus flucytosine), the argument that use of multiple agents routinely results in synergistic or additive effects with a concomitant decrease in toxicity is not well accepted. The combination of β-lactams with aminoglycosides is commonly prescribed. Both of these drugs demonstrate bacteriocidal activity (the β-lactam is thought to cause cell wall injury in such a way that the aminoglycoside can enter and kill the organism). Clinically, the combination of vancomycin or penicillin/ampicillin with an aminoglycoside results in higher cure rates of enterococcal endocarditis than either drug individually.[23] An antipseudomonal penicillin with an antipseudomonal aminoglycoside is more effective than either alone in the treatment of neutropenic gram-negative sepsis.[24] Although the required duration of therapy of *S aureus* and streptococcal endocarditis is shortened, overall cure rates with combination therapy are not improved. Thus, no definitive evidence exists for efficacy of combination antibiotic therapy other than for endocarditis or neutropenic patients with gram-negative sepsis. The most acceptable reason to use a combination of drugs may be to maximally broaden antimicrobial coverage in conditions where suboptimal initial coverage may result in increased mortality.

Dosing Strategies for Antibiotics

Bacteriocidal antibiotics belong to two major groups according to whether the dominant mechanism for bacterial killing is concentration dependent or time dependent. These mechanisms have substantial impact on optimal dosing strategies.[25]

Aminoglycosides, fluoroquinolones, metronidazole, and amphotericin B exhibit concentration-dependent killing for maximum efficacy. Such dosing can be achieved using a schedule that emphasizes large doses administered infrequently. Achievement of a peak concentration of 8 to 20 times the MIC is associated with optimal outcome for aminoglycosides and fluoroquinolones.[26] Many studies and meta-analyses support once-per-day dosing for aminoglycosides. Less frequent dosing with these agents is justified by the presence of a postantibiotic effect, whereby persistent suppression of bacterial growth occurs even when antibiotic concentrations are subtherapeutic. An intact immune system is likely required to continue bacterial killing to take advantage of the postantibiotic effect phase. Drugs from a second category of antibacterial agents exert a bacteriocidal effect independent of the peak concentration. For this class, bacterial kill is related to the proportional duration of time of the dosing interval that the organism is exposed to an antibiotic in excess of the MIC (time-dependent killing). β-lactams and vancomycin fall into this category. In general, intermittent dosing regimens that achieve a serum concentration of two to four times the MIC (approximately two times maximal bactericidal concentration) for 40% to 60% of the dosing interval yield satisfactory results for β-lactams. However, limited human and animal studies demonstrate that optimal (and improved) results can be seen with continuous infusion of β-lactams resulting in time above the MIC values of 100%.[27,28]

Antibiotic Resistance

Antimicrobial resistance to multiple antibiotics has become a major problem in critically ill patients. Methicillin-resistant *S aureus* (MRSA) and vancomycin-resistant *Enterococcus* (VRE) are rapidly advancing problems in the nosocomial setting. Although MRSA can still be treated with vancomycin, intermediate vancomycin-resistant strains have recently been described. At present, VRE and potential vancomycin- and methicillin-resistant species can be treated with the newer antibacterial compounds, including quinipristin-dalfopristin, linezolid, tigecycline, and daptomycin. Plasmid-mediated β-lactamases produced by some gram-negative bacilli mediate resistance to ampicillin, amoxicillin, ticarcillin, piperacillin, mezlocillin, and many cephalosporins. These organisms can be effectively treated with more advanced cephalosporins, β-lactam/β-lactamase inhibitor combinations, and carbapenems. Carbapenems and cefoxitin are potent inducers of chromosomal β-lactamase in some gram-negative bacilli. This effect is rarely a concern for carbapenems because of their potent activity. However, cefoxitin may render concomitantly administered penicillins ineffective by this mechanism.[29] Many third-generation cephalosporins produce chromosomal β-lactamase in *Enterobacter* spp, although carbapenems and fourth-generation cephalosporins still remain active.[30] Clinicians are seeing metallo-β-lactamases rendering gram-negatives resistant to even carbapenems. In treatment of serious gram-negative infections, many ICUs with a high frequency of multiresistant organisms continue two-drug empiric therapy pending identification of the organism's sensitivity pattern. Virtually pan-resistant gram-negative bacilli requiring treatment with marginal agents, such as colistin, are causing serious infections with increasing frequency.

Drug-Level Monitoring

To determine antimicrobial efficacy, clinicians must first monitor clinical response. However, under certain conditions, monitoring of serum antibiotic concentrations is also important. These conditions include cases in which (1) a direct relationship exists between serum levels and efficacy or toxicity; (2) serum concentrations are difficult to predict, as in critically ill patients; and (3) the therapeutic index is low (small difference between the therapeutic and toxic dose). Because all three criteria apply to aminoglycosides, their use in standard dosing regimens, according to recommendations, is a peak serum level of 6 to 8 mg/dL gentamicin or tobramycin with a trough of 0.5 to 1.0 mg/dL for non–life-threatening infections; and peak of 8 to 10 mg/dL with a trough of 1 to 2 mg/dL for life-threatening infections.[31] Due to substantial alterations in volume of distribution and clearance in critically ill patients, close monitoring of aminoglycoside levels is recommended. Therefore, critically ill patients require an average of two to three dosage adjustments during their course of therapy because of constant change of pharmacokinetics and pharmacodynamics.[32,33] It is unnecessary (and cumbersome) to measure β-lactam levels except in very unusual circumstances. In certain infections (primarily endocarditis and osteomyelitis), maintaining serum bactericidal activity above a certain level (1:8 to 1:16) is associated with improved outcome.[34]

FAILURE OF ANTIBIOTIC THERAPY

Clinical deterioration or failure to improve and persistence of fever and high white blood cell counts in an otherwise improved patient are often incorrectly understood as signs that antibiotic therapy has failed.[35] Once severe sepsis has developed, sepsis-associated symptoms can progress independent of eradication of inciting organisms.

Additionally, infectious-appearing clinical symptomatology in the critically ill can frequently be caused by disease other than infection (eg, liver failure, drug or malignancy-related fever, salicylate toxicity, pancreatitis, adrenal insufficiency). The causes of antibiotic failure vary. They include overly delayed administration of appropriate therapy, inappropriate spectrum of activity of the antimicrobial regimen, inadequate antimicrobial blood levels, inadequate penetration of the antimicrobial to the target site, antimicrobial neutralization or antagonism, superinfection or unsuspected secondary bacterial infection, unusual bacterial or nonbacterial infection, and noninfectious source of illness or fever with or without colonization.[10–13,36]

In the critically ill patient, inadequate blood levels of antibiotics most commonly arise because of a lack of appreciation of increased volume of distribution as a consequence of expanded extracellular volume, as when saline resuscitation fluids remain in the extracellular space. In addition, many antibiotics have a significant gradient between serum and the tissue target site even in well-perfused organs. For that reason, maximal recommended dosing should be used in all life-threatening infections, particularly those involving relatively protected or poorly perfused sites. One of the most common causes of apparent failure of antibiotic therapy is inadequate antibiotic penetration. Impaired vascularity of an infected tissue can substantially impede delivery of the antibiotic. Abscesses are an extreme example of this effect, as they have no intrinsic blood supply. Most abscesses require surgical drainage for cure. However, small abscesses (with a decreased area to penetrate), anaerobic lung abscesses, small/multiple brain abscesses, and occasionally renal abscesses can be cured with prolonged antibiotic therapy. Chronic vascular insufficiency (eg, infected diabetic foot ulcer) requires either revascularization or a switch to a more penetrant drug (fluoroquinolones, clindamycin, metronidazole, or rifampin). An infecting organism or its toxins may also impair the vascular supply (eg, *Aspergillus*, *Rhizopus*, *Mucor*, necrotizing fasciitis, or clostridial gangrene), thus requiring aggressive surgical debridement with an appropriate antimicrobial therapy.

Although antibiotic antagonism is an unusual cause of failure of antibiotic therapy, it should always be considered. The potential for antibiotic antagonism is one argument in favor of the use of single agents. It may be better to use single agents with broad activity rather than multiple agents with potentially antagonistic activity. Concurrent unrecognized bacterial infection in a critically ill patient is another possible cause of antibiotic failure. Therefore, each patient should be carefully assessed initially at admission and subsequently. In a critically ill patient on prolonged therapy with broad-spectrum antibiotics, superinfections, such as decubitus ulcers, bacterial sinusitis, line sepsis, and *C difficile* colitis, may occur and should be carefully monitored as possible infectious complications of an ICU stay.

EVIDENCE-BASED RECOMMENDATIONS FOR ANTIMICROBIAL THERAPY IN SEPSIS

Critically ill patients with severe sepsis and septic shock possess unique characteristics that affect the choice of antimicrobial therapy. These characteristics may include altered pharmacokinetics, hepatic and renal dysfunction, unrecognized immune dysfunction, and infection with resistant organisms. In such cases, an adverse outcome is possible, particularly if there is a delay in initiating effective antibiotic therapy (**Figs. 2** and **3**). Management decisions in this patient group must often be made emergently in the absence of data regarding the definitive infecting organism and its sensitivity pattern, or the

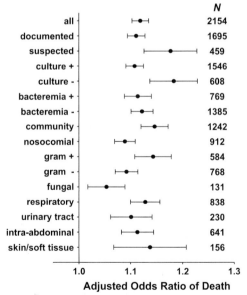

Fig. 3. Relationship of antimicrobial delay to hospital mortality in major subgroups (expressed as adjusted odds ratio of death with time as a continuous variable). For the overall group, mortality risk increases approximately 11% every hour relative to the risk in the previous hour. (*From* Kumar A, Roberts D, Wood KE, et al. Duration of hypotension before initiation of effective antimicrobial therapy is the critical determinant of survival in human septic shock. Crit Care Med 2006;34(6):1593; with permission.)

patient's immune status and organ function. The speed at which an appropriate antimicrobial regimen is administered at first presentation strongly influences outcomes in severe sepsis and septic shock (see **Figs. 2** and **3**). Therefore, a careful and well thought out but expeditious approach to initial empiric antimicrobial therapy is required.[10,11,37]

Empiric Antibiotic Regimens Should Approach 100% Coverage of Pathogens for the Suspected Source of Infection

Administration of inappropriate initial antimicrobials increases morbidity in a wide range of infections.[38–40] The use inappropriate initial antimicrobials may occur in as many as 17.1% of cases involving community-acquired bacteremia and 34.3% of cases involving nosocomial-acquired bacteremia (see **Fig. 1**).[38,39] Similarly, 18.8% and 28.4% of septic shock cases were initially treated with inadequate antimicrobial therapy in another large study of septic shock.[39,40] The risk of death increases from 30%–60% in ICU bacteremia and 70%–100% in gram-negative shock when the initial empiric regimen fails to cover the inciting pathogen.[38,41] Recently, the mortality risk in septic shock increased 5-fold (range 2.5- to 10-fold in selected subgroups) when initial antimicrobial therapy was inappropriate.[40] Consequently, empiric regimens should cover all possible suspected pathogens in a septic patient. Selection of an optimal antimicrobial regimen requires knowledge of (1) the probable anatomic site of infection; (2) the patient's immune status, risk factors, and physical environment; and (3) the local microbiologic flora and organism-resistance patterns. Risk factors for infection with resistant organisms include prolonged hospital stay, prior hospitalization, and prior colonization or infection with multiresistant organisms. Because a majority of patients with septic shock have comorbidities or other factors that make them high risk for resistant organisms, it is recommended that all patients with septic shock be initiated with a broad combination antimicrobial therapy for the first few days.[37]

Broad-Spectrum Antimicrobial Therapy Should be Initiated Immediately (Preferably within First Hour) Following Clinical Diagnosis of Septic Shock

Appropriate intravenous, broad-spectrum empiric antibiotic therapy should be initiated as rapidly as possible for suspected severe infections particularly in the presence of hypotension (ie, presumptive septic shock).[42–45] Data from studies in bacteremia, pneumonia, and meningitis associated with sepsis suggest that mortality in sepsis increases with delay in antimicrobial administration.[42–45] Timing of initial administration of effective antimicrobial therapy is the most important predictor of survival.[42–45] In one study, initiation of effective antimicrobial therapy within the first hour following onset of septic shock–related hypotension was associated with 79.9% survival to hospital discharge.[44] For every additional hour before effective antimicrobial administration following onset of hypotension, survival decreased an average of 7.6% per hour. If antimicrobial therapy is delayed to 5 to 6 hours after onset of septic shock, survival was 42.0%, and a delay of 9 to 12 hours led to 25.4% survival.

Several studies have documented substantial delays before initiation of effective therapy.[41,43–45] Six hours was the median time to delivery of effective antimicrobial therapy following initial resuscitative measures for recurrent or persistent hypotension.[44] Every effort should be made to obtain appropriate site-specific cultures to allow identification and susceptibility testing of the pathogenic organism. However, such efforts should not postpone antimicrobial therapy.

Antimicrobial Therapy Should be Initiated at Maximal Recommended Dosing in all Patients with Life-Threatening Infection

Early optimization of antimicrobial pharmacokinetics can improve the outcome of patients with severe infection, including septic shock. Because cardiac output is elevated in many patients who have early sepsis and septic shock, and increased free drug levels may occur because of decreased serum albumin, drug clearance can be increased transiently. Hence, drug clearance can be transiently increased.[11] As the illness progresses, ICU patients with sepsis or septic shock exhibit substantially increased volumes of distribution and decreased clearance rates. Consequently, suboptimal dosing of antibiotics is common in these conditions.[10,17,18,46,47] Failure to achieve therapeutic levels on initial dosing has been associated with clinical failure with aminoglycosides. Similarly, clinical success rates for treatment of serious infections correlate with higher peak blood levels of fluoroquinolones (nosocomial pneumonia and other serious infections) and aminoglycosides (gram-negative nosocomial pneumonia and other serious infections). A recent study showed improved survival in patients with *Pseudomonas* bacteremia when treated with extended infusion rather than standard intermittent dosing of piperacillin/tazobactam.[48] For aminoglycosides, an appropriate target is a ratio of peak drug concentration to MIC of 12 or more. For β-lactams, the minimum time above MIC in serum should be

60% of dosing interval. Once-daily dosing of aminoglycosides as well as increased frequency of dosing (given identical total daily dose) for β-lactams is recommended. As an example, for piperacillin/tazobactam, 3.375 g every 6 hours for serious infections should be the preferred over 4.5 g every 8 hours. Limited data suggest that continuous infusion of β-lactams and related drugs may be even more effective for relatively resistant organisms.

Multidrug Antimicrobial Therapy Is Preferred for the Initial Empiric Therapy of Septic Shock

Possible pathogens should be covered by at least two antimicrobials with different bactericidal mechanisms. Given that highly resistant organisms are endemic in the critical care environment, multidrug antimicrobial therapy will reduce the probability of failure. In addition, most patients with septic shock (even those without specific pre-existing immune defects) exhibit significant deficits of neutrophil and monocyte function during the course of their illnesses. Septic shock patients likely have reduced ability to clear infection and may be best managed with multidrug therapy similar to that recommended for patients with neutropenic sepsis.

No prospective, controlled study has specifically compared multiple versus single antimicrobial therapy in severe sepsis or septic shock patients. Experts in infectious diseases suggest that there is no advantage to multidrug therapy in serious infections, including bacteremia. However, subgroup analyses of the subset of most critically ill patients with gram-negative bacteremia and shock have suggested that survival improves with the use of two or more antibiotics. Similarly, several studies of the most severe critically ill patients, including those who have bacteremic pneumococcal pneumonia or septic shock, have suggested that outcomes improve if two or more effective agents are used.[49,50]

Empiric Antimicrobial Therapy Should be Adjusted to a Narrower Regimen within 48 To 72 Hours if a Pathogen is Identified or if There is a Resolution of Septic Shock

While several retrospective studies have demonstrated that inappropriate therapy of bacteremic septic shock yields increased mortality, none has suggested that early narrowing of therapy is detrimental if the organism is identified or if the patient is responding well clinically. Such an approach would maximize appropriate antibiotic coverage of inciting pathogens in septic shock while minimizing selection pressure toward resistant organisms. Although it is tempting to continue a broad-spectrum regimen in culture-negative septic patients, such a strategy will only result in the emergence of resistant organisms.

Early Source Control Should be Practiced in Patients with Severe Sepsis, Septic Shock, and Other Life-Threatening Infections

Source control is a critical issue in the optimal management of infection associated with severe sepsis. A wide variety of infections causing sepsis and septic shock in the ICU are amenable to source control (**Box 1**). The need for source control implementation may initially be overlooked in many ICU infections (eg, pneumonia-associated bacterial empyema, decubitus ulcers, and C difficile colitis). Source control may include removal of implanted or tunneled devices, open surgical/percutaneous drainage of infected fluids or abscesses, and surgical resection of infected tissues. Infections requiring source control frequently require rapid (within 2 hours) radiographic imaging or, if clinical status and findings are supportive, immediate surgical intervention. Surgical source control should follow aggressive resuscitative efforts to minimize intraoperative morbidity and mortality. In some cases (eg, rapidly progressive necrotizing soft tissue infections, bowel infarction), optimal management mandates simultaneous aggressive resuscitation and surgical intervention. Earlier surgical intervention has been shown to

have a significant impact on outcome in certain rapidly progressive infections, such as necrotizing fasciitis.[51] Time lapse from hypotension to implementation of source control was found to correlate highly with outcome.[52]

SUMMARY

Every patient with sepsis and septic shock must be evaluated thoroughly at presentation before the initiation of antibiotic therapy. However, in most situations, an abridged initial assessment focusing on critical diagnostic and management planning elements is sufficient. Intravenous antibiotics should be administered as early as possible, and always within the first hour of recognizing severe sepsis and septic shock. Broad-spectrum antibiotics must be selected with one or more agents active against likely bacterial or fungal pathogens and with good penetration into the presumed source. Antimicrobial therapy should be reevaluated daily to optimize efficacy, prevent resistance, avoid toxicity, and minimize costs. Consider combination therapy in *Pseudomonas* infections, and combination empiric therapy in neutropenic patients. Combination therapy should be continued for no more than 3 to 5 days and de-escalation should occur following availability of susceptibilities. The duration of antibiotic therapy typically is limited to 7 to 10 days. Longer duration is considered if response is slow, if surgical source control is inadequate, or if immunologic deficiencies are evident. Antimicrobial therapy should be stopped if infection is not considered the etiologic factor for a shock state.

Box 1
Common sources of severe sepsis/septic shock requiring urgent source control

Toxic megacolon or C difficile colitis with shock

Ischemic bowel

Perforated viscus

Intra-abdominal abscess

Ascending cholangitis

Gangrenous cholecystitis

Necrotizing pancreatitis with infection

Bacterial empyema

Mediastinitis

Purulent tunnel infections

Purulent foreign body infections

Obstructive uropathy

Complicated pyelonephritis/perinephric abscess

Necrotizing soft tissue infections (necrotizing fasciitis)

Clostridial myonecrosis

REFERENCES

1. Angus DC, Linde-Zwirble WT, Lidicker J, et al. Epidemiology of severe sepsis in the United States: analysis of incidence, outcome and associated costs of care. Crit Care Med 2001;29:1303–10.
2. Dombrovskiy VY, Martin AA, Sunderman J, et al. Rapid increase in hospitalization and mortality rates for severe sepsis in the United States: a trend analysis for 1993 to 2003. Crit Care Med 2007;35:1244–50.
3. Martin GS, Mannino DM, Eaton S, et al. The epidemiology of sepsis in the United States from 1979 through 2000. N Engl J Med 2003;348(16):1546–54.
4. Increase in national hospital discharge survey rates for septicemia—United States. 1979–1987. Morb Mortal Wkly Rep 1990;39:31–4.
5. Bone RC, Balk RA, Cerra FB, et al. American College of Chest Physicians/Society of Critical Care Medicine Consensus Conference: definitions for sepsis and organ failure and guidelines for the

use of innovative therapies in sepsis. Chest 1992; 101:1644–55.

6. Rangel-Frausto M, Pittet D, Costigan M, et al. The natural history of the systemic inflammatory response syndrome (SIRS). JAMA 1995;273:117–23.

7. Youkeles LH, Rosen MJ. The epidemiology of sepsis in the immunocompromised host. In: Fein AM, Abraham EM, Balk RA, et al, editors. Sepsis and multiple organ failure. Baltimore (MD): Williams & Wilkins; 1997. p. 35–42.

8. Aube H, Milan C, Blettery B. Risk factors for septic shock in the early management of bacteremia. Am J Med 1992;93:283–8.

9. Christman JW, Wheeler AP, Bernard GR. Cytokines and sepsis: What are the therapeutic implications? J Crit Care 1991;6:172–82.

10. Whipple JK, Ausman RK, Franson T, et al. Effect of individualized pharmacokinetic dosing on patient outcome. Crit Care Med 1991;19(12):1480–5.

11. Pinder M, Bellomo R, Lipman J, et al. Pharmacological principles of antibiotic prescription in the critically ill. Anaesth Intensive Care 2002;30(2):134–44.

12. Solomkin JS, Miyagawa CI. Principles of antibiotic therapy. Surg Clin North Am 1994;74:497–517.

13. Hessen MT, Kaye D. Principles of selection and use of antibacterial agents. Infect Dis Clin North Am 1995;9:531–45.

14. van Dalen R, Vree TB. Pharmacokinetics of antibiotics in critically ill patients. Intensive Care Med 1990;16(Suppl):S235–8.

15. Moore RD, Lietman PS, Smith CR. Clinical response to aminoglycoside therapy: importance of the ratio of peak concentration to minimal inhibitory concentration. J Infect Dis 1987;155(1):93–9.

16. Moore RD, Smith CR, Lietman PS. Association of aminoglycoside plasma levels with therapeutic outcome in gram-negative pneumonia. Am J Med 1984;77(4):657–62.

17. Chelluri L, Jastremski MS. Inadequacy of standard aminoglycoside loading doses in acutely ill patients. Crit Care Med 1987;15(12):1143–5.

18. Joukhadar C, Frossard M, Mayer BX, et al. Impaired target site penetration of beta-lactams may account for therapeutic failure in patients with septic shock. Crit Care Med 2001;29(2):385–91.

19. Levison ME. Pharmacodynamics of antimicrobial agents. Bactericidal and post antibiotic effects. Infect Dis Clin North Am 1995;9:483–95.

20. Schimpff SC. Empiric antibiotic therapy for granulocytopenic cancer patients. Am J Med 1986;80(5C): 13–20.

21. Love LJ, Schimpff SC, Schiffer CA, et al. Improved prognosis for granulocytopenic patients with gram-negative bacteremia. Am J Med 1980;68(5): 643–8.

22. Bartlett JG. Anti-anaerobic antibacterial agents. Lancet 1982;2(8296):478–81.

23. Bryant RE, Alford RH. Treatment of staphylococcal endocarditis. JAMA 1978;239(12):1130–1.

24. Klasterski J. Use of combinations of antibiotics for severe infections in cancer patients. Acta Clin Belg 1977;32(4):271–5.

25. Lepper MH, Dowling HF. Treatment of pneumococcic meningitis with penicillin compared with penicillin plus aureomycin; studies including observations on an apparent antagonism between penicillin and aureomycin. AMA Arch Intern Med 1951;88(4):489–94.

26. Moore GA, Rossi L, Nicotera P, et al. Quinone toxicity in hepatocytes: studies on mitochondrial Ca2+ release induced by benzoquinone derivatives. Arch Biochem Biophys 1987;259(2):283–95.

27. Sande MA. Factors influencing the penetration and activity of antibiotics in experimental meningitis. J Infect 1981;3(1 Suppl):33–8.

28. Bodey GP, Ketchel SJ, Rodriguez V. A randomized study of carbenicillin plus cefamandole or tobramycin in the treatment of febrile episodes in cancer patients. Am J Med 1979;67(4):608–16.

29. Sanders CC, Sanders WE Jr. Microbial resistance to newer generation beta-lactam antibiotics: clinical and laboratory implications. J Infect Dis 1985; 151(3):399–406.

30. Chow JW, Fine MJ, Shlaes DM, et al. Enterobacter bacteremia: clinical features and emergence of antibiotic resistance during therapy. Ann Intern Med 1991;115(8):585–90.

31. Burton ME, Chow MS, Platt DR, et al. Accuracy of Bayesian and Sawchuk-Zaske dosing methods for gentamicin. Clin Pharm 1986;5(2):143–9.

32. Dasta JF, Armstrong DK. Variability in aminoglycoside pharmacokinetics in critically ill surgical patients. Crit Care Med 1988;16(4):327–30.

33. Fuhs DW, Mann HJ, Kubajak CA, et al. Intrapatient variation of aminoglycoside pharmacokinetics in critically ill surgery patients. Clin Pharm 1988;7(3): 207–13.

34. Van Laethem Y, Lagast H, Husson M, et al. Serum bactericidal activity of cefoperazone and ceftazidime at increasing dosages against Pseudomonas aeruginosa. J Antimicrob Chemother 1983;12(5): 475–80.

35. Cunha BA, Ortega AM. Antibiotic failure. Med Clin 1995;79:663–72.

36. Tegeder I, Schmidtko A, Brautigam L, et al. Tissue distribution of imipenem in critically ill patients. Clin Pharmacol Ther 2002;71(5):325–33.

37. Dellinger RP, Levy MM, Carlet JM, et al. Surviving Sepsis Campaign: international guidelines for management of severe sepsis and septic shock: 2008. Crit Care Med 2008;36:296–327.

38. Ibrahim EH, Sherman G, Ward S, et al. The influence of inadequate antimicrobial treatment of bloodstream infections on patient outcomes in the ICU setting. Chest 2000;118(1):146–55.

39. Kollef MH, Sherman G, Ward S, et al. Inadequate antimicrobial treatment of infections: a risk factor for hospital mortality among critically ill patients. Chest 1999;115(2):462–74.

40. Kumar A, Suppes R, Gulati H, et al. The impact of initiation of inadequate antimicrobial therapy on survival in human septic shock. Antimicrobial Agents Chemother 2007;111:271.

41. Kreger BE, Kraven DE, McCabe WR. Gram-negative bacteremia IV. Re-evaluation of clinical features and treatment in 612 patients. Am J Med 1980;68(3): 344–55.

42. Vergis EN, Hayden MK, Chow JW, et al. Determinants of vancomycin resistance and mortality rates in enterococcal bactermia: a prospective multicenter study. Ann Intern Med 2001;135(7):484–92.

43. Miner JR, Heegaard W, Mapes A, et al. Presentation, time to antibiotics, and mortality of patients with bacterial meningitis at an urban county medical center. J Emerg Med 2001;21(4):387–92.

44. Kumar A, Roberts D, Wood KE, et al. Duration of hypotension before initiation of effective antimicrobial therapy is the critical determinant of survival in human septic shock [see comment]. Crit Care Med 2006;34(6):1589–96.

45. Meehan TP, Fine MJ, Krumholz HM, et al. Quality of care, process and outcomes in elderly patients with pneumonia. JAMA 1997;278(23):2080–4.

46. Pimentel FL, Abelha F, Trigo MA, et al. Determination of plasma concentrations of amikacin in patients of an intensive care unit. J Chemother 1995;7(1):45–9.

47. Franson TR, Quebbeman EJ, Whipple J, et al. Prospective comparison of traditional and pharmacokinetic aminoglycoside dosing methods. Crit Care Med 1988;16(9):840–3.

48. Lodise TP, Lomaestro BM, Drusano GL. Piperacillin-tazobactam for Pseudomonas aeruginosa infection: clinical implications of an extended-infusion dosing strategy. Clin Infect Dis 2007;44:357–63.

49. Baddour LM, Yu VL, Klugman KP, et al. Combination antibiotic therapy lowers mortality among severely ill patients with pneumococcal bacteremia. Am J Respir Crit Care Med 2004;170(4):440–4.

50. Rodriguez A, Mendia A, Sirvent JM, et al. Combination antibiotic therapy improves survival in patients with community-acquired pneumonia and shock. Crit Care Med 2007;35(6):1493–8.

51. Moss RL, Musemeche CA, Kosloske AM. Necrotizing fasciitis in children: prompt recognition and aggressive therapy improve survival. J Pediatr Surg 1996; 31(8):1142–6.

52. Kumar A, Wood K, Gurka D, et al. Outcome of septic shock correlates with duration of hypotension prior to source control implementation. ICAAC Proceedings, 350;K-1222. 2004.

Management of Sepsis: Early Resuscitation

Emanuel P. Rivers, MD, MPH[a,b,*], Victor Coba, MD[b],
Alvaro Visbal, MD[c], Melissa Whitmill, MD[b], David Amponsah, MD[a]

KEYWORDS

- Sepsis • Resuscitation • Early goal-directed therapy
- Fluids • Vasopressor • Inotropes

Abbreviations: ARR, Absolute risk reduction; ALI, Acute lung injury; ARDS, Adult respiratory distress syndrome; APACHE II, Acute physiologic and chronic health evaluation score II; CVP, Central venous pressure; CQI, Continuos quality improvement; ED, Emergency department; EDM, Esophageal doppler monitoring; EGDT, Early goal-directed therapy; ESRD, End stage renal disease; GPU, Inpatient general practice unit (medical-surgical floors); HFH, Henry Ford Hospital; ICU, Intensive care unit; IHI, Institute for Health Improvement; IL-8, Interleukin 8; LOS, Length of stay; MB, Maintainance or 24 hour bundle; mmol/L, millimoles per liter; MODS, Multiple organ dysfunction score; NNT, Number needed to treat; OR, Odds ratio; PAC, Pulmonary artery catheter; PAOP, Pulmonary capillary occlusion pressure; PPV, Pulse pressure variation; RR, Relative risk; RRR, Relative risk reduction; SAPS II, Simplified acute physiologic score; SBP, Systolic blood pressure; ScvO$_2$, Central venous oxygen saturation; SvO$_2$, Mixed venous oxygen saturation; SD, Standard deviation; SSC, Surviving Sepsis Campaign.

Key links in the chain of survival for the management of severe sepsis and septic shock are early identification and comprehensive resuscitation of high-risk patients.[1] Multiple studies have shown that the first 6 hours of early sepsis management are especially important from a diagnostic, pathogenic, and therapeutic perspective, and that steps taken during this period can have a significant impact on outcome.[2–7] This period applies to the 700,000 cases per year of sepsis presenting to emergency departments and an equal number of patients on general hospital inpatient floors and intensive care units (ICUs)[8] in the United States. The recognition of this critical period and the robust outcome benefit realized in previous studies provides the rationale for adopting early resuscitation as a distinct intervention.[9] Sepsis joins trauma, stroke, and acute myocardial infarction in having "golden hours," representing a critical opportunity early on in the course of disease for actions that offer the most benefit.

THE PHYSIOLOGIC RATIONALE FOR EARLY HEMODYNAMIC OPTIMIZATION

The hemodynamic picture of sepsis represents a continuum from clinically stable disease to circulatory insufficiency resulting from hypovolemia, myocardial depression, increased metabolic rate, vasoregulatory-perfusion abnormalities leading to inflammation, and cytopathic tissue hypoxia.

Emanuel P. Rivers receives research support from the National Institute of Allergy and Infectious Disease, and from Hutchinson Technologies. In the last 2 years, he has performed as a consultant, delivered lectures, or served as a panelist for Biosite, Edwards Lifesciences, Elan, and Eli Lilly and Co.

[a] Department of Emergency Medicine, Henry Ford Health Systems, 270-Clara Ford Pavilion, 2799 West Grand Boulevard, Detroit, MI 48202, USA
[b] Department of Surgery, Henry Ford Health Systems, 270-Clara Ford Pavilion, 2799 West Grand Boulevard, Detroit, MI 48202, USA
[c] Department of Pulmonary and Critical Care Medicine, Henry Ford Health Systems, 270-Clara Ford Pavilion, 2799 West Grand Boulevard, Detroit, MI 48202, USA
* Corresponding author. Departments of Emergency Medicine and Surgery, Henry Ford Hospital, 270-Clara Ford Pavilion, 2799 West Grand Boulevard, Detroit, MI 48202.
E-mail address: erivers1@hfhs.org (E.P. Rivers).

Clin Chest Med 29 (2008) 689–704
doi:10.1016/j.ccm.2008.06.005
0272-5231/08/$ – see front matter © 2008 Elsevier Inc. All rights reserved.

These hemodynamic combinations create various degrees of systemic imbalance between tissue oxygen supply and demand ranging from global tissue hypoxia to overt shock and multiorgan failure. Increases in oxygen extraction or decreases in central venous oxygen saturation or mixed venous oxygen saturation signal falling venous oxyhemoglobin saturation. These parameters provide a compensatory mechanism for restoring the balance needed to maintain tissue oxygen. When the limits of this compensatory mechanism are reached, however, lactate production ensues as an indicator of anaerobic metabolism. In this delivery-dependency phase, lactate concentration increases and may be inversely correlated with systemic oxygen delivery and mixed or central venous oxygen saturation.[10] This phase, which is characterized as global tissue hypoxia, is an important transition from sepsis to severe disease. Although this phase is associated with increased morbidity and mortality if unrecognized or left untreated, it can occur with normal vital signs.[11–13] The transition to septic shock can range from a hypodynamic state of oxygen delivery dependency (elevated lactate concentrations and low venous oxygen saturations) to the more commonly recognized hyperdynamic state where oxygen consumption is independent of oxygen delivery (normal to increased lactate concentrations and high venous oxygen saturation), depending on the stage of disease presentation and the extent of hemodynamic optimization (**Table 1**).[10,14–17] Comprehensive resuscitation is a way to optimize systemic oxygen delivery (preload, afterload, arterial oxygen content, contractility), balance oxygen delivery with systemic oxygen demands, optimize the microcirculation, and use metabolic end points to verify efficient cellular oxygen use. Although there is much discussion about the components required to accomplish a comprehensive resuscitation, no single component dictates the overall intent of the resuscitation. These components are interrelated and should be considered as a continuum of care and not as isolated variables.

IDENTIFICATION OF THE HIGH-RISK PATIENT

Although hypotension currently is used to define the transition from severe sepsis to septic shock, it is not sufficiently sensitive as a screening tool for tissue perfusion deficits in early sepsis. A number of studies support the employment of lactate equal to or greater than 4 mmol/L as a marker for severe tissue hypoperfusion and as a univariate predictor of mortality.[18–25] Anion gap or base deficit can be helpful when present. However, a normal bicarbonate or anion gap can be observed in over 20% of patients presenting with a lactate level greater than 4.0 mmol/L.[26,27] Serial lactate levels can be used to assess lactate clearance or changes in lactate over time in as little as the first 6 hours of sepsis presentation. Improved lactate clearance is significantly associated with decreased inflammatory response, improved coagulation parameters (**Fig. 1**), preserved organ function, and improved survival.[5,28]

Patients with severe sepsis and septic shock often have elevated brain natriuretic peptide (BNP) and troponin levels, which are significantly associated with organ and myocardial dysfunction, global tissue hypoxia, and mortality.[29] When adjusted for age, gender, history of heart failure, renal function, organ dysfunction, and mean arterial pressure, a BNP greater than 210 pg/mL at 24 hours is a significant independent indicator of increased mortality.[30] Phau and colleagues[31] have shown that elevated baseline lactate levels offer superior prognostic accuracy to baseline procalcitonin levels, which in turn are superior to N-terminal pro-BNP levels. To improve their prognostic utility beyond those of cytokine measurements and clinical severity scores, serial lactate and procalcitonin measurements may be combined.

HEMODYNAMIC MONITORING

The protocol resuscitation components of early goal-directed therapy (EGDT) were largely derived from the practice parameters for the hemodynamic support of sepsis recommended by the American College of Critical Care Medicine in 1999.[32] The EGDT protocol uses central venous pressure measurements instead of pulmonary capillary wedge pressure to address preload (**Fig. 2**). While tools for hemodynamic optimization may vary, the message is that an early-organized approach to hemodynamic optimization improves outcomes. These various tools are discussed in **Table 2**.

FLUID THERAPY

Aggressive fluid resuscitation is required because of hypovolemia resulting from a decreased oral intake and increased insensible losses from vomiting, diarrhea, or sweating. Venodilation and extravasation of fluid into the interstitial space because of increased capillary endothelial permeability results in decreased cardiac preload, decreased cardiac output, and inadequate systemic oxygen delivery. Rapid restoration of fluid deficits not only modulates inflammation but also decreases the need for vasopressor therapy and

Table 1
Hemodynamic patterns of early sepsis

	Mean Arterial Pressure	Central Venous Pressure; Pulmonary Artery Occluded Pressure	Central Venous Oxygen Saturation; Mixed Venous Oxygen Saturation	Lactate	Cardiac Index	Systemic Vascular Resistance	Treatment and Comments
Hypovolemia	Variable	Lower	Lower	Higher	Lower	Higher	Volume: crystalloid or colloid
Compensated and vasodilatory phase	Lower	Normal	Higher	Variable	Higher	Lower	Vasopressors, physiologic vasopressin, low-dose corticosteroids
Myocardial suppression	Variable	Higher	Lower	Higher	Normal or lower	Normal or higher	Increased brain natriuretic peptide levels, inotropic therapy
Impairment of tissue oxygen use	Variable	Normal	Much higher	Higher	Variable	Lower, normal, or higher	Vasodilators, recombinant activated protein C

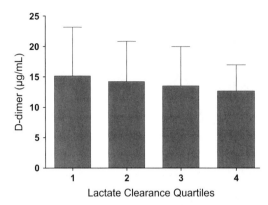

Fig. 1. Lactate clearance and D-dimer. The lactate clearance is defined as the baseline or 0-hour lactate, minus the 6-hour lactate, divided by the baseline lactate. Patients with poor to excellent lactate clearance (quartile 1: −24% [±42%]; quartile 2: 30% [±8%]; quartile 3: 53% [±7%]; quartile 4: 75% [±7%]) are compared. D-dimer levels significantly decrease as lactate clearance increases ($P = .01$).[78]

for subsequent steroid use and invasive monitoring (pulmonary artery catheterization and arterial line placement), which are required when a patient progresses to septic shock.[33,34]

While there is general agreement that volume therapy is an integral component of early resuscitation, there is a lack of consensus for the type of fluid, standards of volume assessment, and end points. The goal of fluid resuscitation in early sepsis is not to achieve a predetermined value, but rather to optimize systemic oxygen delivery (cardiac preload, afterload, arterial oxygen content, contractility, or stroke volume) and ultimately to balance tissue oxygen demands.[35] **Table 1** notes the hemodynamic patterns that must be monitored to help accomplish these goals.[36]

Colloids are high molecular-weight solutions that increase plasma oncotic pressure. Colloids can be classified as either natural (albumin) or artificial (starches, dextrans, and gelatins). Because of their higher molecular weight, colloids stay in the intravascular space significantly longer than crystalloids. For example, the intravascular half-life of albumin is 16 hours versus 30 to 60 minutes for normal saline and lactated Ringer's solution.[37,38] When titrated to the same pulmonary artery occlusion pressure, colloids and crystalloids restore tissue perfusion to the same magnitude, although two to four times more volume of crystalloids are required to achieve the same end point.[39] The required volume obviously depends on the stage of sepsis and capillary permeability. Albumin has the best safety profile of the four aforementioned colloids.[40] No one can yet say whether crystalloids or colloids provide the better outcome advantage in sepsis.[41] **Table 3** compares the most commonly used fluid therapies.

The Fluids and Catheters Treatment Trial isolated the manipulation of volume therapy as a controlled intervention beginning an average of 43 hours after ICU admission and 24 hours after the establishment of acute lung injury.[42] Although there was no difference in 60-day mortality, patients in the conservative strategy group had significantly improved lung and central nervous system function and a decreased need for sedation, mechanical ventilation, and ICU care. However, there was a statistically significant 0.3-day increase in cardiovascular failure–free days in the liberal compared with the conservative fluid group, suggesting that caution should be used in applying a conservative fluid strategy during the resuscitation phase. Even though EGDT has been considered a liberal strategy, there was no difference in ratios of PaO_2 to fraction of inspired oxygen and the use of mechanical ventilation between standard care and EGDT group from baseline to 6 hours in spite of significantly more fluids given. However, over the 7- to 72-hour period, there was a 14.2% higher rate of mechanical ventilation in the standard group. These findings were associated with lower IL-8 levels in the EGDT group during this same period.[7] Others have observed these same increased cardiopulmonary complications in unresolved shock upon admission to the hospital.[43,44] The Fluids and Catheters Treatment Trial is not at odds with EGDT. This study has brought attention to the negative consequences of overzealous fluid administration. These other consequences, which also include intra-abdominal hypertension and increased morbidity and mortality, have been noted, especially in the elderly.[36]

VASOPRESSOR THERAPY

To optimize end-organ perfusion, the second line of intervention after fluid therapy is the administration of vasopressors. LeDoux and colleagues[45] confirmed that the goal of a mean arterial pressure should be at least 65 mm Hg. They found that, when patients were titrated to a mean arterial pressure of 65 mm Hg, 75 mm Hg, and 85 mm Hg, there was no difference in urine output, lactate clearance, and skin capillary blood flow. De Backer and colleagues[46] examined the effects of different doses of various vasopressors in septic shock with a goal mean arterial pressure of at least 65 mm Hg. The administration of adrenergic agents resulted in unpredictable plasma concentrations and these concentrations did not correlate with their pharmacologic effects.[46] In addition, the severity of

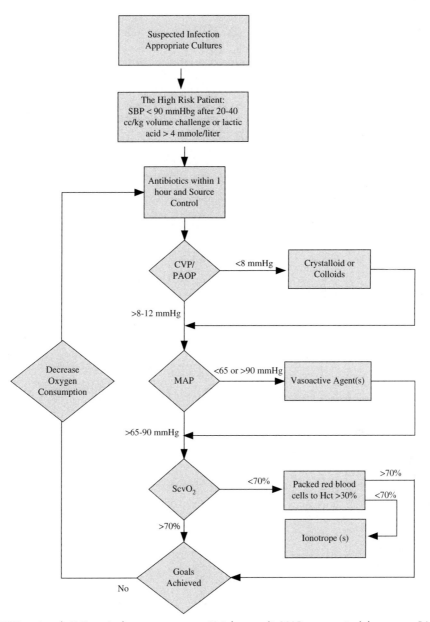

Fig. 2. The EGDT protocol. CVP, central venous pressure; Hct, hemocrit; MAP, mean arterial pressure; PAOP, pulmonary artery occluded pressure; SBP, systolic blood pressure; ScvO$_2$, central venous oxygen saturation.

septic shock did not identify a minimal or maximal therapeutic dose range to maintain perfusion for norepinephrine, dopamine, phenylephrine, epinephrine, and vasopressin.

The optimal vasopressor should be selected based on the pharmacologic properties that best augment the physiologic status of the patient. The various adrenergic receptors are alpha adrenergic receptors, B1 receptors, B2 receptors, and dopaminergic receptors. Alpha adrenergic receptors are located in the peripheral circulation leading to vasoconstriction. B1 receptors have both chronotropic and inotropic effects. B2 receptors activate vasodilatation and brochodilation. Dopaminergic receptors are located throughout the cardiovascular, mesenteric, and renal systems.[47] For example, a patient with severe tachycardia would be best served by an agent with more alpha selective activity and less beta to avoid tachycardia and increased myocardial oxygen consumption. There is no evidence to suggest superiority or inferiority when using a "high dose" single agent compared with using "modest" dosages of two or more vasopressors. However, when very high doses of

Table 2
Tools for hemodynamic monitoring

Tool	Notes on Use
Invasive blood pressure monitoring	Intra-arterial pressure measurement is preferable because vasoactive drugs may cause rapid swings in blood pressure and multiple blood samplings are typically required. Radial artery pressure may underestimate central pressure in hypotensive septic patients receiving high-dose vasopressor therapy. Clinical management based on radial pressures may lead to excessive vasopressor administration. Awareness of this phenomenon may help minimize adverse effects of these potent agents by enabling dosage reduction.[79]
Pulse pressure variation and pulse contour analysis of stroke volume variation	Measures of stroke volume variation made using arterial pulse contour analysis estimate cardiac output and can demonstrate fluid responsiveness if cardiac output increases after volume loading and stroke volume variation during positive-pressure ventilation decreases.[80]
Central venous pressure	Central venous pressure may not reliably reflect the left ventricular filling pressure in clinical states that produce pulmonary hypertension or compliance changes in the right or left heart. Common iliac venous pressure can approximate central venous pressure.[35,81]
Static measures of fluid responsiveness	Static measures of fluid responsiveness include central venous pressure, right atrial pressure, wedge pressure, pulmonary artery occlusion pressure, right ventricular end-diastolic volume index, left ventricular end-diastolic area, global end-diastolic volume, and intrathoracic blood volume. One of the disadvantages of this diagnostic approach in unstable patients is that it is definitive in only 50% of unstable patients.[82]
Dynamic measures of fluid responsiveness	Dynamic measures of fluid responsiveness include inspiratory decrements of right atrial pressure, pulse pressure variation, peak aortic blood flow velocity variation, respiratory variation in vena cava diameter, and after passive leg raising.[83] A pulse pressure variation of 13% or more in septic patients breathing with a tidal volume of 8 mL/kg is highly sensitive and specific for detecting preload responsiveness.[82]
Fluid challenge or fluid responsiveness	Measures related to fluid challenge or fluid responsiveness include the fall in systolic pressure compared with end-expiratory baseline; the intrathoracic blood volume index; variation in aortic peak flow velocity; the global end-diastolic volume index; inferior vena cava collapsibility; superior venal cava diameter; strike volume variation; and plethysmographic pulse wave variation.[36,84]
Central and mixed venous oximetry	Central venous oxygen saturation closely approximates mixed venous oxygen saturation and can be monitored continuously using infrared oximetry. This technology enables the clinician to detect clinically unrecognized global tissue hypoperfusion in the treatment of myocardial infarction, general medical shock, trauma, hemorrhage, septic shock, hypovolemic shock, end-stage heart failure, and cardiogenic shock during and after cardiopulmonary arrest.[85]
Systemic arterial–venous carbon dioxide difference	Increased arterial–mixed venous carbon dioxide gradients are seen in acute circulatory failure, and inversely correlate with the cardiac index. Central venous and pulmonary artery carbon dioxide values can be interchanged to determine cardiac index.[86]

Gastric tonometry and sublingual capnography	Serial measurements of gastric and sublingual mucosal blood flow are based on hydrogen ion diffusion and carbon dioxide elimination. Inadequate visceral perfusion, as evidenced by persistently low intramucosal pH or increased sublingual carbon dioxide concentration after resuscitation, is associated with subsequent organ dysfunction and death.[87,88]
Pulmonary artery catheterization	Pulmonary artery catheterization is useful for obtaining measurements of left-sided heart filling, pulmonary artery occlusion pressure, cardiac output, and mixed venous oxygen saturation. Pulmonary artery catheterization enables calculation of hemodynamic and oxygen transport variables. Special catheters can measure the right ventricular end-diastolic volume index calculated from the right ventricular ejection fraction.
Ultrasound and echocardiography	Ultrasound and echocardiography can be used for assessing volume status by measuring intracardiac diameters, vena caval diameters and left ventricular end-diastolic area after a fluid challenge or passive leg raising. Controlled-compression sonography is a valuable tool for measuring venous pressure in peripheral veins and allows reliable indirect assessment of central venous pressure. Ultrasound can also be used to assist in line placement.[89]
Noninvasive cardiac output	Cardiac output can be measured by pulse pressure variation, pulse contour analysis, transesophageal Doppler, thoracic cutaneous bioimpedance, lithium dilution, or transpulmonary thermodilution.[90]
Metabolic cart or direct calorimetry	Metabolic cart or direct calorimetry can directly measure VO_2 using systemic gas exchange. A reduction in VO_2 correlates with poor outcome.[91]
Near-infrared spectroscopy	Near-infrared spectroscopy has been used to find lower values in patients with severe sepsis (versus healthy volunteers) in tissue oxygen saturation, in the tissue oxygen saturation recovery slope, in the tissue hemoglobin index, and in the total tissue hemoglobin increase on venous occlusion. Patients with severe sepsis had longer tissue oxygen saturation recovery times and lower near-infrared spectroscopy–derived local oxygen consumption values versus healthy volunteers.[92]
Orthogonal polarization spectral imaging	Disordered microcirculatory flow can now be associated with systemic inflammation, acute organ dysfunction, and increased mortality. Using new technologies, such as orthogonal polarization spectral imaging, to directly image microcirculatory blood flow will help define the role of microcirculatory dysfunction in oxygen transport and circulatory support in severe sepsis.[93]

Table 3
Fluid therapies for sepsis

Fluid	Notes on Use
Normal saline	Normal saline is a slightly hyperosmolar solution containing 154 mEq/L of both sodium and chloride. Due to the relatively high chloride concentration, normal saline carries a risk of inducing hyperchloremic metabolic acidosis when given in large amounts.[38]
Lactated Ringer's solution	Lactate can accept a proton and subsequently be metabolized to carbon dioxide and water by the liver, leading to release of carbon dioxide in the lungs and excretion of water by the kidneys. Lactated Ringer's solution results in a buffering of the acidemia, which is advantageous over normal saline. Because lactated Ringer's solution contains potassium, albeit a very small amount, there is a risk of inducing hyperkalemia in patients with renal insufficiency or renal failure. Another potential downside to using lactated Ringer's solution for resuscitation is the significant immune activation and induction of cellular injury caused by the D-isomer of lactated Ringer's solution. Replacement of the lactate with ethyl pyruvate or β-hydroxybutyrate or using only the L-isomer of lactate in Ringer's solution decreases this adverse effect.[38]
Albumin	Albumin is a protein derived from human plasma. It is available in strengths varying from 4% to 25%. The Saline Versus Albumin Fluid Evaluation study compared fluid resuscitation with albumin or saline on mortality and found similar 28-day mortalities and secondary outcomes in each arm.[94] However, a subset analysis of septic patients resuscitated with albumin showed a decrease in mortality, although statistically the decrease was insignificant.[38]
Hydroxyethyl starch	Hydroxyethyl starch, a synthetic colloid derived from hydrolyzed amylopectin, has been found to be harmful, causing renal impairment at recommended doses and impairing long-term survival at high doses.[95] Hydroxyethyl starch can also cause coagulopathy and bleeding complications from reduced factor VIII and von Willebrand factor levels, as well as impaired platelet function. Hydroxyethyl starch increases the risk of acute renal failure among patients with sepsis and reduces the probability of survival. Hydroxyethyl starch should be avoided in sepsis.[95–97]
Dextrans and gelatins	Dextrans, other examples of artificial colloids, are glucose polymers synthesized by *Leuconostoc mesenteroides* bacteria grown in sucrose media. Dextrans are not frequently used for rapid plasma expansion, but rather to lower blood viscosity. This class can cause renal dysfunction, as well as anaphylactoid reactions. Gelatins, which are also artificial colloids, are produced from bovine collagen. Because they have a much smaller molecular weight, they are not as effective for expanding plasma volume. However, they cost less.[98] They too have been reported to cause renal impairment, as well as allergic reactions ranging from pruritus to anaphylaxis. Gelatins are not currently available in North America.

a single vasopressor are required, clinicians should consider changing the vasopressor agent and evaluating for confounding factors that may limit maximal effect.[47] There is insufficient evidence proving that one particular vasopressor is superior to others.[35,48] The clinical caveat is to minimize vasopressor use (**Table 4**). The delayed use of vasopressor has outcome implications. Levy and colleagues[49] noted that the delayed need for vasopressors (cardiovascular insufficiency) has the strongest association with increased mortality when compared to any other organ failure.

In January 2008, the Surviving Sepsis Campaign Recommendations were published with six evidence-graded statements for vasopressor use in septic shock:[35]

1. The mean arterial pressure should be maintained at 65 mm Hg or higher (grade 1C).
2. Either norepinephrine or dopamine is the first choice vasopressor agent to correct hypotension in septic shock (administered through a central catheter as soon as one is available) (grade 1C).
3. Epinephrine, phenylephrine, or vasopressin should not be administered as the initial vasopressor in septic shock (grade 2C). Vasopressin 0.03–0.04 U/min may be added to norepinephrine subsequently with anticipation of an effect equivalent to that of norepinephrine alone.
4. Epinephrine is the first chosen alternative agent in septic shock that is poorly responsive to norepinephrine or dopamine (grade 2B).
5. Low-dose dopamine should not be used for renal protection (grade 1A).
6. All patients requiring vasopressors should have an arterial catheter placed as soon as practicable if resources are available (grade 1D).

VASODILATOR THERAPY AND MICROCIRCULATORY MANIPULATION

It is becoming increasingly evident that disordered microcirculatory flow is associated with systemic inflammation, acute organ dysfunction, and increased mortality. New technologies that directly image microcirculatory blood flow may help define the role of microcirculatory dysfunction in oxygen transport and circulatory support.[50] Cerra and colleagues[51] provided vasodilator therapy to sepsis patients with low cardiac output and observed physiologic improvement. Sprong and colleagues[52] examined eight volume-resuscitated septic patients (mean arterial pressure >60 mm Hg) and observed increased microvascular perfusion in response to a loading dose and infusion of

nitroglycerin every 7 hours. Of the eight patients observed, seven survived. Thus, although these agents may be prohibitive early in sepsis, once blood pressure is stabilized, vasodilating drugs may improve outcomes. There is evidence that the recombinant activated protein C improved microcirculatory flow and further evidence suggests improved outcome with early administration.[53]

OPTIMAL HEMOGLOBIN

After correcting for central venous pressure and mean arterial pressure, the EGDT protocol addresses arterial oxygen content as the next step if the central venous oxygen saturation is less than 70%. The combination of anemia and global tissue hypoxia provides the physiologic rationale for transfusion of red blood cells during this delivery-dependent (low central venous oxygen saturation) phase. This anemia is also exacerbated by the large volume resuscitation during the first 6 hours of resuscitation. It is this particular phase that has gone unstudied in previous trials of conservation hemoglobin strategies. While transfusion therapy has received increasing scrutiny in critical illness, recent data are conflicting.[54] Furthermore, some findings suggest that the sublingual microcirculation is globally unaltered by red blood cell transfusion in septic patients and can improve in patients with altered capillary perfusion at baseline.[55]

INOTROPIC THERAPY

Myocardial dysfunction in sepsis manifests as a decrease in ejection fraction. Ventricular dilation is one of the likely compensatory mechanisms to maintain cardiac output. However, it may be insufficient to provide adequate systemic oxygen delivery.[14] This may be seen particularly in patients with premorbid cardiovascular disease, which may compromise the host response to the increased cardiac output commonly seen in the latter stages of sepsis.

Inotropic support is recommended in the setting of low cardiac output and venous oxygen saturation where adequate fluid resuscitation and blood pressure have been achieved.[35] Elevated BNP levels may also indicate myocardial dysfunction and the need for inotropic therapy.[30] Given the failure of large, prospective trials to demonstrate benefit from the use of inotropic support to increase oxygen delivery and cardiac output to supranormal levels, this practice is discouraged.[56]

Dobutamine is one of the more commonly used inotropes in sepsis. Its effects are mostly due to its

Table 4
Vasopressor therapies for sepsis

Drug	Side Effects and Comments
Norepinephrine	Norepinephrine, which has the physiologic properties of an inotrope, causes vasoconstriction.[47] Researchers have found favorable outcomes in 7- and 28-day mortality while the other vasopressors did not extrapolate to have either a negative or positive association in mortality with multivariant analysis.[99] A comparison of norepinephrine with dopamine showing improved splanchnic oxygen use with norepinephrine.[100]
Dopamine	Most of the effects of dopamine <5 ug/kg/min are seen in the dopaminergic receptors in renal, mesenteric, and coronary cells. Some effects may also be found in other cells throughout the body At doses of 5–10 ug/kg/min, β-adrenergic effects are seen that increase cardiac contractility. At doses >10 ug/kg/min, α-adrenergic effects predominate with arterial vasoconstriction. A randomized clinical trial of low-dose dopamine in septic shock patients showed no protective effects from renal insufficiency.[101] Increased splanchnic oxygen consumption reduces overall hepatosplanchnic impairment even in the face of increase splanchnic blood flow.[47,102] Observational study suggests that dopamine administration may be associated with increased mortality rates in shock.[103]
Phenylephrine	Phenylephrine has primary selectivity for alpha-1 receptors in increasing peripheral resistance.[47] It is best in patients who present with tachycardia. Phenylephrine lacks significant inotropic or chronotropic effects and should be used with caution in cases of cardiac dysfunction in sepsis. One concern is the increase in oxygen consumption, decrease in splanchnic blood flow, and decrease in cardiac output for septic shock patients.[104]
Ephedrine	An indirect-acting central nervous system stimulant, ephedrine causes palpitations, hypertension, and cardiac arrhythmias. It has limited long-term value as therapy for shock.
Vasopressin	Septic shock patients have reduced vasopressin levels and respond to exogenous vasopressin infusion.[105] Also, the addition of dobutamine dosed at 5–10 µg/kg/min reverses the vasopressin impairment in the cardiac index, oxygen delivery index, and venous oxygen saturation, and even increases the mean arterial pressure.[106] A trial investigating vasopressin as an adjunctive and alternative therapy to norepinephrine found no statistical 28-day or 90-day mortality difference.[104,107]
Epinephrine	An investigation of the splanchnic circulation in septic shock patients compared epinephrine with other vasopressors and found a dose-dependent redistribution phenomenon away from the hepatosplanchnic system, lowering splanchnic blood flow despite a higher cardiac output.[46] Hyperlactatemia has been described as a detrimental effect of epinephrine. However, this effect has been described as transient with a 24-hour recovery independent of hypoxemia and likely an adaptive physiologic response to maintain carbohydrate metabolism under an aggressive circulatory insult. Epinephrine, in addition to offering antithrombotic properties, may attenuate excessive activity of inflammatory cytokines during infections. In persistent hypotensives on dopamine, the addition of epinephrine was not a significant factor for prediction of mortality.[99] An investigation into the management of septic shock with either epinephrine alone or norepinephrine plus dobutamine found no significance in mortality.[35,99]

β_1 agonist properties, even though it has some α_1 and β_2 agonist effects. Its effects on blood pressure are variable, with the most concerning one being hypotension. The administration of 5μg/kg/min dobutamine can improve but not restore capillary perfusion in patients with septic shock. Dobutamine may also exert salutary effects on the microcirculation independent of its systemic effects on hemodynamic variables.[57] Dobutamine challenges have also been used diagnostically and prognostically.[58,59] Dopamine at intermediate doses (10μg/kg/min) improves cardiac function, with the added effect of improved mesenteric blood flow. However, it may produce a greater increase in heart rate than that produced by other drugs. Phosphodiesterase inhibitors, such as milrinone, also have positive inotropic effects, but have a longer half-life and have been less studied in the early phases of septic shock. Norepinephrine has both α and β effects, with vasoconstriction being more prominent. It is the vasopressor of choice in septic patients with hypotension and may be used in combination with dobutamine when patients have an impaired cardiac output. Lastly, epinephrine stimulates both α and β effects. At low doses, the β-adrenergic effects are predominant. Levosimendan increases the sensitivity of troponin C to calcium, thus providing an inotropic effect. It has been targeted primarily to patients with heart failure, but recent prospective studies have not shown an improvement in mortality. Its role in the management of sepsis and septic shock is not clearly known, and is limited to case reports and small case series. One recent study compared levosimendan to dobutamine in patients with severe left ventricular dysfunction in the setting of septic shock. It showed an improvement in hemodynamics and regional perfusion when compared with dobutamine at a dose of 5 μg/kg/min. Its side effect profile is similar to that of other inotropic drugs, and is contraindicated in severe hepatic or renal dysfunction. Further studies are needed to clarify its potential benefits.[60]

Side effects of inotropic drugs include tachycardia and other arrhythmias, which may limit their use. Because of the vasodilatory activity associated with inotropic drugs, hypotension is also a concern. Inotropic drugs usually require the addition of a vasopressor, such as norepinephrine. These medications cause an increase in myocardial oxygen consumption and may precipitate cardiac ischemia, especially in patients with coronary artery disease. Epinephrine has been shown to worsen lactic acidosis and impair gut perfusion as compared with dobutamine and norepinephrine.[46] Digoxin can be used for rate control and has been shown to increase contractility even in patients on other adrenergic agents.[61]

EARLY RESUSCITATION EFFECTS ON INFLAMMATION

A pathologic link exists between the clinical presence of global tissue hypoxia, the generation of inflammatory mediators, and the mitochondrial impairment of oxygen use seen in septic ICU patients.[62–64] EGDT results in a statistically significant modulation of proinflammatory, anti-inflammatory, and coagulation biomarkers in patients treated with EGDT versus standard therapy.[7] In early severe sepsis and septic shock, distinct biomarker patterns emerge in response to hemodynamic optimization strategies within the first 3 hours of hospital presentation. A significant association exists among temporal biomarker patterns in the first 72 hours: severity of global tissue hypoxia, organ dysfunction, and mortality (**Fig. 3**). This biomarker activity closely relates to and corresponds with organ dysfunction.[65–67]

EARLY RESUSCITATION EFFECTS ON ORGAN FUNCTION

EGDT resulted in a 100% reduction in sudden cardiopulmonary complications during the first 72 hours, which was associated with a decreased need for cardiopulmonary support, including mechanical ventilation and pulmonary artery catheterization.[17] Consistent with these findings, Estenssoro and colleagues[43] found that the presence of shock on ICU admission day was the only factor, even adjusting for severity of illness and hypoxemia, that predicted prolonged mechanical ventilation.

THE OUTCOME EVIDENCE OF EARLY RESUSCITATION

Eleven peer-reviewed publications (1569 patients) and 28 abstracts (4429 patients) after the original EGDT study have been identified from academic, community, and international settings. These publications total 5998 patients (3042 before and 2956 after EGDT). The mean age, sex, Acute Physiology and Chronic Health Evaluation II scores, and mortality were similar across all studies. The mean relative and absolute risk reduction was 46% (±26%) and 20.3% (±12.7%), respectively. These findings are superior to those from the original EGDT trial, which showed figures of 34% and 16%, respectively. When peer-reviewed publications are compared, the relative risk reduction exceeded 25% and absolute risk reduction exceeds 9% in all studies. This evidence shows

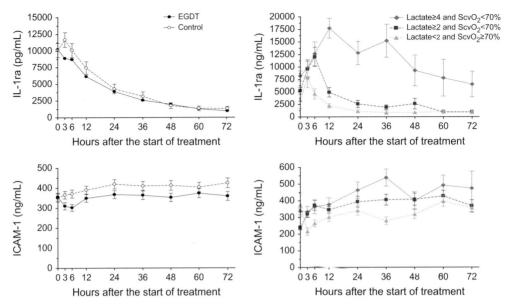

Fig. 3. The influence of resuscitation and severity of global tissue hypoxia on IL-1 receptor antagonists (IL-1ra) and intracellular adhesion molecules (ICAM-1). ScvO₂, central venous oxygen saturation.

effectiveness across a broad range of mortality risks.[9]

DECREASED HEALTH CARE RESOURCE CONSUMPTION

Hospital costs for severe sepsis and septic shock account for over $54 billion of the Medicare and Medicaid budget. Reports in the literature have noted reductions in ICU length of stay, hospital length of stay, duration of mechanical ventilation, renal replacement therapy, vasopressor therapy, and pulmonary artery catheterization with early hemodynamic optimization.[68,69] These studies have shown that sepsis-related hospital costs can be reduced up to 20%.[70,71]

IMPLEMENTATION STRATEGIES AND CONTINUOUS QUALITY IMPROVEMENT

Logistical issues regarding early hemodynamic optimization limit its generalizability because of resources. However, to alleviate this problem several approaches have been taken. To achieve a consistent level of quality at various locations within the hospital, multiple models may be required. The first model of sepsis management is based in the emergency department, with the emergency department team performing the initial algorithmic resuscitation. A second and increasingly popular model uses a multidisciplinary rapid response team trained to efficiently mobilize resources to resuscitate an unstable sepsis patient irrespective of location.[72] A third model is

ICU-based, emphasizing rapid transfer of critically ill sepsis patients from their initial location (emergency department, medical or surgical floor, operating room) to the ICU, where the ICU team initiates EGDT.[73] Each of these models can be tailored to the unique needs of individual institutions, but each has the potential to be implemented in a clinical and cost-effective manner. As with acute myocardial infarction, stroke, and trauma, continuous quality improvement is required to realize the best outcomes. Nguyen and colleagues[74–77] showed that a continuous quality initiative is important to realize the outcome benefit and is directly associated with improved outcomes. Thus, the effectiveness of EGDT as with any life-saving intervention is significantly related to a critical compliance effort.

SUMMARY

Early resuscitation in severe sepsis and septic shock modulates inflammation and results in significant reductions in morbidity, mortality, and health care resource consumption. While the diagnostic components, therapeutic components, and monitoring methods of resuscitation evolve and continue to be debated, EGDT has been externally validated and has consistently shown to be generalizable. Further emphasis should be placed on overcoming logistical, institutional, and professional barriers to the implementation.

REFERENCES

1. Kern JW, Shoemaker WC. Meta-analysis of hemo-dynamic optimization in high-risk patients. Crit Care Med 2002;30(8):1686–92.
2. Engoren M. The effect of prompt physician visits on intensive care unit mortality and cost. Crit Care Med 2005;33(4):727–32.
3. Kumar A, Roberts D, Wood KE, et al. Duration of hypotension before initiation of effective antimicrobial therapy is the critical determinant of survival in human septic shock. Crit Care Med 2006;34(6): 1589–96.
4. Lundberg JS, Perl TM, Wiblin T, et al. Septic shock: an analysis of outcomes for patients with onset on hospital wards versus intensive care units. Crit Care Med 1998;26(6):1020–4.
5. Nguyen HB, Rivers EP, Knoblich BP, et al. Early lactate clearance is associated with improved outcome in severe sepsis and septic shock. Crit Care Med 2004;32(8):1637–42.
6. Varpula M, Tallgren M, Saukkonen K, et al. Hemo-dynamic variables related to outcome in septic shock. Intensive Care Med 2005;31:1066–71.
7. Rivers EP, Kruse JA, Jacobsen G, et al. The influence of early hemodynamic optimization on bio-marker patterns of severe sepsis and septic shock. Crit Care Med 2007;35(9):2016–24.
8. Wang HE, Shapiro NI, Angus DC, et al. National estimates of severe sepsis in United States emergency departments. Crit Care Med 2007;35(8): 1928–36.
9. Rivers EP, Coba V, Whitmill M. Early goal-directed therapy in severe sepsis and septic shock: a contemporary review of the literature. Volume therapy and innate immune response during systemic inflammation or sepsis. Curr Opin Anaesthesiol 2008;21:128–40.
10. Astiz ME, Rackow EC, Weil MH. Oxygen delivery and utilization during rapidly fatal septic shock in rats. Circ Shock 1986;20(4):281–90.
11. Rady MY, Rivers EP, Nowak RM. Resuscitation of the critically ill in the ED: responses of blood pressure, heart rate, shock index, central venous oxygen saturation, and lactate. Am J Emerg Med 1996;14(2):218–25.
12. Brun-Buisson C, Doyon F, Carlet J, et al. Incidence, risk factors, and outcome of severe sepsis and septic shock in adults. A multicenter prospective study in intensive care units. French ICU group for severe sepsis. J Am Med Assoc 1995;274(12): 968–74.
13. Vincent JL, De Backer D. Oxygen uptake/oxygen supply dependency: fact or fiction? Acta Anaesthesiol Scand Suppl 1995;107:229–37.
14. Parrillo JE, Parker MM, Natanson C, et al. Septic shock in humans. Advances in the understanding of pathogenesis, cardiovascular dysfunction, and therapy [see comments]. Ann Intern Med 1990; 113(3):227–42.
15. Silance PG, Vincent JL. Oxygen extraction in patients with sepsis and heart failure: another look at clinical studies. Clin Intensive Care 1994; 5(1):4–14.
16. Astiz ME, Rackow EC, Kaufman B, et al. Relationship of oxygen delivery and mixed venous oxygenation to lactic acidosis in patients with sepsis and acute myocardial infarction. Crit Care Med 1988; 16(7):655–8.
17. Rivers E, Nguyen B, Havstad S, et al. Early goal-directed therapy in the treatment of severe sepsis and septic shock. N Engl J Med 2001;345(19): 1368–77.
18. Aduen J, Bernstein WK, Khastgir T, et al. The use and clinical importance of a substrate-specific electrode for rapid determination of blood lactate concentrations. J Am Med Assoc 1994;272(21): 1678–85.
19. Broder G, Weil MH. Excess lactate: an index of reversibility of shock in human patients. Science 1964;143:1457–9.
20. Cady LD Jr, Weil MH, Afifi AA, et al. Quantitation of severity of critical illness with special reference to blood lactate. Crit Care Med 1973;1(2):75–80.
21. Shapiro NI, Howell MD, Talmor D, et al. Serum lactate as a predictor of mortality in emergency department patients with infection. Ann Emerg Med 2005;45(5):524–8.
22. Middleton P, Kelly AM, Brown J, et al. Agreement between arterial and central venous values for pH, bicarbonate, base excess, and lactate. Emerg Med J 2006;23(8):622–4.
23. Younger JG, Falk JL, Rothrock SG. Relationship between arterial and peripheral venous lactate levels. Acad Emerg Med 1996;3(7):730–4.
24. Garcia AJ, Sherwin RL, Bilkovski RN. Point-of-care lactate testing as a predictor of mortality in a hetero-geneous emergency department population. Acad Emerg Med 2006;13(5 Suppl 1):S152.
25. Trzeciak S, Dellinger RP, Chansky ME, et al. Serum lactate as a predictor of mortality in patients with infection. Intensive Care Med 2007;33(6): 970–7.
26. Wira C, Rivers E, Donnino M, et al. Surrogate markers for lactic acidosis in patients with severe sepsis and septic shock. Crit Care Med 2004; 32(12):A151.
27. James JH, Luchette FA, McCarter FD, et al. Lactate is an unreliable indicator of tissue hypoxia in injury or sepsis. Lancet 1999;354(9177):505–8.
28. De Backer D. Lactic acidosis. Minerva Anestesiol 2003;69(4):281–4.
29. Maeder M, Fehr T, Rickli H, et al. Sepsis-associated myocardial dysfunction: diagnostic and prognostic

impact of cardiac troponins and natriuretic peptides. Chest 2006;129(5):1349–66.

30. Rivers EP, McCord J, Otero R, et al. Clinical utility of B-type natriuretic peptide in early severe sepsis and septic shock. J Intensive Care Med 2007; 22(6):363–73.

31. Phua J, Koay ES, Lee KH. Lactate, procalcitonin, and amino-terminal pro-B-type natriuretic peptide versus cytokine measurements and clinical severity scores for prognostication in septic shock. Shock 2008;29(3):328–33.

32. Practice parameters for hemodynamic support of sepsis in adult patients in sepsis. Task force of the American College of Critical Care Medicine, Society of Critical Care Medicine. Crit Care Med 1999; 27(3):639–60.

33. Dorresteijn MJ, van Eijk LT, Netea MG, et al. Iso-osmolar prehydration shifts the cytokine response towards a more anti-inflammatory balance in human endotoxemia. J Endotoxin Res 2005;11(5): 287–93.

34. Packman MI, Rackow EC. Optimum left heart filling pressure during fluid resuscitation of patients with hypovolemic and septic shock. Crit Care Med 1983;11(3):165–9.

35. Dellinger RP, Levy MM, Carlet JM, et al. Surviving sepsis campaign: international guidelines for management of severe sepsis and septic shock: 2008. Crit Care Med 2008;36(1):296–327.

36. Durairaj L, Schmidt GA. Fluid therapy in resuscitated sepsis: less is more. Chest 2008;133(1): 252–63.

37. Shoemaker WC. Relation of oxygen transport patterns to the pathophysiology and therapy of shock states. Intensive Care Med 1987;13(4):230–43.

38. Vincent JL, Gerlach H. Fluid resuscitation in severe sepsis and septic shock: an evidence-based review. Crit Care Med 2004;32(11 Suppl):S451–4.

39. Rackow EC, Falk JL, Fein IA, et al. Fluid resuscitation in circulatory shock: a comparison of the cardiorespiratory effects of albumin, hetastarch, and saline solutions in patients with hypovolemic and septic shock. Crit Care Med 1983;11(11): 839–50.

40. Barron ME, Wilkes MM, Navickis RJ. A systematic review of the comparative safety of colloids. Arch Surg 2004;139(5):552–63.

41. Evidence-based colloid use in the critically ill: American Thoracic Society consensus statement. Am J Respir Crit Care Med 2004;170(11):1247–59.

42. Wiedemann HP, Wheeler AP, Bernard GR, et al. Comparison of two fluid-management strategies in acute lung injury. N Engl J Med 2006;354(24): 2564–75.

43. Estenssoro E, Gonzalez F, Laffaire E, et al. Shock on admission day is the best predictor of prolonged mechanical ventilation in the ICU. Chest 2005;127(2):598–603.

44. Rivers EP. Fluid-management strategies in acute lung injury—liberal, conservative, or both? N Engl J Med 2006.

45. LeDoux D, Astiz ME, Carpati CM, et al. Effects of perfusion pressure on tissue perfusion in septic shock. Crit Care Med 2000;28(8):2729–32.

46. De Backer D, Creteur J, Silva E, et al. Effects of dopamine, norepinephrine, and epinephrine on the splanchnic circulation in septic shock: Which is best? Crit Care Med 2003;31(6):1659–67.

47. Marini JJ, Wheeler AP, editors. Critical care medicine: the essentials. 3rd edition. Philadelphia: Lippincott Williams & Wilkins; 2006. No. 1.

48. Mullner M, Urbanek B, Havel C, et al. Vasopressors for shock. Cochrane Database Syst Rev 2004;(3): CD003709.

49. Levy MM, Macias WL, Vincent JL, et al. Early changes in organ function predict eventual survival in severe sepsis. Crit Care Med 2005;33(10): 2194–201.

50. Trzeciak S, Rivers EP. Clinical manifestations of disordered microcirculatory perfusion in severe sepsis. Crit Care 2005;9(Suppl 4):S20–6.

51. Cerra FB, Hassett J, Siegel JH. Vasodilator therapy in clinical sepsis with low output syndrome. J Surg Res 1978;25(2):180–3.

52. Spronk PE, Ince C, Gardien MJ, et al. Nitroglycerin in septic shock after intravascular volume resuscitation. Lancet 2002;360(9343):1395–6.

53. Vincent J-L, O'Brien J, Wheeler A, et al. Use of an integrated clinical trial database to evaluate the effect of timing of drotrecogin alfa (activated) treatment in severe sepsis. Critical Care 2006;10(3):1–10.

54. Vincent JL, Sakr Y, Sprung C, et al. Are blood transfusions associated with greater mortality rates? Results of the Sepsis Occurrence in Acutely Ill Patients study. Anesthesiology 2008;108(1):31–9.

55. Sakr Y, Chierego M, Piagnerelli M, et al. Microvascular response to red blood cell transfusion in patients with severe sepsis. Crit Care Med 2007.

56. Heyland DK, Cook DJ, King D, et al. Maximizing oxygen delivery in critically ill patients: a methodologic appraisal of the evidence [see comments]. Crit Care Med 1996;24(3):517–24.

57. De Backer D, Creteur J, Dubois MJ, et al. The effects of dobutamine on microcirculatory alterations in patients with septic shock are independent of its systemic effects. Crit Care Med 2006; 34(2):403–8.

58. Qiu HB, Yang Y, Zhou SX, et al. Prognostic value of dobutamine stress test in patients with septic shock. Acta Pharmacol Sin 2001;22(1):71–5.

59. Rhodes A, Lamb FJ, Malagon I, et al. A prospective study of the use of a dobutamine stress test to identify outcome in patients with sepsis, severe

sepsis, or septic shock. Crit Care Med 1999; 27(11):2361–6.

60. Morelli A, De Castro S, Teboul JL, et al. Effects of levosimendan on systemic and regional hemodynamics in septic myocardial depression. Intensive Care Med 2005;31(5):638–44.

61. Nasraway SA, Rackow EC, Astiz ME, et al. Inotropic response to digoxin and dopamine in patients with severe sepsis, cardiac failure, and systemic hypoperfusion. Chest 1989;95(3):612–5.

62. Boulos M, Astiz ME, Barua RS, et al. Impaired mitochondrial function induced by serum from septic shock patients is attenuated by inhibition of nitric oxide synthase and poly(ADP-ribose) synthase. Crit Care Med 2003;31(2):353–8.

63. Karimova A, Pinsky DJ. The endothelial response to oxygen deprivation: biology and clinical implications. Intensive Care Med 2001;27(1):19–31.

64. Benjamin E, Leibowitz AB, Oropello J, et al. Systemic hypoxic and inflammatory syndrome: an alternative designation for "sepsis syndrome". Crit Care Med 1992;20(5):680–2.

65. Goodman RB, Strieter RM, Martin DP, et al. Inflammatory cytokines in patients with persistence of the acute respiratory distress syndrome. Am J Respir Crit Care Med 1996;154(3 Pt 1):602–11.

66. Webert KE, Blajchman MA. Transfusion-related acute lung injury. Curr Opin Hematol 2005;12(6): 480–7.

67. Bernard GR, Vincent JL, Laterre PF, et al. Efficacy and safety of recombinant human activated protein C for severe sepsis. N Engl J Med 2001;344(10): 699–709.

68. Shapiro NI, Howell MD, Talmor D, et al. Implementation and outcomes of the Multiple Urgent Sepsis Therapies (MUST) protocol. Crit Care Med 2006; 34(4):1025–32.

69. Trzeciak S, Dellinger RP, Abate NL, et al. Translating research to clinical practice: a 1-year experience with implementing early goal-directed therapy for septic shock in the emergency department. Chest 2006;129(2):225–32.

70. Talmor D, Greenberg D, Howell MD, et al. The costs and cost-effectiveness of an integrated sepsis treatment protocol. Crit Care Med 2008;36(4):1168–74.

71. Shorr AF, Micek ST, Jackson WL Jr, et al. Economic implications of an evidence-based sepsis protocol: can we improve outcomes and lower costs? Crit Care Med 2007;35(5):1257–62.

72. Frank ED. A shock team in a general hospital. Anesth Analg 1967;46(6):740–5.

73. Sebat F, Johnson D, Musthafa AA, et al. A multidisciplinary community hospital program for early and rapid resuscitation of shock in nontrauma patients. Chest 2005;127(5):1729–43.

74. Nguyen HB, Corbett SW, Steele R, et al. Implementation of a bundle of quality indicators for the early management of severe sepsis and septic shock is associated with decreased mortality. Crit Care Med 2007;35(4):1105–12.

75. Mullon J, Subramanian S, Haro L, et al. Sepsis order set improves adherence to evidence-based practices. Scientific highlights: abstracts of original investigations and case reports. Chest 2006; 130(4 Suppl):134S–5S.

76. Becker ML. LIFE campaign: implementation of sepsis bundle results in significant cost savings. Ann Emerg Med 2007;50(3):S82.

77. McGrath ME, Lada P, Rebholz CM, et al. Does introduction of a sepsis protocol reduce time to antibiotics or improve outcomes for critical septic patients? A before and after study. Ann Emerg Med 2007;50(3):S19–20.

78. Otero RM, Nguyen HB, Huang DT, et al. Early goal-directed therapy in severe sepsis and septic shock revisited: concepts, controversies, and contemporary findings. Chest 2006;130(5):1579–95.

79. Dorman T, Breslow MJ, Lipsett PA, et al. Radial artery pressure monitoring underestimates central arterial pressure during vasopressor therapy in critically ill surgical patients. Crit Care Med 1998; 26(10):1646–9.

80. Pinsky MR, Teboul JL. Assessment of indices of preload and volume responsiveness. Curr Opin Crit Care 2005;11(3):235–9.

81. Osman D, Ridel C, Ray P, et al. Cardiac filling pressures are not appropriate to predict hemodynamic response to volume challenge. Crit Care Med 2007; 35(1):64–8.

82. Michard F, Lopes M, Auler J-O. Pulse pressure variation: beyond the fluid management of patients with shock. Critical Care 2007;11(3):131.

83. Hadian M, Pinsky MR. Functional hemodynamic monitoring. Curr Opin Crit Care 2007;13(3): 318–23.

84. Michard F, Teboul JL. Predicting fluid responsiveness in ICU patients: a critical analysis of the evidence. Chest 2002;121(6):2000–8.

85. Reinhart K, Bloos F. The value of venous oximetry. Curr Opin Crit Care 2005;11(3):259–63.

86. Cuschieri J, Rivers EP, Donnino MW, et al. Central venous-arterial carbon dioxide difference as an indicator of cardiac index. Intensive Care Med 2005;31(6):818–22.

87. Weil MH, Nakagawa Y, Tang W, et al. Sublingual capnometry: a new noninvasive measurement for diagnosis and quantitation of severity of circulatory shock. Crit Care Med 1999;27(7):1225–9.

88. Marik PE. Regional carbon dioxide monitoring to assess the adequacy of tissue perfusion. Curr Opin Crit Care 2005;11(3):245–51.

89. Beaulieu Y. Bedside echocardiography in the assessment of the critically ill. Crit Care Med 2007;35(5 Suppl):S235–49.

90. Prentice D, Sona C. Esophageal Doppler monitoring for hemodynamic assessment. Crit Care Nurs Clin North Am 2006;18(2):189–93, x.

91. Houtchens BA, Westenskow DR. Oxygen consumption in septic shock: collective review. Circ Shock 1984;13(4):361–84.

92. Skarda DE, Mulier KE, Myers DE, et al. Dynamic near-infrared spectroscopy measurements in patients with severe sepsis. Shock 2007;27(4):348–53.

93. Verdant C, De Backer D. How monitoring of the microcirculation may help us at the bedside. Curr Opin Crit Care 2005;11(3):240–4.

94. Finfer S, Bellomo R, Boyce N, et al. A comparison of albumin and saline for fluid resuscitation in the intensive care unit. N Engl J Med 2004;350(22):2247–56.

95. Brunkhorst FM, Engel C, Bloos F, et al. Intensive insulin therapy and pentastarch resuscitation in severe sepsis. N Engl J Med 2008;358(2):125–39.

96. Wiedermann CJ. Systematic review of randomized clinical trials on the use of hydroxyethyl starch for fluid management in sepsis. BMC Emerg Med 2008;8:1–8.

97. Sriskandan S, Altmann DM. The immunology of sepsis. J Pathol 2008;214(2):211–23.

98. Vincent JL, Weil MH. Fluid challenge revisited. Crit Care Med 2006.

99. Martin C, Viviand X, Leone M, et al. Effect of norepinephrine on the outcome of septic shock. Crit Care Med 2000;28(8):2758–65.

100. Marik PE, Mohedin M. The contrasting effects of dopamine and norepinephrine on systemic and splanchnic oxygen utilization in hyperdynamic sepsis. J Am Med Assoc 1994;272(17):1354–7.

101. Beale RJ, Hollenberg SM, Vincent JL, et al. Vasopressor and inotropic support in septic shock: an evidence-based review. Crit Care Med 2004;32(11 Suppl):S455–65.

102. Jakob S. Clinical review: splanchnic ischaemia. Critical Care 2002;6(4):306–12.

103. Sakr Y, Reinhart K, Vincent JL, et al. Does dopamine administration in shock influence outcome? Results of the Sepsis Occurrence in Acutely Ill Patients (SOAP) study. Crit Care Med 2006;34(3):589–97.

104. Parrillo JE, Dellinger RP, editors. Critical care medicine: principles of diagnosis and management in the adult, 3rd edition. Philadelphia: Mosby Elsevier; 2008. p. 1.

105. Landry DW, Levin HR, Gallant EM, et al. Vasopressin deficiency contributes to the vasodilation of septic shock. Circulation 1997;95(5):1122–5.

106. Ertmer C, Morelli A, Bone HG, et al. Dobutamine reverses the vasopressin-associated impairment in cardiac index and systemic oxygen supply in ovine endotoxemia. Crit Care 2006;10(5):1–9.

107. Russell JA, Walley KR, Singer J, et al. Vasopressin versus norepinephrine infusion in patients with septic shock. N Engl J Med 2008;358(9):877–87.

Corticosteroids and Human Recombinant Activated Protein C for Septic Shock

Gwenhaël Colin, MD, Djillali Annane, MD, PhD*

KEYWORDS

- Clinical trials • Cardiovascular system
- Inflammation • Cytokines • Survival • Metaanalysis

Septic shock remains a deadly disease that places a burden on the health care system.[1] Recent advances in the understanding of the pathomechanisms of sepsis have highlighted the complex interplay among the immune, coagulation, and neuroendocrine systems in response to severe infection. The discovery that the imbalance between pro- and anti-inflammatory pathways may have a role has led to the notion that treatment should be aimed at modulating these systems, rather than blocking key steps in the complex cascade of events triggered by an infection. Meanwhile, interest in the use of low-dose corticosteroids has revived and a new class of drugs—recombinant human activated protein C—has been developed. Both therapeutic approaches have shown a promising benefit/risk profile in clinical studies.[2,3] However, more recent studies in different populations failed to confirm findings from initial studies of survival benefits from these treatments. This review summarizes the current knowledge on the benefit/risk profile from low-dose corticosteroids and activated protein C.

CORTICOSTEROIDS
Summary of Putative Effects of Corticosteroids

Corticosteroids interfere with almost all the components of the inflammatory chain (**Table 1**). These effects have been described elsewhere.[4] Briefly, at the molecular level, corticosteroids have very rapid (within minutes) nongenomic effects via interaction with membrane sites or the release of chaperone proteins from the glucocorticoid receptor. These effects include mainly a modulation of cellular responses with a decrease in cell adhesion and phosphotyrosine kinases, and an increase in annexin 1 externalization. Then, in a few hours, mainly through sequestration of transcription factors in the cytosol, corticosteroids induce transrepression, resulting in inhibition of cell trafficking and a decrease in synthesis of proinflammatory mediators, such as cytokines, adhesion molecules, and receptors. Finally, in a few days, corticosteroids induce transactivation with up-regulation of phagocytosis, chemokinesis, and antioxidant

Djillali Annane received funding support through grants from the French Ministry of Health for research related to (1) the prognostic value of corticotropin tests in septic shock, (2) the French multicenter randomized controlled trial on a combination of hydrocortisone and fludrocortisone, (3) the ongoing French multicenter 2×2 factorial study that compares strict glucose control versus conventional treatment for steroid-treated septic shock, and that compares hydrocortisone alone versus a combination of hydrocortisone and fludrocortisone, and (4) the French multicenter 2×2 factorial trial that compares a combination of hydrocortisone and fludrocortisone with activated protein C; with a combination of hydrocortisone, fludrocortisone, and activated protein C; and with placebos for the treatment of septic shock.

Assistance Publique Hôpitaux de Paris, General Intensive Care Unit, Hôpital Raymond Poincaré (AP-HP), Université de Versailles SQY (UniverSud Paris), 104 Boulevard Raymond Poincaré, 92380 Garches, France

* Corresponding author.

E-mail address: djillali.annane@rpc.aphp.fr (D. Annane).

Clin Chest Med 29 (2008) 705–712
doi:10.1016/j.ccm.2008.06.009

Table 1
Putative effects of corticosteroids and activated protein C

	Corticosteroids	Activated Protein C
Inflammation	Reduce inflammation by decreasing cytokines, adhesion molecules, and receptor synthesis; modulating expression of Toll-like receptors 2 and 4; promoting shift toward Th-2 immune response; and stimulating activation of mechanisms for resolving inflammation	Reduces inflammation by inhibiting NF-κB nuclear translocation; and restoring haemostatic balance (leading to indirect anti-inflammatory effects)
Coagulation and fibrinolysis	Promote coagulation by increasing levels of factor VIII and von Willebrand factor; inhibit fibrinolysis by increasing plasminogen activator inhibitor–1 activity; inhibit coagulation by inhibiting platelet aggregation and decreasing tissue factor–mediated procoagulant activity	Inhibits coagulation by inhibiting factors Va and VIIIa; up-regulates fibrinolysis by inactivating plasminogen activator inhibitor–1
Apoptosis	Provide proapoptotic effects upon T-lymphocytes, eosinophils, osteoblasts, osteocysts, fibroblasts; provide antiapoptotic effects on neutrophils, erythroblasts, and cells of the mammary gland, ovaries, and liver	Prevents endothelial cell apoptosis
Haemodynamics	Help maintain vascular tone, endothelium integrity, capillary permeability, myocardial inotropic activity	As consequences of other effects, helps maintain endothelium integrity, vascular permeability

processes, and of various mechanisms of resolution of inflammation. In addition, corticosteroid effects may vary with cell activation state. For example, they can increase or decrease the expression of innate immunity proteins, such as Toll-like receptors 2 and 4.

Glucocorticoids interact with myochardial fibers and smooth muscle in blood vessels, maintaining vascular tone, endothelium integrity, capillary permeability, and myocardial inotropic activity. Glucocorticoids act in synergy with norepinephrine and angiotensin II. The mechanisms of these cardiovascular effects are still unclear. It is likely that very early effects (within minutes) are nongenomic and may result from a direct action of corticosteroids on vascular smooth muscles as well as up-regulation of endothelial nitric oxide synthase. More sustained effects are likely genomic through inhibition of the transcription of the genes' encoding for the inducible nitric oxide synthase and cyclooxygenase type II.

Glucocorticoids have two effects on the coagulation system. In one hand, they inhibit platelet aggregation and attenuate tissue factor–mediated procoagulant activity.[5,6] On the other hand, glucocorticoids increase plasma levels of factors VIII and von Willebrand,[7] thus inhibiting physiologic fibrinolysis as a result of an increase in plasma plasminogen activator inhibitor–1 activity.[8]

Finally, corticosteroids may induce or foster apoptosis in different cells and tissues: T lymphocytes, eosinophils, osteoblasts, osteocytes, the hippocampus, and fibroblasts.[9] They may also prevent premature death of neutrophils, erythroblasts, and cells of the mammary gland, ovaries, and liver.[9]

Summary of Findings in Randomized Controlled Trials

The effects of corticosteroids in patients with severe sepsis or septic shock have been investigated in controlled clinical trials for about half a century. Two meta-analyses highlighted more than a decade ago the unfavorable benefit/risk ratio of a short course of high-dose corticosteroids in sepsis.[10,11] In the 90s, the demonstration that an inappropriate endogenous neuroendocrine response to infection plays a role in the pathomechanisms and prognosis of sepsis has prompted renewed interest in the use of corticosteroids at lower doses and for a longer period.[12,13] Recently, the term *critical illness–related corticosteroid insufficiency* (CIRCI) has been introduced to help recognize this complication of sepsis. Briefly, CIRCI can result from impaired cortisol synthesis or tissue resistance to corticosteroids.

Several small studies have reported a decrease in the duration of vasopressor therapy withdrawal with low doses of corticosteroids.[14–18] Two of these studies suggested a survival benefit from a long course of low-dose corticosteroids.[14,16] There are two large, multicenter, randomized, placebo-controlled, double-blind studies[2,19] evaluating the efficacy and safety of a low dose of corticosteroids in septic shock. In the first study, 300 vasopressor- and ventilator-dependent septic shock patients were randomized within the first 8 hours to receive 50 mg hydrocortisone as intravenous bolus every 6 hours and 50 µg of fludrocortisone via the gastric tube once a day for 7 days. More patients in the corticosteroid group than in the placebo group had shock reversed (57% versus 40%). Also, among those patients whose shock was reversed, reversal occurred faster in the corticosteroid group than in the placebo group (approximately 2 days earlier). Twenty-eight-day mortality was significantly decreased in the experimental group (61% versus 55%). Corticosteroid effects were mostly seen in the group of patients who did not respond to a short corticotrophin test (63% versus 53%). No evidence was found for an increased risk of gastroduodenal bleeding, superinfection, or neuromuscular weakness. Subsequently, two updates of the systematic review on the use of corticosteroids in septic shock[20,21] and the Surviving Sepsis Campaign[22] have recommended that low-dose hydrocortisone should be considered in the management of septic shock, although corticosteroid therapy may favor onset of critical illness polyneuromyopathy.[23,24]

More recently, the European Corticosteroid Therapy of Septic Shock (Corticus) trial reported conflicting results.[19] In that study, patients were included if they met all of the following criteria: clinical evidence of infection, two of the four signs of systemic inflammatory response syndrome, a systolic blood pressure less than 90 mm Hg despite adequate fluid replacement or need for vasopressors for at least 1 hour within the previous 72 hours, and at least one sign of hypoperfusion or organ dysfunction attributable to sepsis. Five hundred patients were randomized to receive 50 mg of intravenous hydrocortisone every 6 hours for 5 days, then every 12 hours for 3 days and once daily for 3 days. Fludrocortisone was not used in this study. This study confirmed that hydrocortisone treatment accelerated shock reversal, though at 28 days the proportion of patients with shock reversed was not significantly greater in the treated patients versus those receiving a placebo. In addition, though the rate of specific superinfection was the same for groups, some patients in the hydrocortisone group experienced new episodes of shock. Finally, the corticosteroid therapy increased the risk of hyperglycemia and hypernatremia. The main limitations of the Corticus study included (1) a lack of power with only 500 patients out of the expected 800 and a lower baseline risk of death than expected (observed placebo mortality in the nonresponders 36% versus expected mortality of 50%); and (2) a selection bias with a very slow recruitment rate following the loss of equipoise among the investigators, resulting in predominantly surgical sepsis with an intra-abdominal source.

Thus, the French study and Corticus came to opposite conclusions with some similarities and major differences between the two studies. Similarities between the two studies included the findings that steroids offer beneficial effects in shortening the time to shock reversal, that the use of steroids did not increase risk of neuromuscular weakness, and that steroids increased the risk of hyperglycemia. Differences between the two studies included:

Differences in timing: time window allowed for inclusion (8 versus 72 hours) resulting in only early septic shock in the French study and both early and late septic shock in the Corticus study

Difference in types, duration, and doses of corticosteroids: fludrocortisone versus no fludrocortisone; treatment duration (7 versus 11 days); weaning (none versus tapering in 6 days)

Differences in populations: severity of shock—systolic blood pressure <90 mm Hg (>1 hour versus <1 hour); general severity of illness—simplified acute physiology II scores (59 versus 49); proportion of nonresponders to corticotrophin (77% versus 47%); proportion of medical patients (66% versus 36%); primary source of infection (lung versus abdomen)

Differences in context: practice guidelines not recommending steroids versus guidelines recommending use of hydrocortisone

Summary of Current Recommendations

A recent update of the Cochrane systematic review of corticosteroids for severe sepsis and septic shock suggested that a prolonged (>5 days) treatment with low-dose hydrocortisone (200 mg per day of hydrocortisone or equivalent) is associated with survival benefit. This meta-analysis included 12 trials accounting for 1230 patients. The relative risk of death was 0.86 (95% CI: 0.75–0.98) in favor of corticosteroids. There was no evidence for heterogeneity across the studies (heterogeneity: $\chi^2_{11} = 11.29$ ($P = .42$); $I^2 = 3\%$).

The Surviving Sepsis Campaign has recently updated the guidelines for the use of corticosteroids on the basis of the most recent data, including Corticus findings.[25] In these guidelines, the Grading of Recommendations Assessment, Development and Evaluation (GRADE) system was used to quantify the strength of the recommendation. Given that the two largest trials had conflicting results, the grade could only be 2 (ie, a suggestion) and not a 1 (ie, a recommendation). Given that the two trials focused on very different populations, the recommendation tried to limit the use of corticosteroids to those patients mimicking entry criteria in the French trial:

We suggest intravenous hydrocortisone should be given only to adult septic shock patients after blood pressure is identified to be poorly responsive to fluid resuscitation and vasopressor therapy (2C).

The guidelines did not recommend the use of fludrocortisones, nor did they recommend guiding corticosteroid therapy on the results of the Synacthen test.

Subsequently, given the broad use of corticosteroids and the remaining uncertainty surrounding their benefit/risk profile in different septic shock populations, further adequately powered clinical trials are needed. Such trials are ongoing. Two large randomized controlled trials, NCT00320099 and NCT00368381, are comparing the efficacy and safety of hydrocortisone alone versus hydrocortisone plus fludrocortisone in septic shock. Another randomized trial, NCT00625209, has a 2×2 factorial design to compare hydrocortisone and fludrocortisone with each other, with a recombinant human activated protein C, with a combination of these, and with placebos.

HUMAN RECOMBINANT ACTIVATED PROTEIN C
Summary of Putative Effects

An imbalance from an increased activation of coagulation and a decrease in fibrinolysis is the hallmark of sepsis (see **Table 1**). The subsequent generation of thrombi in the vessels may impair organ perfusion and may activate the endothelium and immune cells. The protein C pathway plays a key role in preventing microvascular thrombosis. Indeed, the thrombin-thrombomodulin complex activates protein C, which in turn binds to protein S and inhibits the coagulation factors Va and VIIIa, which are necessary for thrombin formation. Moreover, activated protein C up-regulates fibrinolysis mainly by inactivating plasminogen activator inhibitor–1. Additionally, activation of endothelial cell protein C receptor (EPCR) increases protein C activation.[26]

By restoring the haemostatic balance in sepsis, activated protein C has indirect anti-inflammatory effects. Indeed, thrombin fosters the release of inflammatory mediators. Activated protein C is also likely to have direct effects on inflammation. For example, the binding of activated protein C to EPCR prevents the translocation of nuclear factor κ B to the nucleus.[27]

A growing body of evidence indicates that activated protein C favorably modulates endothelial cell apoptosis. In fact, activation of EPCR up-regulates endothelial protease activated receptor–1, the phosphorylation rate of mitogen-activated protein kinases, and Bcl2-homolog protein (inhibiting apoptosis); and down-regulates p53, a well-known proapoptotic factor.[28–30]

Summary of Findings in Randomized Clinical Trials

The Recombinant Human Protein C Worldwide Evaluation in Severe Sepsis (Prowess) study[3] was a phase III randomized, double-blind, placebo-controlled, multicenter trial that investigated the efficacy and safety of a recombinant human activated protein C, drotrecogin alpha activated (Drot-AA). The study included 1690 patients with a known or suspected infection, three or four criteria of the systemic inflammatory response syndrome, and one or more sepsis-induced organ dysfunction. The treatment was infused at a dose of 24 μg/kg/h for 96 hours and was initiated within 24 hours after the patients met inclusion criteria. The dose was previously defined in a phase II trial as the dose associated with the best effects on serum D-dimer and IL-6 levels.[31] The primary endpoint was 28-day mortality. The study was stopped prematurely after the second interim analysis for treatment efficacy. The mortality rate was 30.8% in the placebo group and 24.7% in the Drot-AA group ($P = .005$). The relative risk of death was 0.80 (95% CI: 0.69–0.94). The absolute reduction of mortality was 6.1% (1.9%–10.4%).

The treatment effect on survival was unrelated to serum levels of activated protein C. The study drug was associated with an increased risk of serious bleeding (3.5% versus 2%, $P = .06$), with 0.2% of patients with intracranial bleeding. The study had some limitations, including amendment of the protocol after enrolment of 720 patients to modify exclusion criteria and to change the placebo (0.9% sodium chloride solution was replaced by 0.1% human serum albumin) and, 5 months later, a modification in the manufacturing of the study drug. Interestingly, regulatory agencies in the United States and in Europe approved the marketing of Drot-AA in Prowess subgroups. The US Food and Drug Administration defined the subgroup as those with an Acute Physiology and Chronic Health Evaluation (APACHE) II score of 25 or more. The European Agency for the Evaluation of Medical Products defined the subgroup according to the presence of two or more organs with sepsis-induced dysfunctions. It was thought that the benefit/risk profile was best in the sickest patients.[32] Indeed, post hoc analyses of the Prowess study showed a trend toward higher mortality rates in Drot-AA–treated patients whose APACHE II score was below 20 (15.1% versus 12.1% for placebo), and no evidence for patients whose APACHE II score was between 20 and 24, or for those who had a single organ dysfunction.

Regulatory agencies requested additional randomized controlled trials to evaluate the benefit/risk profile of Drot-AA in (1) patients with mild to moderate sepsis (ie, APACHE II score of less than 25 or one organ dysfunction), (2) children with sepsis, and (3) patients with concomitant heparin treatment.

The efficacy and safety of Drot-AA, at a dose of 24 μg/kg/h for 96 hours, in mild to moderate sepsis was investigated in the Administration of Drotrecogin Alfa (Activated) in Early Stage Severe Sepsis (Address) study group.[33] This was a randomized, double-blind, placebo-controlled, multicenter clinical trial. Patients were included if they had a suspected or known infection, a sepsis-induced organ dysfunction, and were not eligible for commercially available Xigris (ie, they had an APACHE II score of less than 25 if they were United States patients, or, if they were European patients, they had two or more organ dysfunctions). The study was stopped for futility after the second interim analysis and inclusion of 2640 patients. There was no evidence for a difference in 28-day mortality between placebo and Drot-AA (17.0% versus 18.5%). There was a significant increase in the rate of serious bleeding with Drot-AA (3.9% versus 2.2%, $P = .02$). Interestingly enough, in the United States, patients with an APACHE II score of less

than 25 and two or more organ dysfunctions could have been enrolled in this study. Similarly, in Europe, patients with one organ dysfunction and an APACHE II score of more than 25 could have been enrolled in the Address trial. Then, post hoc analysis in patients with an APACHE II score of more than 25 showed a 28-day mortality of 24.7% and 29.5% in the placebo and Drot-AA groups, respectively. In patients with two or more organ dysfunctions, 28-day mortality rates were 21.9% and 20.7% in the placebo and Drot-AA groups, respectively. Nevertheless, in these two populations with severe sepsis among the Address population, the basal risk of death was much lower than in the corresponding subgroups from the Prowess trial. In the subgroup of patients with APACHE II scores of 25 or more, placebo mortality was 27.4% versus 43.7% in the Address and Prowess trials, respectively. In the subgroup of patients with two or more organ dysfunctions, it was 21.9% versus 33.9%, respectively.

In both the Prowess and Address trials, exploratory analysis suggested an increased 28-day mortality in patients who had one organ dysfunction and a recent surgery before Drot-AA treatment.

One phase III randomized controlled trial (the Researching Severe Sepsis and Organ Dysfunction in Children: A Global Perspective [Resolve] trial) investigated the benefit/risk profile of Drot-AA at a dose of 24 μg/kg/h for 96 hours in 477 children with severe sepsis.[34] Children were eligible if they were between 38 weeks corrected gestational age and 17 years old; had suspected or proven infection; showed signs of systemic inflammation; and had cardiovascular and respiratory organ dysfunctions. The primary objective was to calculate a composite score called the Composite Time to Complete Organ Failure Resolution (CTCOFR). There was no evidence for a difference in CTCOFR or in 28-day mortality (17.5% versus 17.2%). Drot-AA treatment was associated with an increase in the risk of intracranial bleeding (4.6% versus 2.6% of episodes), particularly in the youngest patients.

The interaction between Drot-AA and heparin was tested in the Xigris and Prophylactic Heparin Evaluation in Severe Sepsis (X-Press) randomized controlled trial. In this trial, 1994 patients eligible for commercially available Xigris were randomized to receive heparin or a placebo every 12 hours during Drot-AA infusion. This was an equivalence-design trial. Twenty-eight–day mortality rates were 28.3% versus 31.9% ($P = .09$) in the heparin and placebo-treated patients, respectively. There was no evidence for an increased proportion of serious bleeding events with the use of prophylactic heparin (3.8% versus 5.2%, $P = .06$). There were fewer

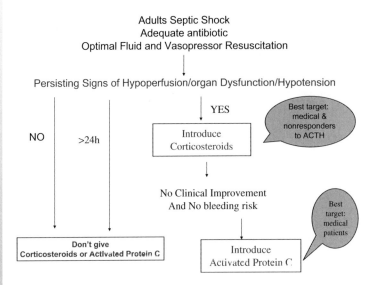

Fig. 1. Treatment plan for patients with vasopressor-dependent septic shock with persistent signs of hypoperfusion, organ dysfunction, or hypotension. ACTH, corticotropin.

ischemic strokes in the heparin-treated patients (0.5% versus 1.8%, $P = .01$). Interestingly enough, patients who were receiving heparin before randomization and were allocated to heparin had a lower 28-day mortality rate than the placebo-treated patients (26.9% versus 35.6%, $P = .03$).

Recommendations

A recent Cochrane systematic review[35] suggested that the use of Drot-AA be suspended pending the results of additional trials. This systematic review included four studies accounting for 4911 patients. In the group of patients with an APACHE II score of less than 25, the relative risk of death was 1.04 (95% CI: 0.89–1.21, $P = .70$). In the group of patients with an APACHE II score of 25 or more, the relative risk of death was 0.90 (95% CI: 0.54–1.49).

The recent update of the Surviving Sepsis Campaign yielded different conclusions.[25] The panel of experts suggested:

that adult patients with sepsis-induced organ dysfunction associated with a clinical assessment of high risk of death, most of whom will have Acute Physiology and Chronic Health Evaluation (APACHE) II of 25 or more, or multiple organ failure, receive rhAPC [recombinant activated protein C] if there are no contraindications (grade 2B except for patients within 30 days of surgery, for whom it is grade 2C).

They also recommended

that adult patients with severe sepsis and low risk of death, most of whom will have

APACHE II <20 or one organ failure, do not receive rhAPC (grade 1A).

The benefit/risk profile of Drot-AA is likely inversely related to the time elapsed from onset of the first sepsis-induced organ dysfunction, with maximal benefit if administered within the first 24 hours.[36] In addition, its benefit/risk profile may be greater in the medical population than among surgical patients. Finally, prophylactic heparin should not be stopped when initiating Drot-AA.

Given the very low rate of prescription of Xigris in practice, and given the uncertainty surrounding the criteria to identify the population with the optimal benefit/risk profile, additional trials are needed. Upon the request of the European Agency for the Evaluation of Medical Products, drug maker Eli Lilly and Co. has launched a new multinational, randomized, placebo-controlled, double-blind trial (NCT00604214) to clarify the efficacy and safety of a treatment with 24 µg/kg/h for 96 hours with Drot-AA in 1500 patients with severe septic shock. Another trial (NCT00625209), this one academic-driven, has been launched in France and will compare, in a 2×2 factorial design, the efficacy and safety of low doses of corticosteroids, Drot-AA, their combination, and placebos, in 1280 cases of severe septic shock.

SUMMARY

In addition to antibiotic therapy and symptomatic treatment, low doses of corticosteroids and activated protein C should still be considered as valuable adjuvant therapies in patients with septic shock. For both therapies, good experimental and clinical evidence shows their efficacy in decreasing septic shock morbidity and mortality. Both drugs may have serious adverse events. Therefore, ongoing investigations aim at defining the optimal target population for corticosteroids and activated protein C. In the meantime, physicians should consider using low-dose corticosteroids and Drot-AA in the treatment of patients with vasopressor-dependent septic shock with persistent signs of hypoperfusion, organ dysfunction, or hypotension (**Fig. 1**). The optimal timing for initiating these treatments is from 6 to 24 hours from onset of shock. When patients are receiving these drugs, physicians should systematically screen for superinfection and serious bleeding events.

REFERENCES

1. Angus DC, Linde-Zwirble WT, Lidicker J, et al. Epidemiology of severe sepsis in the United States: analysis of incidence, outcome, and associated costs of care. Crit Care Med 2001;29(7):1303–10.
2. Annane D, Sebille V, Charpentier C, et al. Effect of treatment with low doses of hydrocortisone and fludrocortisone on mortality in patients with septic shock. JAMA 2002;288(7):862–71.
3. Bernard GR, Vincent JL, Laterre PF, et al. Efficacy and safety of recombinant human activated protein C for severe sepsis. N Engl J Med 2001;344(10): 699–709.
4. Galon J, Franchimont D, Hiroi N, et al. Gene profiling reveals unknown enhancing and suppressive actions of glucocorticoids on immune cells. FASEB J 2002;16(1):61–71.
5. Muhlfelder TW, Niemetz J, Kang S. Glucocorticoids inhibit the generation of leukocyte procoagulant (tissue factor) activity. Blood 1982;60(5):1169–72.
6. van Giezen JJ, Jansen JW. Inhibition of fibrinolytic activity in-vivo by dexamethasone is counterbalanced by an inhibition of platelet aggregation. Thromb Haemost 1992;68(1):69–73.
7. Jorgensen KA, Sorensen P, Freund L. Effect of glucocorticosteroids on some coagulation tests. Acta Haematol 1982;68(1):39–42.
8. Patrassi GM, Sartori MT, Livi U, et al. Impairment of fibrinolytic potential in long-term steroid treatment after heart transplantation. Transplantation 1997; 64(11):1610–4.
9. Schmidt S, Rainer J, Ploner C, et al. Glucocorticoid-induced apoptosis and glucocorticoid resistance: molecular mechanisms and clinical relevance. Cell Death Differ 2004;11(Suppl 1):S45–55.
10. Lefering R, Neugebauer EA. Steroid controversy in sepsis and septic shock: a meta-analysis. Crit Care Med 1995;23(7):1294–303.
11. Cronin L, Cook DJ, Carlet J, et al. Corticosteroid treatment for sepsis: a critical appraisal and meta-analysis of the literature. Crit Care Med 1995; 23(8):1430–9.
12. Annane D, Sebille V, Troche G, et al. A 3-level prognostic classification in septic shock based on cortisol levels and cortisol response to corticotropin. JAMA 2000;283(8):1038–45.
13. Briegel J, Schelling G, Haller M, et al. A comparison of the adrenocortical response during septic shock and after complete recovery. Intensive Care Med 1996;22(9):894–9.
14. Bollaert PE, Charpentier C, Levy B, et al. Reversal of late septic shock with supraphysiologic doses of hydrocortisone. Crit Care Med 1998;26(4):645–50.
15. Briegel J, Forst H, Haller M, et al. Stress doses of hydrocortisone reverse hyperdynamic septic shock: a prospective, randomized, double-blind, single-center study. Crit Care Med 1999;27(4):723–32.
16. Cicarelli DD, Vieira JE, Bensenor FE. Early dexamethasone treatment for septic shock patients: a prospective randomized clinical trial. Sao Paulo Med J 2007;125(4):237–41.
17. Keh D, Boehnke T, Weber-Cartens S, et al. Immunologic and hemodynamic effects of "low-dose" hydrocortisone in septic shock: a double-blind, randomized, placebo-controlled, crossover study. Am J Respir Crit Care Med 2003;167(4):512–20.
18. Oppert M, Schindler R, Husung C, et al. Low-dose hydrocortisone improves shock reversal and reduces cytokine levels in early hyperdynamic septic shock. Crit Care Med 2005;33(11):2457–64.
19. Sprung CL, Annane D, Keh D, et al. Hydrocortisone therapy for patients with septic shock. N Engl J Med 2008;358(2):111–24.
20. Annane D, Bellissant E, Bollaert PE, et al. Corticosteroids for severe sepsis and septic shock: a systematic review and meta-analysis. BMJ 2004; 329(7464):480.
21. Minneci PC, Deans KJ, Banks SM, et al. Meta-analysis: the effect of steroids on survival and shock during sepsis depends on the dose. Ann Intern Med 2004;141(1):47–56.
22. Dellinger RP, Carlet JM, Masur H, et al. Surviving Sepsis Campaign guidelines for management of severe sepsis and septic shock. Crit Care Med 2004;32(3):858–73.
23. De Jonghe B, Sharshar T, Lefaucheur JP, et al. Paresis acquired in the intensive care unit: a prospective multicenter study. JAMA 2002;288(22): 2859–67.
24. Herridge MS, Cheung AM, Tansey CM, et al. One-year outcomes in survivors of the acute respiratory distress syndrome. N Engl J Med 2003;348(8): 683–93.
25. Dellinger RP, Levy MM, Carlet JM, et al. Surviving sepsis campaign: international guidelines for management of severe sepsis and septic shock: 2008. Crit Care Med 2008;36(1):296–327.

26. Haley M, Cui X, Minneci PC, et al. Activated protein C in sepsis: emerging insights regarding its mechanism of action and clinical effectiveness. Curr Opin Infect Dis 2004;17(3):205–11.

27. Yuksel M, Okajima K, Uchiba M, et al. Activated protein C inhibits lipopolysaccharide-induced tumor necrosis factor–alpha production by inhibiting activation of both nuclear factor–kappa B and activator protein–1 in human monocytes. Thromb Haemost 2002;88(2):267–73.

28. Cheng T, Liu D, Griffin JH, et al. Activated protein C blocks p53-mediated apoptosis in ischemic human brain endothelium and is neuroprotective. Nat Med 2003;9(3):338–42.

29. Domotor E, Benzakour O, Griffin JH, et al. Activated protein C alters cytosolic calcium flux in human brain endothelium via binding to endothelial protein C receptor and activation of protease activated receptor–1. Blood 2003;101(12):4797–801.

30. Mosnier LO, Griffin JH. Inhibition of staurosporine-induced apoptosis of endothelial cells by activated protein C requires protease-activated receptor-1 and endothelial cell protein C receptor. Biochem J 2003;373(Pt 1):65–70.

31. Bernard GR, Ely EW, Wright TJ, et al. Safety and dose relationship of recombinant human activated protein C for coagulopathy in severe sepsis. Crit Care Med 2001;29(11):2051–9.

32. Ely EW, Laterre PF, Angus DC, et al. Drotrecogin alfa (activated) administration across clinically important subgroups of patients with severe sepsis. Crit Care Med 2003;31(1):12–9.

33. Abraham E, Laterre PF, Garg R, et al. Drotrecogin alfa (activated) for adults with severe sepsis and a low risk of death. N Engl J Med 2005;353(13):1332–41.

34. Nadel S, Goldstein B, Williams MD, et al. Drotrecogin alfa (activated) in children with severe sepsis: a multicentre phase III randomised controlled trial. Lancet 2007;369(9564):836–43.

35. Marti-Carvajal A, Salanti G, Cardona A. Human recombinant activated protein C for severe sepsis. Cochrane Database Syst Rev 2008;(1):CD004388.

36. Vincent JL, Bernard GR, Beale R, et al. Drotrecogin alfa (activated) treatment in severe sepsis from the global open-label trial ENHANCE: further evidence for survival and safety and implications for early treatment. Crit Care Med 2005;33(10):2266–77.

Glucose Control in Sepsis

B. Taylor Thompson, MD

KEYWORDS

- Insulin therapy • Critical illness

Hyperglycemia is common in critically ill patients and is associated with increased morbidity and mortality.[1–3] Intravenous insulin therapy (IIT), adjusted to target the range of 80 to 110 mg/dL, reduces mortality in critically ill adult surgical and medical patients but not in a follow-up trial focuses solely on patients who have septic shock.[4–6] A recent consensus statement on the treatment of patients who have severe sepsis recommended a target blood glucose level of less than 150 mg/dL.[7] This is a lower level than prior usual care practices that generally began insulin therapy for blood glucose values exceeding the 180 to 200 mg/dL range during critical illness. A review of published protocols for insulin titration during critical illness showed marked variability in approaches, and the protocols used in the aforementioned trials were paper-based guidelines rather than explicit protocols. Thus it is difficult to know exactly how insulin was dosed during these trials. Furthermore, the nursing effort required to interpret an adequately explicit protocol can be substantial, and IIT increases the risk of hypoglycemia.[4–6,8,9] It remains unclear if self-limited episodes of hypoglycemia contribute to short-term mortality and long-term neurocognitive complications or both. It is increasingly clear, however, that patients who have severe sepsis are at increased risk for hypoglycemia during IIT.[10–12] In this article, the evidence supporting tight glycemic control and the tools available to accomplish it are reviewed.

STRESS HYPERGLYCEMIA AND MORTALITY

Hyperglycemia has been defined as blood glucose levels greater than 120 mg/dL in healthy fasting children, greater than 106 mg/dL (95th percentile) in healthy fasting adults, and greater than 110 in critically ill adults.[13] Plasma and serum levels of glucose are approximately 12% higher than whole blood. Arterial (and capillary) blood glucose concentrations are 2 to 5 mg/dL higher than venous blood, and this gradient is larger after a glucose load.[13] Plasma, capillary, and whole blood glucose measurements often are used interchangeably in ordinary care ICU practices, although caution is warranted. Glucose values determined by point-of-care testing of capillary blood glucose may overestimate arterial blood glucose when values are low, and the degree of overestimation can impact clinical decision making.[14]

Stress-induced hyperglycemia during critical illness is common.[3,15] In one study, septic patients without underlying diabetes had average plasma glucose values of 194 plus or minus 66 mg/dL in the absence of nutritional support, and more than 50% of all patients developed stress-induced hyperglycemia.[16] Stress hyperglycemia is common in critically ill children also, and the magnitude of the hyperglycemia is associated with mortality.[1,2] Stress hyperglycemia is a physiologic response caused by insulin resistance, glycogenolysis, and increased hepatic gluconeogenesis from the release of catecholamines, cortisol, and glucagon.[15,17,18] In the setting of sepsis or endotoxemia, stress hyperglycemia is promoted by the production of inflammatory cytokines (interleukin [IL]-6, tumor necrosis factor α [TNF-α]).[15,19]

Long-term hyperglycemia is associated with complications that can be improved with better glycemic control. In addition, there is increasing observational evidence that short-term hyperglycemia is deleterious in critically ill and injured patients. For instance, the incidence of postoperative wound infections is increased significantly in diabetic patients with hyperglycemia, and glycemic control in diabetic patients has reduced post-surgical infections.[20,21] Gore and colleagues[22] demonstrated that hyperglycemic pediatric burn patients had an increased rate of bacteremia and fungemia and an increase in the failure rate of

Department of Medicine, Pulmonary and Critical Care Unit, Medical Intensive Care Unit, Massachusetts General Hospital, Harvard Medical School, 55 Fruit Street, Boston, MA 02114, USA
E-mail address: tthompson1@partners.org

Clin Chest Med 29 (2008) 713–720
doi:10.1016/j.ccm.2008.06.002

skin grafts compared with nonhyperglycemic patients. Stress-induced hyperglycemia also is associated with an increase in the risk of death, congestive heart failure, and cardiogenic shock after myocardial infarction and an increase in mortality after ischemic stroke.[15,20,23] Higher glucose concentrations have been reported in patients who have infections than in uninfected controls.[24] Hyperglycemia was an independent predictor of poor outcome in 267 patients who had severe head injury.[25] In children who had head injury and hyperglycemia, and its persistence over time, were important predictors of poor outcome.[26–28] These observational studies demonstrate strong associations between hyperglycemia and poor clinical outcomes, but they do not demonstrate a cause–effect relationship. The association could be expected given that the degree of stress hyperglycemia appears to be proportional to the severity of critical illness and the intensity of treatment.

INTENSIVE INSULIN THERAPY FOR STRESS HYPERGLYCEMIA

Van den Berghe and colleagues[6] reported reduced mortality with IIT (continuous insulin infusions to target an arterial blood glucose concentration of 80 to 110 mg/dL (or 4.4 to 6.1 mmol/L) in a single-center study of patients in a cardiac surgical ICU (CSICU). IIT was compared with a representative usual care practice that began insulin therapy when blood glucose concentrations exceeded 180 to 200 mg/dL. In the intention- to-treat analysis, IIT resulted in a 3.4% absolute reduction in mortality. For patients who required intensive care for more the 5 days, there was a relative reduction in mortality of 48% (9.6% absolute), giving a number needed to treat (NNT) of approximately 10. The intensive insulin group also had decreased length of ICU stay, shorter duration of ventilator support, less renal impairment and need for dialysis, less electrophysiologic evidence for critical illness polyneuropathy, fewer bloodstream infections, fewer transfusions, and lower TISS-28 scores (a measure of how many interventions a patient requires). The survival benefit lasted through the hospital stay and persisted to 4 years in the cardiac surgical subset.[6,29]

In a subsequent quality improvement effort from a mixed medical and surgical ICU in a community hospital, Krinsley[30] reported that mortality was reduced by 29% (P = .002) in 800 consecutive patients managed with a paper-based insulin protocol that lowered mean plasma glucose to 133 mg/dL (target less than 140 mg/dL), when compared with 800 consecutive historical controls in whom mean plasma glucose was 152 mg/dL (P<.001). The proportion of plasma glucose values less than 40 mg/dL was 0.35% in the historical controls and 0.34% during the intervention. Furthermore, the subset of patients who had severe sepsis appeared to benefit from improved glucose control. Finney and colleagues[31] demonstrated an association with better outcome and glucose levels in a prospective cohort study of 531 adult ICU patients treated with insulin. Gore and colleagues[22] also demonstrated that improved glucose control reduced mortality from 27% to 4% in a prospective study of pediatric burn patients.

Based on these observations, intensivists changed their practices in an attempt to better control glucose during critical illness. In a recent editorial, Krinsley[32] commented that the first Van den Berghe study was the study that "launched a thousand protocols." Change likely was driven by the large effect size in the longer stay CSICU patients, plausibility given the strong association with hyperglycemia and poor outcomes in prior observational trials, and the strong pathophysiologic rationale for benefit. Subsequent trials, however, have left clinicians less enthusiastic.

One such trial was a follow-up study of 1200 patients enrolled from three medical intensive care units.[5] Medical ICU patients with an expected ICU length of stay of 3 or more days were randomized to IIT using the same Leuven guidelines used in the CSICU cohort. The control group received less intensive therapy with the same targets for blood glucose used in the earlier trial in surgical patients.[6] Overall, there was no mortality benefit with IIT in the intention-to-treat analysis, yet the duration of mechanical ventilation was reduced. Additionally, the development of new acute kidney injury was less frequent with insulin therapy. In a secondary analysis of patients requiring medical ICU stays more than 7 days, IIT reduced the incidence of critical illness polyneuropathy or myopathy, and patients required prolonged mechanical ventilation less frequently.[33] In the targeted population with a medical ICU length of stay of 3 or more than days, IIT was associated with a similarly large effect size as in the CSICU cohort (10% absolute reduction in mortality from 53% to 43%, P = .009). This subset, however, was difficult to identify a priori as 433 of the 1200 enrolled patients expected to require a medical ICU stay of more than 3 days did not. For this subgroup with a short length of stay, hospital mortality was higher in absolute numbers, either because of an adverse treatment effect or an imbalance favoring the control group (fewer patients randomized to control therapy had support withdrawn).[5]

The first trial to focus exclusively on IIT for patients who had severe sepsis was conducted by the German Competence Network Sepsis investigators as part of a two-by- two factorial design testing crystalloid versus hydroxyethyl starch (HES) in the other factorial.[4] The trial, titled Efficacy of Volume Substitution and Insulin Therapy in Severe Sepsis (VISEP), was stopped early, because IIT was associated with a significant increased rate of hypoglycemic events and trend suggesting an increased ICU length of stay. In the 537 evaluable patients, those randomized to IIT using the Leuven guidelines had a mean glucose of 112 mg/dL versus a mean glucose of 151 mg/dL in the control arm. There was no difference in mortality or organ failures with IIT, although there was a possible interaction of insulin therapy, HES, and the development of renal failure (interaction $P = .06$). The risk of acute renal failure was higher in the HES group overall, and was higher yet in IIT group versus control (odds ratio [OR] 1.69; 95% CI, 1.01 to 3.83). Hypoglycemia (less than or equal to 40 mg/dL) occurred in 17% of IIT patients versus 4% of controls ($P<.001$).[4]

TIMING OF GLUCOSE CONTROL: EARLIER THE BETTER?

One single prospective cohort study observed a significantly better outcome when stress hyperglycemia was controlled earlier during critical illness.[34] After adjusting for severity of illness and comorbidities, patients started on IIT within 48 hours of admission had lower mortality compared than those with delayed initiation of therapy (OR adjusted 0.29, 95% CI .11 to .77). ICU length of stay was shorter, and ventilator free days were greater in the early treatment group. A randomized controlled trial of immediate versus delayed glucose control is underway.

MECHANISM OF THE PUTATIVE BENEFICIAL EFFECTS: INSULIN DOSE OR BLOOD GLUCOSE LEVEL?

The decreased rates of sepsis and blood stream infections noted in the first Van den Berghe[35–39] study may be attributed to improved neutrophil and macrophage function, modulation of the systemic inflammatory response, modulation of circulating lipids, decreased endothelial activation, or counteracting the adverse effects of low mannose-binding lectin levels. The decreased need for dialysis and hemofiltration may reflect prevention of apoptosis in renal cells as result of strict glucose control, the effect of exogenous insulin, or both.[39] Modeling of this CSICU cohort suggested that glucose control per se resulted in the mortality reduction, although insulin dose was associated with the prevention of renal failure. A secondary analysis of two large Van den Berghe[39] trials also indicated that IIT was renoprotective, a finding confirmed by others.[40,41] Normalization of blood glucose (less than 110 mg/dL) was associated with the greatest mortality benefit.

HYPOGLYCEMIA: NUISANCE OR MENACE?

The normal lower bound for blood glucose is dependent on age, ranging from 30 mg/dL in full-term neonates and 60 mg/dL in children to 74 mg/dL (95th percentile) in adults.[13] Values of 50 mg/dL are not uncommon 2 hours after a glucose load, and values as low as 30 mg/dL may be observed in healthy premenopausal women after a 72- hour fast.[13]

The major known risk of insulin infusion is hypoglycemia, and the most feared complication is permanent brain injury. Severe hypoglycemia leads to neuronal cell death caused by an increase in extracellular glutamate, glutamate receptor activation, and resultant excitotoxicity.[42] Extracellular glutamate increases because of a reduction in energy-dependent glutamate reuptake, complicating a reduction in brain metabolism from hypoglycemia. Neuronal death requires blood glucose levels to very low levels for an extended period of time.[42,43] This has led some to question the clinical significance of less severe and presumably less prolonged hypoglycemia during IIT as monitoring of blood glucose in the ICU every 1 to 2 hours is thought to detect hypoglycemia well before injury. Critically ill patients, however, often are sedated heavily, and detection of hypoglycemic symptoms can be difficult.

Astrocyte glycogen stores appear to be a key factor in maintaining neuronal energetics in the absence of glucose.[42,44] Astrocyte glycogen stores are depleted during prolonged hypoglycemia, suggesting that a patient may be particularly vulnerable to permanent central nervous system injury from a second episode shortly following the first. Furthermore, astrocyte glycogen stores are depleted more quickly during anoxia; thus a patient's ability to tolerate hypoglycemia may be impaired significantly after brain ischemic events, such as cardiopulmonary resuscitation or prolonged hypoxemia.[42]

Rates of hypoglycemia vary substantially among studies of insulin therapy in the ICU. Gore and colleagues [22] reported no episodes of hypoglycemia with attempts at glycemic control in pediatric burn patients. Van den Berghe and colleagues[6] reported hypoglycemia (blood glucose less than or equal to 40 mg/dL) in 5% (39 of 765) of the patients who received IIT and in 1% (6 of 783) of the ordinary blood glucose control group in the CSICU study. Of the 39 patients who experienced hypoglycemia in the IIT group, two developed symptomatic hypoglycemia with sweating and agitation. None experienced convulsions or hemodynamic deterioration. Rates of hypoglycemia, however, were much higher (18.7%) in the IIT arm of the follow-up trial of medical ICU patients, and as noted previously, excessive rates of hypoglycemia resulted in the premature termination of the VISEP trial.[4,5] More episodes of hypoglycemia were judged to be serious (19 versus 7 patients, $P = .005$), life-threatening (in 13 versus 6 patients, $P = .05$), or requiring prolonged hospitalization (six patients versus one patient, $P = .05$). No deaths were attributed directly to hypoglycemia.[4]

Long-term neurocognitive complications of hypoglycemia complicating critical illness have not been studied extensively. One trial showed that the combination of hypoxemia and hypoglycemia was associated with impaired neurocognitive outcomes.[11] Hyperglycemia (greater than 180 mg/dL), however, also was associated with impaired visual and spatial abilities, visual memory, slow mental processing, and executive dysfunction following recovery from acute respiratory distress syndrome (ARDS).[10,11] Potential mechanisms of brain injury from hyperglycemia include free radical production, reduction in cerebral blood flow, injury to vascular endothelium, and alterations in blood–brain barrier permeability.[10] Neurocognitive outcomes associated with hyperglycemia have been observed up to 1 year after recovery from ARDS, suggesting they may be permanent.[10,11]

In a nested case–control study of 320 patients, Viesenthorp and colleagues[45] found no association between hypoglycemia and early (5-day) and later (hospital) mortality after controlling for prognostic covariates. Another case–control study of 102 patients who had hypoglycemia matched with 306 controls found that hypoglycemia was associated independently with risk of death (OR adjusted 2.27; 95% CI 1.4 to 3.68).[12] The beneficial effect of controlling blood glucose, however, was far greater that the risk of death from hypoglycemia. A sensitivity analysis suggested that a fourfold increase in the rate of hypoglycemia coupled with a doubling of the attributable mortality risk would be needed to offset the benefit of IIT in this cohort.[12] The rate of hypoglycemia was relatively low in this study, and rates approaching fourfold higher in the IIT versus control arms of recent negative clinical trials bring this risk–benefit question into sharp focus.

Thus clinicians must balance the potential risks of both uncontrolled hyperglycemia and hypoglycemia at a time when there is incomplete information about this trade off. Renal failure, interruption of caloric intake, vasoactive infusions, and continuous venovenous hemofiltration with a bicarbonate replacement solution have been identified as risk factors for hypoglycemia during critical illness,[12,45] Thus judging the risk–benefit ratio for IIT during sepsis is challenging, as many of these risk factors for developing hypoglycemia are commonly present. Furthermore, in multivariate analyses, severe sepsis per se emerges as an independent risk factor for hypoglycemia during IIT.[12] Thus IIT in patients who have severe sepsis requires added vigilance and the use of protocols demonstrated to be safe and effective in this high-risk population.

VARIABILITY OF PROTOCOLS FOR GLUCOSE CONTROL

Wilson and colleagues[46] recently reviewed 12 published insulin therapy protocols for critically ill patients and compared the insulin dosing rules for each protocol. Most simply compare the current and recent glucose values and recommend insulin dose adjustments based on the rate of change of blood glucose. Few use insulin sensitivity factors or calibrate insulin dose based on caloric intake. Wilson managed one patient using the Leuven guidelines, then used this patient's glucose values over a 9-hour period to simulate what 11 additional protocols would have done when presented with this same sequence of glucose values.

The initial insulin dose varied from 2 to 18 U/h for initial blood glucose of 459. Some but not all protocols used bolus dosing initially and for subsequent attempts at glucose control. Protocols also varied in how insulin dose was adjusted when blood glucose was falling. For example, the Leuven protocol, which delivered 115 U of insulin over 9 hours, did not recommend an insulin dose reduction as blood glucose values approached the lower bound of the target range (80 to 110 mg/dL) and a negligible dose reduction when glucose fell through the bottom of the range from 83 to 61 mg/dL (insulin dose reduced from 15 to 14.5 U/h). These differences combined to generate 9-hour total doses of insulin that varied from a low of 27 U to a high of 115 U (mean 67 U). The wide variability in insulin dosing approaches led the authors to the sensible recommendation that clinicians should pay close attention to the choice of a protocol.[46]

It is unclear why such marked variability in insulin dosing approaches has evolved. Presumably, these protocols reflect usual care practices put to paper, with some iterative refinement along the way. There does not appear to be a convergence around a single method of insulin titration during critical illness, in contrast to the standardized approach to titration of unfractionated heparin. This lack of standardization may be because of the complexity of glucose control during critical illness. Insulin sensitivity may vary hour-to-hour as a result of bolus corticosteroids, titration or catecholamines, or changes in severity of illness and the magnitude of the stress response. Certainly, caloric intake can be quite variable over the course of severe sepsis.

Other possible explanations for insulin protocols with such disparate approaches are differences in patient demographics and ICU practices where these protocols were developed. For example, varying prevalence of diabetes or obesity or different approaches to nutrition or corticosteroid use may have shaped insulin dosing practices, and thus local protocols, differently. If these are the reasons behind the variability, then protocol performance would depend on and be linked to the population and clinical environment in which the protocol was developed and tested. The Leuven guideline may be one example with ICU- or practice-specific performance. This protocol was developed and refined in a single CSICU where relatively high rates of parenteral dextrose were used routinely, which may have protected patients from hypoglycemia.[6] When this protocol was exported to three medical ICUs or a consortium of German ICUs participating in the VISEP trial, however, the rates of hypoglycemia tripled.[4,5] The degree to which this difference was caused by differences in interpretation of the protocol, ICU practices, or patient-specific factors is unclear.

It is unlikely that all these protocols are equally safe and effective given the wide variation in approaches.[46] Clinician oversight probably acts to correct deficiencies of these protocols. For example, ICU nurses or physicians may decline or modify a protocol instruction they find troublesome, especially if they have knowledge of the patient's condition that is not accounted for by the protocol's rules. Such an example would be a recent intolerance of enteral feeding, leading clinicians to reduce the insulin infusion rate when the protocol may not have accounted for such a clinical event. It is unclear how often the 12 protocols reviewed by Wilson and colleagues generate troublesome instructions and what the overall override rate for these protocols is.

COMPUTERIZED PROTOCOLS FOR INTRAVENOUS INSULIN THERAPY

Recently, the performance of a few open-loop computerized protocols has been published, and some are commercially available.[47–55] In general, these tools appear to be superior to paper-based IIT protocols for glucose control.[47,48] Unfortunately, with some exceptions, the insulin titration algorithms have not been published. Thus analysis of the protocol rules in the higher-performing protocols for evidence of convergence around a more universal insulin dosing approach is not possible. The percent of protocol overrides has been reported for only one of the many computerized approaches to IIT, and such information is important for judging just how carefully these protocols must be watched to perform as well as they are reported to do.[48,54,56] A rigorous comparison of different protocols likely will require a randomized comparison.

ASSESSING GLUCOSE CONTROL

It is not understand how to assess a given protocol's potential for optimally improving important clinical outcomes. Obviously, a protocol that reduces blood glucose but does not cause hypoglycemia is a start. The optimal target range for blood glucose during an episode of severe sepsis is controversial, however, and cannot be determined for patients who have severe sepsis from the available evidence. Furthermore, it is not clear how one should determine successful glucose control.

One report suggested superiority of reducing the glycemic index, a time-weighted average of values above the normal range as the superior metric versus mean glucose.[57] Another observational cohort study of 7049 critically ill patients suggested that reduced variability in blood glucose, measured by the standard deviation, was equally predictive of adverse outcomes as the mean glucose.[58] This raises the possibility that two protocols that produce the same mean glucose or glycemic index but produce different levels of glucose fluctuation may have different clinical effects. If reduction of glucose variability should be the goal, then perhaps one should seek to limit the spikes in blood glucose that complicate the administration of intravenous medications mixed in dextrose.

More recently, the glycemic penalty index was proposed to be the ideal metric for comparing the effectiveness of different IIT approaches.[59] Founded on a smooth penalty function, this approach assigns weights to high and low glucose values and overcomes confounding by the variation in glucose sampling frequencies recommended by various protocols.[59] Further research is needed to determine the optimal strategy and timing for control of stress hyperglycemia.

GLUCOSE CONTROL AND NURSE WORK

IIT requires a change in clinical behavior and resource use in the ICU.[60] Aragon and colleagues[8] observed 21 ICU nurses performing scheduled blood glucose monitoring and making adjustments in insulin therapy. Nurses spent a median of 4.67 minutes per blood work titration cycle, with more time spent when glucose-monitoring supplies were not available or functioning properly. Malesker and colleagues[9] performed a time–motion survey of 452 blood glucose determinations for 38 patients cared for by 47 nurses. The mean time to find a glucometer and measure capillary glucose was 5.18 minutes, and another 10.65 minutes were needed to interpret a paper-based protocol and change the insulin infusion rate. Of 60 nurses responding to a workload survey, 70% indicated that the paper-based protocol increased their workload, and identified the frequency of blood glucose monitoring as the main reason.[9] In contrast, Vogelzag and colleagues [57] surveyed nurses before and after implementation of a computerized IIT system and reported time savings; specifically, time was saved by not needing to call the physician with each blood glucose result and treatment change. Nurses reported that the time saved was devoted to other patient care activities. Additional and more comprehensive evaluations of the impact of IIT approaches on nursing care are needed.

SUMMARY

Patients who have severe sepsis are at increased risk for hypoglycemia during IIT, and the evidence supporting strict normalization of blood glucose in this subset of critically ill patients is conflicting. The recent surviving sepsis guidelines recommend that blood glucose should be controlled with intravenous insulin to achieve levels below 150 mg/dL after initial stabilization of the patient with severe sepsis (a level 2B recommendation). The 150 mg/dL target represents a compromise between the traditional approach and the intensive approach pending the results of adequately powered studies. The guidelines further recommend the use of a validated insulin titration protocol, glucose monitoring every 1 to 2 hours, and the provision of a caloric source while on insulin therapy.

A protocol that is simple, easy to use, limits nurse work, and reduces blood glucose levels without causing hypoglycemia is the current goal, and computerized open-loop systems appear to be better able to accomplish most of these aims. If future research confirms that strict normalization of blood glucose, avoidance of

hypoglycemia, and minimal minute-to-minute variation all are needed for optimal outcomes, then continuous glucose monitoring and closed-loop insulin titration systems likely will be needed to accomplish such precision. For now, clinicians should evaluate the performance of their insulin-dosing approaches for patients with severe sepsis carefully, given the increased risk and uncertain consequence of hypoglycemia in this subset.

REFERENCES

1. Srinivasan V, Spinella PC, Drott HR, et al. Association of timing, duration, and intensity of hyperglycemia with intensive care unit mortality in critically ill children. Pediatr Crit Care Med 2004;5(4):329–36.
2. Faustino EV, Apkon M. Persistent hyperglycemia in critically ill children. J Pediatr 2005;146(1):30–4.
3. Vanhorebeek I, Langouche L, Vanden Berghe G. Tight blood glucose control: what is the evidence. Crit Care Med 2007;35(9):S496–502.
4. Brunkhorst FM, Engel C, Bloos F, et al. Intensive insulin therapy and pentastarch resuscitation in severe sepsis. N Engl J Med 2008;358(2):125–39.
5. Van den Berghe G, Wilmer A, Hermans G, et al. Intensive insulin therapy in the medical ICU. N Engl J Med 2006;354(5):449–61.
6. Van den Berghe G, Wouters P, Weekers F, et al. Intensive insulin therapy in the critically ill patients. N Engl J Med 2001;345(19):1359–67.
7. Dellinger RP, Levy MM, Carlet JM, et al. Surviving Sepsis Campaign: international guidelines for management of severe sepsis and septic shock. Intensive Care Med 2008;34:17–60.
8. Aragon D. Evaluation of nursing work effort and perceptions about blood glucose testing in tight glycemic control. Am J Crit Care 2006;15(4):370–7.
9. Malesker MA, Foral PA, McPhillips AC, et al. An efficiency evaluation of protocols for tight glycemic control in intensive care units. Am J Crit Care 2007;16(6):589–98.
10. Herridge MS, Batt J, Hopkins RO. The pathophysiology of long-term neuromuscular and cognitive outcomes following critical illness. Crit Care Clin 2008;24(1):179–99.
11. Hopkins RO, Suchyta MR, Jephson A, et al. Hyperglycemia and neurocognitive outcomes in ARDS survivors. Proceedings of the American Thoracic Society 2005;A36 [abstracts].
12. Krinsley JS, Grover A. Severe hypoglycemia in critically ill patients: risk factors and outcomes. Crit Care Med 2007;35(10):2262–7.
13. Burtis CA, Aswood E, editors. Tietz textbook of clinical chemistry. 3rd edition. Philadelphia: WP Saunders; 1999.
14. Kanji S, Singh A, Tierney M, et al. Standardization of intravenous insulin therapy improves the efficiency

and safety of blood glucose control in critically ill adults. Intensive Care Med 2004;30(5):804–10.

15. McCowen KC, Malhotra A, Bistrian BR. Stress-induced hyperglycemia. Crit Care Clin 2001;17(1):107–24.

16. Frankenfield DC, Omert LA, Badellino MM, et al. Correlation between measured energy expenditure and clinically obtained variables in trauma and sepsis patients. JPEN J Parenter Enteral Nutr 1994;18(5):398–403.

17. Montori VM, Bistrian BR, McMahon MM. Hyperglycemia in acutely ill patients. JAMA 2002;288(17):2167–9.

18. Michie HR. Metabolism of sepsis and multiple organ failure. World J Surg 1996;20(4):460–4.

19. Marette A. Mediators of cytokine-induced insulin resistance in obesity and other inflammatory settings. Curr Opin Clin Nutr Metab Care 2002;5(4):377–83.

20. Golden SH, Peart-Vigilance C, Kao WH, et al. Perioperative glycemic control and the risk of infectious complications in a cohort of adults with diabetes. Diabetes Care 1999;22(9):1408–14.

21. Fietsam R Jr, Bassett J, Glover JL. Complications of coronary artery surgery in diabetic patients. Am Surg 1991;57(9):551–7.

22. Gore DC, Chinkes D, Heggers J, et al. Association of hyperglycemia with increased mortality after severe burn injury. J Trauma 2001;51(3):540–4.

23. Capes SE, Hunt D, Malmberg K, et al. Stress hyperglycemia and prognosis of stroke in nondiabetic and diabetic patients: a systematic overview. Stroke 2001;32(10):2426–32.

24. Kudsk KA, Laulederkind A, Hanna MK. Most infectious complications in parenterally fed trauma patients are not due to elevated blood glucose levels. JPEN J Parenter Enteral Nutr 2001;25(4):174–9.

25. Rovlias A, Kotsou S. The influence of hyperglycemia on neurological outcome in patients with severe head injury. Neurosurgery 2000;46(2):335–42.

26. Chiaretti A, De Benedictis R, Langer A, et al. Prognostic implications of hyperglycaemia in paediatric head injury. Childs Nerv Syst 1998;14(9):455–9.

27. Wass CT, Lanier WL. Glucose modulation of ischemic brain injury: review and clinical recommendations. Mayo Clin Proc 1996;71(8):801–12.

28. Paret G, Tirosh R, Lotan D, et al. Early prediction of neurological outcome after falls in children: metabolic and clinical markers. J Accid Emerg Med 1999;16(3):186–8.

29. Ingles C, Debaveye Y, Milants I, et al. Strict blood glucose control with insulin during intensive care after cardiac surgery: impact on 4-years survival, dependency on medical care, and quality of life. Eur Heart J 2006;27:2716–24.

30. Krinsley JS. Effect of an intensive glucose management protocol on the mortality of critically ill adult patients. Mayo Clin Proc 2004;79(8):992–1000.

31. Finney SJ, Zekveld C, Elia A, et al. Glucose control and mortality in critically ill patients. JAMA 2003;290(15):2041–7.

32. Krinsley J. Glycemic control in critically ill patients: leuven and beyond. Chest 2007;132(1):1–2.

33. Hermans G, Wilmer A, Meersseman W, et al. Impact of intensive insulin therapy on neuromuscular complications and ventilator dependency in the medical intensive care unit. Am J Respir Crit Care Med 2007;175:480–9.

34. Honiden S, Schultz A, Im SA, Nierman DM, et al. Early versus late intravenous insulin administration in critically ill patients. Intensive Care Med 2008; [Epub ahead of print].

35. Hansen TK, Thiel S, Wouters PJ, et al. Intensive insulin therapy exerts anti-inflammatory effects in critically ill patients and counteracts the adverse effect of low mannose-binding lectin levels. J Clin Endocrinol Metab 2003;88(3):1082–8.

36. Langouche L, Vanhorebeek I, Vlasselaers D, et al. Intensive insulin therapy protects the endothelium of critically ill patients. J Clin Invest 2005;115(8):2277–86.

37. Mesotten D, Swinnen JV, Vanderhoydonc F, et al. Contribution of circulating lipids to the improved outcome of critical illness by glycemic control with intensive insulin therapy. J Clin Endocrinol Metab 2004;89(1):219–26.

38. Rassias AJ, Marrin CA, Arruda J, et al. Insulin infusion improves neutrophil function in diabetic cardiac surgery patients. Anesth Analg 1999;88(5):1011–6.

39. Van den Berghe G, Wouters PJ, Bouillon R, et al. Outcome benefit of intensive insulin therapy in the critically ill: insulin dose versus glycemic control. Crit Care Med 2003;31(2):359–66.

40. Schetz M, Vanhorebeek I, Wouters PJ, Wilmer A, et al. Tight blood glucose control is renoprotective in critically ill patients. J Am Soc Nephrol 2008;19:571–8.

41. Thomas G, Rojas MC, Epstein SK, et al. Insulin therapy and acute kidney injury in critically ill patients: a systematic review. Nephrol Dial Transplant 2007;22(10):2849–55.

42. Suh SW, Hamby AM, Swanson RA. Hypoglycemia, brain energetics, and hypoglycemic neuronal death. Glia 2007;55(12):1280–6.

43. Suh SW, Aoyama K, Chen Y, et al. Hypoglycemic neuronal death and cognitive impairment are prevented by poly(ADP-ribose) polymerase inhibitors administered after hypoglycemia. J Neurosci 2003;23:10681–90.

44. Suh SW, Gum ET, Hamby AM, et al. Hypoglycemic neuronal death is triggered by glucose reperfusion and activation of neuronal NADPH oxidase. J Clin Invest 2007;117(4):910–8.

45. Vriesendorp TM, van Santen S, DeVries JH, et al. Predisposing factors for hypoglycemia in the intensive care unit. Crit Care Med 2006;34(1):96–101.

46. Wilson M, Weinreb J, Hoo GW. Intensive insulin therapy in critical care: a review of 12 protocols. Diabetes Care 2007;30(4):1005–11 [Epub ahead of print, January 1009, 2007].

47. Boord JB, Sharifi M, Greevy RA, et al. Computer-based insulin infusion protocol improves glycemia control over manual protocol. J Am Med Inform Assoc 2007;14(3):278–87.

48. Morris A, Orme J, Truwit J, et al. A replicable method for blood glucose control in critically ill patients. Critical Care Medicine 2008;36:1787–95.

49. Juneja R, Roudebush C, Kumar N, et al. Utilization of a computerized intravenous insulin infusion program to control blood glucose in the intensive care unit. Diabetes Technol Ther 2007;9:232–40.

50. Wong X, Singh-Levett I, Hollingsworth L, et al. A novel, model-based insulin and nutrition delivery controller for glycemic regulation in critically ill patients. Diabetes Technol Ther 2006;8:174–90.

51. Davidson PC, Steed RD, Bode BW. Glucommander: a computer-directed intravenous insulin system shown to be safe, simple, and effective in 120,618 h of operation. Diabetes Care 2005;28(10):2418–23.

52. Dortch MJ, Mowery NT, Ozdas A, et al. A computerized insulin infusion titration protocol improves glucose control with less hypoglycemia compared to a manual titration protocol in a trauma intensive care unit. JPEN J Parenter Enteral Nutr 2008;32(1):18–27.

53. Rood E, Bosman RJ, van der Spoel JI, et al. Use of a computerized guideline for glucose regulation in the intensive care unit improved both guideline adherence and glucose regulation. J Am Med Inform Assoc 2005;12(2):172–80.

54. Thompson BT, Orme J, Truwit JD, et al. Multicenter validation of a computer-based clinical decision support tool for glucose control in adult and pediatric intensive care units. Journal of Diabetes Science and Technology 2008;2:357–68.

55. Vogelzang M, Zijlstra F, Nijsten MW. Design and implementation of GRIP: a computerized glucose control system at a surgical intensive care unit. BMC Med Inform Decis Mak 2005;5.38.

56. Morris AH. Rational use of computerized protocols in the intensive care unit. Crit Care 2001;5(5):249–54.

57. Vogelzang M, van der Horst IC, Nijsten MW. Hyperglycaemic index as a tool to assess glucose control: a retrospective study. Crit Care 2004;8(3):R122–7.

58. Egi M, Bellomo R, Stachowski E, et al. Variability of blood glucose concentration and short-term mortality in critically ill patients. Anesthesiology 2006;105(2):244–52.

59. Van Herpe T, De Brabanter J, Beullens M, et al. Glycemic penalty index for adequately assessing and comparing different blood glucose control algorithms. Crit Care 2008;12(1):R24.

60. Ingle S, Underwood C, Blunt M, et al. Tight glycaemic control: impact on nursing staff. Proc Am Thorac Soc 2005;2:A38.

Reducing Mortality in Severe Sepsis: The Surviving Sepsis Campaign

Sean R. Townsend, MD[a],*, Christa Schorr, RN[b],
Mitchell M. Levy, MD[c,d], R. Phillip Dellinger, MD[b]

KEYWORDS

- Sepsis • Bundles • Guidelines • Mortality • Compliance
- Improvement

When the Surviving Sepsis Campaign (SSC) set about its work in 2002, establishing a goal to decrease mortality caused by severe sepsis and septic shock by 25% by 2009, the investigators who began the effort did not know what the future would hold for the project. In many ways, the campaign has become a phenomenon in critical care, attracting supporters and detractors alike. The campaign probably is understood best as something other than a movement in and of itself in the world of critical care medicine. Instead, the campaign is an epiphenomenon of the larger phenomenon of quality improvement that aims to translate clinical science into bedside practice. That phenomenon is revolutionary in its scope.

As the campaign has sought to wend a path toward lower mortality in severe sepsis, varieties of methods, organizational structures, funding sources, and new knowledge itself have evolved. In this article, the history and evolution of the campaign as a public health initiative is traced through its several stages of development. The literature that has characterized clinical experiences with interventions related to the campaign is reviewed and conclusions discussed.

THE SURVIVING SEPSIS CAMPAIGN RATIONALE

Through collaboration of members of the European Society of Intensive Care Medicine (ESICM), International Sepsis Forum (ISF), and the Society of Critical Care Medicine (SCCM), the SSC is aimed at improving the diagnosis, survival, and management of patients who have sepsis by addressing the challenges associated with it. At the outset of the campaign, the clinical leaders involved with the project began with a few premises about severe sepsis as a disease state and the prevailing treatments for severe sepsis:

- Mortality associated with sepsis is unacceptably high and is increasing.
- Physicians may be unaware of all treatment/intervention options.
- Physicians are managing severe sepsis suboptimally; improvements can be made.
- There is hope for new exciting therapies through continuing innovation and research.
- There is no consensus on an outcome target in the care of septic patients.

[a] Division of Pulmonary and Critical Care Medicine, Rhode Island Hospital, Brown University, 593 Eddy Street, APC 756, Providence, RI 02903, USA
[b] Division of Critical Care Medicine, Cooper University Hospital, Robert Wood Johnson Medical School at Camden, University of Medicine and Dentistry of New Jersey Camden, One Cooper Plaza, Camden, NJ 08103, USA
[c] Division of Pulmonary and Critical Care Medicine, Brown University, 593 Eddy Street, Main 7, Providence, RI, USA
[d] Medical Intensive Care Unit, Rhode Island Hospital, 593 Eddy Street, Providence, RI 02903, USA
* Corresponding author.
E-mail address: sean_townsend@brown.edu (S.R. Townsend).

Clin Chest Med 29 (2008) 721–733
doi:10.1016/j.ccm.2008.06.011

- Debate continues on the relative importance and risks/benefits of specific interventions in severe sepsis, but physicians should not lose sight of the fact that these strategies are likely to improve care.
- Severely septic patients do not stop presenting for care while studies are ongoing and/or debated.

In light of those circumstances, the campaign leaders resolved to work with available resources to modify care patterns and elevate physicians' level of knowledge about the disease and treatment options.

The project was aptly named a campaign. In creating the project, the leaders speculated that the development of a successful health care program would necessitate a mobilization of a groundswell of multidisciplinary health care professionals, hospital leaders, administrators, patients, and their families. The campaign was built to provide coordination with experts from the critical care organizations (ESICM, ISF, and SCCM). Funding for the enterprise necessarily began with unrestricted industry educational grants, including those from Edwards Life-Sciences, Eli Lilly and Company, and Baxter. The campaign also received funding from Philips Medical Systems and the Coalition for Critical Care Excellence of the Society of Critical Care Medicine later. Today, the campaign strives to become self-sustaining through nonindustry support, perhaps involving third-party payers or the assistance of grant-making agencies.

A THREE-PHASE CAMPAIGN

The campaign evolved into its present form through three phases. Phase 1 was the introduction of the campaign at several major international critical care medicine conferences, beginning with the ESICM meeting in Barcelona in 2002, and followed by the SCCM meeting in 2003. Viewed in retrospect, the undertaking as conceptualized in phase 1 was a groundbreaking venture into transforming the delivery of health care for severely septic and septic shock patients. Campaign literature from this time highlighted an ambitious mission not commonly seen in health care initiatives, including:

Changing perceptions and behavior
Increasing the pace of change in patterns of care
Influencing public policy
Defining standards of care in severe sepsis

Improving the management of sepsis through targeted initiatives[1]

These aims, which set out to challenge the prevailing standard of care, predated even the 100K Lives Campaign launched by the Institute for Health care Improvement (IHI).[2]

The next most pressing concern for the campaign was the development and publication of guidelines for managing severe sepsis and septic shock (phase 2 of the campaign). Phase 2 consisted of convening an international consensus committee representing 11 international organizations with interest and expertise in sepsis to create evidence-based guidelines for managing severe sepsis and septic shock. These guidelines first were published in March 2004 in *Critical Care Medicine* and April 2004 in *Intensive Care Medicine*.[3,4] Phase 2 recently was revisited with the reconvening of a similarly composed committee to review updates to evidence since the initial publications in 2004. The renewed effort was sponsored by 16 international organizations with interest and expertise in sepsis. After extensive deliberation and with the benefit of an updated evidence-based grading system used to weight the recommendations (the GRADE system), the committee agreed on updated guidelines recommendations, which were published in 2008msimultaneously in the two journals.[5,6]

The evolution of the guidelines from 2004 to 2008 reflected the arc of the campaign as a movement dedicated to improving care, and substantial effort was devoted to improving the way in which the guidelines were funded, evaluated, and ultimately published. The two aspects of the new guidelines that most reflect this maturation were the absence of industry funding in the guidelines development process and the adoption of the GRADE system. The 2008 guidelines revision was sponsored in 2006 by SCCM and ESICM directly and through the courtesy of meeting space provided at the SCCM's Annual Congress (San Francisco, 2006 and Orlando, Florida, 2007) and the International Symposium on Intensive Care and Emergency Medicine (Brussels, Belgium, 2007). The previous guidelines had been criticized for employing an evidence-based grading system that relied on randomized–control trials to a detriment, without providing deference to the consensus opinion of experts and accepted clinical actions not amenable to study.[7] The evidence-based ranking system used for the initial guidelines was chosen, however, because it was the approach most widely accepted by professional critical care societies at that time. For the revision, the campaign leadership chose to adopt the

GRADE system to reflect the most current thinking on evidence-based medicine grading systems.

The adoption of the GRADE system allowed the campaign to expand its consideration of additional factors important to rating the quality of the evidence for or against an intervention. The GRADE system is based on an assessment of the quality of evidence on a topic, followed by assessment of the risks, benefits, burden, and cost. The assessment begins with a rating of the quality of the evidence.[8–10] Generally, randomized control trials are of higher value than observational trials, but if especially well done or if there are limitations in the trial, either may be credited or discredited. The quality of the evidence may be rated high, moderate, low, or very low (grades A, B, C, and D, respectively). Next, the GRADE system classifies recommendations as strong or weak (grades 1 and 2, respectively). The strength of the recommendation includes an assessment of quality of evidence plus other important deliberations and is considered more important than the quality of evidence alone. A strong or weak recommendation reflects the panel's opinion that the beneficial effects of an intervention outweigh the harmful risks.

Once the 2004 guidelines were published, the campaign opened phase 3, an effort to actually implement the care recommended in the guidelines. The campaign, working with the IHI, constructed a set of user-friendly tools to assist clinicians in the challenge of incorporating the new recommendations into bedside care. These tools included educational programs designed to increase awareness and agreement with the recommendations, care bundles to help ensure patients receive the appropriate interventions, and a set of quality indicators designed to assess compliance with the therapies included in the bundles. The campaign designed and deployed a database, downloadable at no cost from the SSC Web site, which enabled participating hospitals to collect data about their performance in management of severe sepsis and review that performance in real time. In concert with its stated mission, the campaign facilitated the formation of networks of hospitals throughout the world to participate in the goals of the campaign.

Fundamental to the creation of the performance improvement program, a set of core changes was distilled from the campaign guidelines and incorporated into two smaller packages. These packages represented key elements of severe sepsis management and are referred to as the sepsis bundles (**Box 1**). Elements of quality care were derived from the guidelines recommendations and included in the bundles if they were (1) likely to impact outcomes in a positive fashion, (2)

> **Box 1**
> **Severe sepsis bundles**
>
> *Sepsis resuscitation bundle*
>
> Serum lactate measured
>
> Blood cultures obtained before antibiotic administration
>
> From the time of presentation, broad-spectrum antibiotics administered within 3 hours for emergency department admissions and 1 hour for non-emergency department ICU admissions
>
> In the event of hypotension and/or lactate greater than 4 mmol/L (36 mg/dL):
>
> > Deliver an initial minimum of 20 mL/kg of crystalloid (or colloid equivalent)
> >
> > Apply vasopressors for hypotension not responding to initial fluid resuscitation to maintain mean arterial pressure (MAP) greater than 65 mm Hg
>
> In the event of persistent hypotension despite fluid resuscitation (septic shock) and/or lactate greater than 4 mmol/L (36 mg/dL):
>
> > Achieve central venous pressure (CVP) of greater than 8 mm Hg
> >
> > Achieve central venous oxygen saturation (ScvO2) of greater than 70%
>
> *Sepsis management bundle*
>
> Low-dose steroids administered for septic shock in accordance with a standardized hospital policy
>
> Drotrecogin alfa (activated) administered in accordance with a standardized hospital policy
>
> Glucose control maintained greater than the lower limit of normal, but less than 150 mg/dL (8.3 mmol/L)
>
> Inspiratory plateau pressures maintained less than 30 cm H_2O for mechanically ventilated patients

---

currently infrequently accomplished, and (3) susceptible to scoring from a review of medical records. The intent in establishing sepsis bundles was to eliminate the piecemeal application of published guidelines that characterizes most clinical environments today and to make it easier for clinicians to bring the thrust of the guidelines into practice.

The sepsis resuscitation bundle has three to seven indicators depending on the presence or absence of hypotension and the presence or absence of persistent hypotension (following initial fluid resuscitation) or lactate greater than 4 mmol/L. For patients without hypotension or a lactate greater than 4 mmol/L, the three indicators for the first 6 hours of treatment are:

> Measure serum lactate
> Obtain blood cultures before antibiotic administration
> Administration of broad-spectrum antibiotics within 3 hours of emergency department triage time and 1 hour for nonemergency department ICU admissions

Time to antibiotics correlates strongly with survival in severe sepsis.[11] Measuring serum lactate is an important component of the 6 hour bundle as it (1) qualifies patients for the bundles if elevated, and (2) if it is greater than 4 mmol/L qualifies the patient for indicators 4, 5, 6, and 7. Indicator 4 is the delivery of an initial minimum of a 20 mL/kg of crystalloid (or colloid equivalent) in the presence of hypotension (systolic pressure less than 90 mm Hg) or lactate greater than 4 mmol/L. The fifth indicator is, in the presence of hypotension, the use of vasopressors as needed to maintain mean arterial pressure greater than 65 mm Hg. In the event of hypotension persisting after the initial fluid therapy or lactate greater than 4 mmol/L, two final indicators in the 6-hour resuscitation bundle are achieved, with insertion of a central venous catheter in the neck or chest to achieve a central venous pressure of greater than 8 mm Hg, and a central venous oxygen saturation of greater than 70% (measured in the superior vena cava). This is in line with the early goal-directed therapy (EGDT) protocol demonstrated to improve survival in sepsis-induced tissue hypoperfusion.[12] In patients who have septic shock, maintaining a mean arterial pressure greater than or equal to 65 mm Hg and achieving normal central venous oxygen saturation have been demonstrated to be the two greatest predictors of survival.[13]

The 24-hour sepsis management bundle consists of four indicators. The first is low-dose steroids administered for septic shock in accordance with a standardized hospital policy. The current guidelines' recommendation for use of steroids in septic shock is for use only in patients whose blood pressure is poorly responsive to adequate fluid resuscitation and vasopressor therapy.[14,15]

The second indicator is drotrecogin alfa (recombinant activated protein C, rhAPC) administered in accordance with a standardized hospital policy. The current guidelines' recommendation for use of drotrecogin alfa is in patients who have severe sepsis with a clinical assessment of high risk of death, typically with Acute Physiology and Chronic Health Evaluation (APACHE) II greater than or equal to 25 and multiple organ

failure, and is in line with United States and European regulatory agencies. For these first two indicators of the management bundle, each hospital is asked to create its own criteria for steroids and drotrecogin alfa and to grade performance based on that policy. Therefore, the bundles do not mandate administration of steroids and rhAPC. The bundles direct clinicians to establish and be incompliance with their institutional criteria for administration of these agents. Documentation is critical for judging compliance with these two indicators.

Indicator three of the sepsis management bundle is glucose control maintained greater than lower limit of normal, but less than 150 mg/dL. This is scored by selecting the median glucose value between 6 and 24 hours. It is recommended that glycemic control efforts begin only after the first 6 hours of therapy. There is recent controversy concerning tight glycemic control (80 to 110 mg/dL) as originally proposed by Van den Berghe,[16,17] which showed improved survival in surgical ICU patients and decreased organ dysfunction in medical ICU patients. A subsequent study has raised concerns about the untoward effects of hypoglycemia when using this degree of glycemic control.[18] The position of the SSC both in the 2004 and 2008 guidelines, is to target the threshold of less than 150 mg/dL to limit hypoglycemic episodes.

The final indicator of the management bundle is maintaining inspiratory plateau pressures less than 30 cm H_2O for mechanically ventilated patients, in line with the ARDSnet strategy for acute lung injury.[19] This is recommended for all patients, as applying the indicators only to patients who have acute lung injury would require another set of screening tool criteria. This indicator should be applied to all patients who have sepsis-induced acute lung injury and patients without acute lung injury. It is certainly appropriate to maintain inspiratory plateau pressures less than 30 cm H_2O in patients without acute lung injury, as data indicate that high tidal volumes in patients without acute lung injury are also problematic.

EARLY RESULTS

A review of the literature about the experience of some of the representative hospitals and networks involved in the campaign offers some context to understand the typical methods used in the campaign and the early results. To date, no published experience that relied on care patterns approximating the campaign guidelines or the bundles has shown a negative result in terms of increased mortality. Experiences have varied regarding evidence of an effect on the processes of care and on length of stay, with no study showing a deleterious effect on length of stay for severe sepsis or septic shock.[12,20–27]

The first evidence of an effect of sepsis bundles on patient care came from Birmingham, England. Gao and colleagues[20] conducted a prospective observational study on 101 consecutive adult patients who had severe sepsis or septic shock on medical or surgical wards or presenting from emergency care at two acute National Health Service Trust teaching hospitals in England. The main outcome measures were the rate of compliance with the sepsis resuscitation and management bundles and the difference in hospital mortality between the compliant and the noncompliant groups. The rate of full compliance with all elements of the 6-hour resuscitation bundle was 52%. Compared with the compliant group, the noncompliant group had a more than twofold increase in hospital mortality (49% versus 23%, relative risk [RR] 2.12, 95% CI1.20 to 3.76, $P = .01$), with similar ages and severity of sepsis. Compliance with the 24-hour sepsis bundle was achieved in only 30% of eligible candidates (21 of 69 patients). Hospital mortality was increased in the noncompliant group from 29% to 50%, with a 76% increase in risk for death, although the difference did not reach statistical significance (RR 1.76, 95% CI 0.84 to 3.64, $P = .16$).

The Gao analysis did not compare compliance with all elements, resuscitation and management combined, with partial compliance. The study was limited further in that it did not measure other risk factors for death, such as the severity of sepsis using a sequential organ failure assessment (SOFA) score, or assess patients' comorbidities, which may have had an impact on decisions regarding withholding or withdrawal of care. Gao also did not assess patients who were not admitted to the ICU despite the presence of severe sepsis (some patients were admitted to medical wards). Despite the limitations, these data suggested for the first time that the sepsis bundles had a positive effect on outcomes measured in terms of mortality.

In the United States, the Colorado Critical Care Collaborative (C4), a coalition of 14 hospitals affiliated with the Colorado Hospital Association, was among the first networks to develop. C4 is a multiprofessional, statewide 14-hospital collaborative with a mission to implement critical care best practices. In 2005, C4 members agreed to join the campaign and implement the care as set forth in the sepsis bundles. In early 2007 at the SCCM Congress (Orlando), the group made an initial report of its results. Of 509 evaluable adult severely septic patients from 10 hospitals accumulated over 16 months, 72% had septic shock and an associated 22% hospital mortality, compared with the remainder without shock, who had 13% hospital mortality.[21]

The C4 analysis compared adherence to the entire bundle, either resuscitation or management, with partial compliance. Overall bundle adherence was low, with 5% for all bundle elements (resuscitation and management combined), and did not change significantly over time. Mortality, however, was decreased by 65% for the 8.6% of patients treated with all applicable resuscitation and management bundle elements (9.1% versus 26% for partial bundle adherence, $P<.025$). Mortality was halved for the 15% of patients treated with all resuscitation bundle elements (13% versus 26% for partial bundle adherence, $P<.05$). Complete management bundle care (117 patients, 23%) also was associated with a trend to reduced mortality (18% versus 26% for partial bundle adherence, $P = .2$).[21] C4 presently has more than 1500 patient charts contributing to the campaign database and is preparing to report additional results.

Subsequent observational trials moved beyond the model of comparing complete bundle adherence with partial bundle compliance. In 2006, four observational trials were published that compared either bundle care as described by the campaign or a similar variant containing many of the same elements. Kortgen and colleagues performed a retrospective cohort study to assess the impact of standard operating procedure (SOP) algorithms, including EGDT, glycemic control, administration of stress doses of hydrocortisone, and use of rhAPC on measures of organ dysfunction and outcome in septic shock. Sixty patient charts in a 10-bed academic ICU at the University of Saarland, Homburg/Saar, Germany, were analyzed, 30 of which were consecutively collected patient charts.

Thirty patients fulfilling criteria for septic shock, treated from September 2002 until December 2003 after implementation of the SOP for severe sepsis and septic shock, were compared with 30 patients who had septic shock treated from January until August 2002 in the same unit as controls. Sequential Organ Failure Assessment (SOFA) scores were calculated, and 28-day survival was assessed. With implementation of the SOP, use of dobutamine (12 out of 30 versus 2 out of 30), insulin (blood glucose less than 150 mg/dL, day 4: 26 out of 28 versus 13 out of 25), hydrocortisone (30 out of 30 versus 13 out of 30), and rhAPC (7 out of 30 versus 0 out of 30) significantly increased, whereas volume for resuscitation and use of packed red blood cells were unaffected. Mortality was 53% in the historical control group and 27% after implementation of the SOP ($P<.05$). The authors concluded that implementation of a sepsis bundle comprised of EGDT, intensive insulin therapy, hydrocortisone administration, and additional application of rhAPC in selected cases seems to influence outcome favorably and can be facilitated by a standardized protocol.[23]

Trzeciak and colleagues[23] aimed to determine if EGDT end points could be achieved reliably in real-world clinical practice. A retrospective analysis was performed of emergency department patients who had persistent sepsis-induced hypotension (systolic blood pressure [BP] less than 90 mm Hg despite 1.5 L of intravenous fluid) treated with EGDT during the first year of the initiative. Primary outcome measures included successful achievement of EGDT end points and time to achievement. EGDT included intravenous fluid administration targeting central venous pressure greater than or equal to 8 mm Hg, vasopressors targeting mean arterial pressure greater than or equal to 65 mm Hg, and packed red blood cells (PRBCs) as needed or dobutamine infusion to target a central venous oxygen saturation greater than or equal to 70%. A secondary analysis was performed comparing EGDT cases with historical control cases (nonprotocolized control subjects without invasive monitoring). All end points were achieved in 20 of 22 cases (91%). The median time to reach each end point was less than 6 hours. In the secondary analysis, patients (n = 38; EGDT, n = 22; pre-EGDT, n = 16) had similar age, do-not-resuscitate status, severity scores, hypotension duration, and vasopressor requirement (P = not significant). With effective emergency medicine/critical care collaboration, the authors concluded that EGDT end points can be achieved reliably in real-world sepsis resuscitation.

Micek and colleagues evaluated a standardized hospital order set for managing septic shock in the emergency department using a before-and-after study design with prospective consecutive data collection. The study was conducted from the emergency department of Barnes–Jewish Hospital (St. Louis), a 1200-bed academic medical center. One hundred-twenty consecutive patients who had septic shock were evaluated. Sixty patients (50.0%) were managed before the implementation of the standardized order set, constituting the before group, and 60 (50.0%) were evaluated after the implementation of the standardized order set, making up the after group. Demographic variables and severity of illness measured by APACHE II were similar for both groups.

Patients in the after group received statistically more intravenous fluids while in the emergency department (2825 plus or minus 1624 mL versus 3789 plus or minus 1730 mL, P = .002), were more likely to receive intravenous fluids of greater than 20 mL/kg body weight before vasopressor administration (58.3% versus 88.3%, $P<.001$), and were more likely to be treated with an appropriate initial antimicrobial regimen (71.7% versus 86.7%, P = .043) compared with patients in the before group. Patients in the after group were less likely to require vasopressor administration at the time of transfer to the ICU (100.0% versus 71.7%, $P<.001$), had a shorter hospital length of stay (12.1 plus or minus 9.2 days versus 8.9 plus or minus 7.2 days, P = .038), and a lower risk for 28-day mortality (48.3% versus 30.0%, P = .040). The authors concluded that the implementation of a standardized order set for the management of septic shock in the emergency department was associated with statistically more rigorous fluid resuscitation of patients, greater administration of appropriate initial antibiotic treatment, and lower 28-day mortality.[24]

Shapiro and colleagues sought to describe the effectiveness of a comprehensive, interdisciplinary sepsis treatment protocol with regard to both implementation and outcomes and to compare the mortality rates and therapies of patients who had septic shock with similar historical controls. The study design was a prospective, interventional cohort study with a historical control comparison group and was undertaken at Beth Israel Deaconess Medical Center (Boston). Patients in the interventional cohort were recruited from the emergency department from November 10, 2003, through November 9, 2004, and historical controls were drawn from patient records from February 1, 2000, through January 31, 2001. The intervention consisted of a sepsis treatment protocol including antibiotics, EGDT, rhAPC, steroids, intensive insulin therapy, and lung-protective ventilation.

Shapiro and colleagues[25] enrolled 116 protocol patients, with a mortality rate of 18% (11% to 25%), of whom 79 patients had septic shock. Comparing these patients with 51 historical controls, protocol patients received:

- More fluid (4.0 versus 2.5 L crystalloid, $P<.001$)
- Earlier antibiotics (90 versus 120 minutes, $P<.013$)
- More appropriate empiric coverage (97% versus 88%, $P<.05$)
- More vasopressors in the first 6 hours (80% versus 45%, $P<.001$)

Tighter glucose control (mean morning glucose, 123 versus 140, $P<.001$)

More frequent assessment of adrenal function (82% versus 10%, $P<.001$), with a nonstatistically significant increase in dobutamine use (14% vs. 4%, $P = .06$) and red blood cell transfusions (30% vs. 18%, $P = .07$) in the first 24 hours

For protocol patients who had septic shock, 28-day in-hospital mortality was 20.3% compared with 29.4% for historical controls ($P = .3$). The authors concluded that implementation of a comprehensive sepsis treatment protocol was feasible and was associated with changes in therapies such as time to antibiotics, intravenous fluid delivery, and vasopressor use in the first 6 hours. No statistically significant decrease in mortality was demonstrated, although a trend toward lower mortality was suggested.

In 2007, Nguyen and colleagues examined the effect of implementing a severe sepsis bundle in the emergency department at Loma Linda University Medical Center (Loma Linda, California). The bundle was introduced as a quality indicator, and regular feedback to modify physician behavior in the early management of severe sepsis and septic shock was provided routinely. Three hundred-thirty patients who met criteria for severe sepsis or septic shock were enrolled in the 2-year prospective observational cohort study. Patients were exposed to five elements of a sepsis bundle including:

1. Initiation of central venous pressure (CVP)/central venous oxygen saturation (ScvO2) monitoring within 2 hours
2. Delivery of broad-spectrum antibiotics within 4 hours
3. Completion of an EGDT trial at 6 hours
4. Delivery of corticosteroids to vasopressor-dependent patients or if adrenal insufficiency was suspected
5. Ongoing monitoring for lactate clearance

Patients had a mean age of 63.8 plus or minus 18.5 years, APACHE II score 29.6 plus or minus 10.6, emergency department length of stay 8.5 plus or minus 4.4 hours, hospital length of stay 11.3 plus or minus 12.9 days, and in-hospital mortality 35.2%. Bundle compliance increased from zero to 51.2% at the end of the study period. During the emergency department stay, patients who had the bundle completed received more CVP/ScvO2 monitoring (100.0 versus 64.8%, $P<.01$), more antibiotics (100.0 versus 89.7%, $P = .04$), and more corticosteroids (29.9 versus16.2%,

$P = .01$) compared with patients with the bundle not completed. In a multivariate regression analysis including the five quality indicators, completion of EGDT was associated significantly with decreased mortality (odds ratio, 0.36; 95% CI, 0.17 to 0.79; $P = .01$). In-hospital mortality was less in patients who had the bundle completed compared with patients with the bundle not completed (20.8 versus 39.5%, $P<.01$). The authors concluded that implementation of a severe sepsis bundle as a quality indicator, with regular feedback to modify physician behavior in the emergency department, was feasible and associated with decreased in-hospital mortality.[26]

Also in 2007, Jones and colleagues[28] published results of a prospective interventional study trial in which they sought to determine the clinical effectiveness of implementing EGDT as a routine protocol in the emergency department. The study was conducted during the course of 2 years at Carolinas Medical Center (Charlotte, North Carolina). Jones prospectively recorded preintervention clinical and mortality data on consecutive, eligible patients for 12 months. Next, an EGDT protocol was introduced, and clinical data including mortality rates were collected for an additional 12 months. Prior to the first year, the investigators defined a 33% relative reduction in mortality (relative mortality reduction that was found in the original EGDT trial) to indicate clinical effectiveness of the intervention.[12]

In the 12 months before intervention, 79 patients were enrolled in the study, and 77 patients were added during the 12 months immediately after intervention. Compared with the preintervention period, patients in the postintervention period received significantly greater crystalloid volume (2.54 L versus 4.66 L, $P<.001$) and frequency of vasopressor infusion (34% versus 69%, $P<.001$) during the initial resuscitation. In-hospital mortality was 21 of 79 patients (27%) before intervention compared with 14 of 77 patients (18%) after intervention (absolute difference, - 9%; 95% CI, + 5% to - 21%). Jones and colleagues[28] concluded that implementation of EGDT was associated with a 9% absolute (33% relative) mortality reduction, providing external validation of the clinical effectiveness of EGDT to treat sepsis and septic shock in the emergency department.

In the most recent analysis of sepsis bundles, the Spanish SSC Network completed the Edusepsis Study and reported results in May of 2008. Ferrer and colleagues used a before-and-after study design to determine whether a national educational program based on the SSC guidelines affected processes of care and hospital mortality for severe sepsis. In 59 medical–surgical ICUs throughout

Table 1
Study characteristics

Author	Year of Publication	Country	Number of Hospitals or ICUs Included	Patient Recruitment Location	Study Design	Patient Types	Intervention	Total Enrollment
Gao	2005	England	2 Acute National Health Service teaching hospitals	Critical care unit	Prospective, observational; intracohort comparison of SSC bundle compliant versus non-compliant groups	Medical, surgical[a]	Modified SSC resuscitation[b] and management bundles	101
Douglas	2006, abstract only	United States (Colorado)	10 community hospitals	Emergency and critical care units	Prospective, observational; intracohort comparison of SSC bundle compliant versus non-compliant groups	Medical, surgical	SSC bundles	509
Kortgen	2006	Germany	1 hospital; academic university hospital	Critical care unit admissions	Retrospective, cohort study	Medical, surgical	Non-SSC sepsis bundle[c]	60
Trzeciak	2006	United States (New Jersey)	1 hospital; academic university hospital	Emergency department	Retrospective cohort with historical controls	Medical, surgical	Early goal-directed therapy (EGDT) only[d]	38
Micek	2006	United States (Missouri)	1 hospital; academic medical center	Emergency department	Before/after design	Medical, surgical, trauma	Three admission order sets based on the SSC guidelines[e]	120

Shapiro	2006	US (Massachusetts)	1 hospital; academic medical center	Emergency Department	Prospective, interventional cohort study with historical controls	Medical, surgical	Non-SSC bundle: "MUST protocol"	167
Jones	2007	United States (North Carolina)	1 hospital; academic medical center	Emergency department with critical care admission	Prospective interventional cohort study	Medical, surgical	EGDT only	156
Nguyen	2007	United States (California)	1 hospital; academic medical center	Emergency department with critical care admission	Prospective observational cohort; intracohort comparison of emergency department bundle compliant versus non-compliant groups	Medical, surgical	6-hour modified SSC bundle completed in the emergency department	330
Ferrer	2008	Spain	77 ICUs throughout Spain	Patients admitted to critical care from emergency department or wards	Before/after design;	Medical, surgical	2-month standardized educational program at each hospital based on SSC guidelines	2566

[a] Only severely septic or septic shock patients ultimately admitted to critical care units were included (71 of 100 of patients).

[b] The modified resuscitation bundle used here differed from the SSC bundle employing a hemoglobin of 7 to 9 g/dL as a threshold for transfusion, versus no threshold in the SSC resuscitation bundle, and used persistent hypotension after fluid resuscitation as a trigger for administration of inotropes rather than central venous oxygen saturation (ScVO2).

[c] EGDT, glycemic control, administration of stress doses of hydrocortisone, and use of recombinant human activated protein C in septic shock patients only.

[d] Although lactate elevation is a trigger for EGDT in the SSC bundles, the only criteria to initiate EGDT evaluated was persistent hypotension despite volume repletion, because the author reported not previously checking lactate routinely in practice.

[e] Although lactate elevation is a trigger for EGDT in the SSC bundles, the only criterion to initiate EGDT was restricted to vasodilatory shock requiring fluid resuscitation plus vasopressor administration in the emergency department. Patients not admitted to the hospital (ie, dying in the emergency department) were excluded.

Table 2 Outcomes				
Author	**Year of Publication**	**Country**	**Bundle Compliance**	**Mortality**
Gao	2005	England	Resuscitation: 52%	Resuscitation: full compliance: 23% partial compliance: 49%
			Management: 30%	Management: full compliance: 29% partial compliance: 50%
Douglas	2006, abstract only	United States (Colorado)	Resuscitation:15%	Resuscitation: full compliance: 13% partial compliance: 26%
			Management: 23%	Management:[a] full compliance: 18% partial compliance: 26%
			Both bundles: 8.6%	Both bundles: full compliance: 9.1% partial compliance: 26%
Kortgen	2006	Germany	Compliance with use of the modified bundle not reported; individual process measures cited reporting significant improvements.	Before: 53% after: 27%
Trzeciak	2006	United States (New Jersey)	No bundle	Not reported
Micek	2006	United States (Missouri)	Compliance with use of the order set not reported; individual process measures cited reporting significant improvements.	Before: 48% after: 30%
Shapiro	2006	United States (Massachusetts)	Compliance with use of the MUST protocol not reported; individual process measures cited reporting significant improvements.	Historical controls: 29.4% protocol: 20.3%[b]
Jones	2007	United States (North Carolina)	No bundle	Before: 27% after: 18%
Nguyen	2007	United States (California)	Emergency department 6-h bundle: 51.2%	Full compliance: 20.8% partial compliance: 39.5%
Ferrer	2008	Spain	Resuscitation: before: 5.3% after: 10% management: before: 10.9% after: 15.7%	Before: 44% after: 39.7%

[a] Management bundle mortality statistics not reaching statistical significance.
[b] Mortality statistics not reaching statistical significance.

Spain, patients were screened daily and enrolled if they fulfilled severe sepsis or septic shock criteria. Eight hundred fifty-four patients were enrolled in the preintervention period (November to December 2005), 1465 patients during the postintervention period (March to June 2006), and 247 additional patients were enrolled during a long-term follow-up period 1 year later (November to December 2006) in a subset of 23 ICUs.

The educational program consisted of training physicians and nursing staff from the emergency department, wards, and ICU in the definition, recognition, and treatment of severe sepsis and septic shock as outlined in the 2004 campaign guidelines. Both the campaign resuscitation and management bundles were introduced to the participating sites after the educational program was complete. Hospital mortality, differences in adherence to the bundles' process-of-care variables, ICU mortality, 28-day mortality, hospital length of stay, and ICU length of stay were calculated. Patients in the postintervention cohort had a lower risk of hospital mortality (44.0% versus 39.7%, $P = .04$). The compliance with process-of-care variables also improved after the intervention in the sepsis resuscitation bundle (5.3%, 95%CI, 4% to 7%) versus 10.0% (95% CI, 8% to 12%; $P<.001$) and in the sepsis management bundle (10.9%; 95% CI, 9% to 13% versus 15.7%; 95% CI, 14% to18%; $P = .001$). Hospital length of stay and ICU length of stay did not change after the intervention. During long-term follow-up, compliance with the sepsis resuscitation bundle returned to baseline, but compliance with the sepsis management bundle and mortality remained stable with respect to the postintervention period. Overall, the study demonstrated that a national educational effort to promote bundles of care for severe sepsis and septic shock was associated with improved guideline compliance and lower hospital mortality. Notably, compliance rates, although statistically significant for improvement, were low, and the observed improvement in the resuscitation bundle lapsed at 1 year.[27]

Comparing these studies in terms of individual characteristics, it becomes clear that although they share many features, they are divergent in important ways (**Table 1**). Notably, not all studies included a bundle strategy, and others studied only EGDT. Those studies that did include a bundle strategy modified the bundle from SSC specifications, and most of the studies employed varied EGDT specifications. Moreover, the designs of the studies were substantially different, including purely retrospective designs, before/after designs, prospective designs with historical controls, and entirely prospective studies. Nevertheless, the degree of compliance with the chosen strategies and their results in terms of mortality were favorable (**Table 2**). All told, these observational trials suggest that the interventions in the SSC bundles are likely to reduce mortality caused by severe sepsis and septic shock. These studies provide confidence that clinical trials showing benefits in the care of severely septic patients can be brought to the bedside.

One final study is of interest with regard to the effect of implementing the sepsis bundles in caring for severely septic and shock patients. Shorr and colleagues reported on the financial cost savings associated with the experience of adopting the standardized order set described by Micek and colleagues at Barnes-Jewish Hospital. The authors compared patients treated before the protocol with those cared for after the protocol was implemented. Overall hospital costs represented the primary end point, whereas hospital length of stay served as a secondary end point. All hospital costs were calculated based on charges after conversion to costs based on department-specific cost-to-charge ratios. The authors employed linear regression to measure the independent impact of the protocol on costs and conducted a sensitivity analysis assessing end points in the subgroup of subjects who survived their hospitalization.

The total cohort included 120 subjects (60 before, 60 after) with a mean age of 64.7 plus or minus 18.2 years and median APACHE II score of 22.5 plus or minus 8.3. There were more survivors following the protocol's adoption (70.0% versus 51.7%, $P = .040$). Median total costs were significantly lower with use of the protocol ($16,103 versus $21,985, $P = .008$). The length of stay was also on average 5 days less among the postintervention population ($P = .023$). A Cox proportional hazard model indicated that the protocol was associated with less per-patient cost. Restricting the analysis to only survivors did not alter the cost savings. Shorr and colleagues[29] concluded that use of a sepsis protocol can result, not only in improved mortality, but also in substantial savings for institutions and third-party payers.

SUMMARY

In the *Structure of Scientific Revolutions,* Thomas S. Kuhn[30] challenged the logical empiricist view of science as an objective progression toward the truth. Kuhn viewed science as heavily influenced by nonrational procedures. As described by Nicholas Wade in *Science,* Kuhn casts science not as the cumulative acquisition of knowledge, but rather as "a series of peaceful interludes punctuated by intellectually violent revolutions," where the prevailing paradigm is usurped by another.

The SSC has applied experts' collectively determined best estimations of the import of the scientific literature, improvement and bundle technologies (viewed as controversial and unproven by some), unconventional funding sources for a scientific and public health enterprise, and partnerships among professional societies to achieve unprecedented results in the care of septic patients. The campaign has advocated a balance of proscriptive behavior and simultaneously allowed key decisions in care to be tempered by clinician caution. The means, methods, and strategies adopted by the campaign have created a network of 250 hospitals dedicated to testing new approaches in the care of septic patients. It is no surprise that in challenging the assumptions and beliefs of many in the health profession, the campaign has generated as much controversy as enthusiasm. Nevertheless, as more trials are published showing positive results in terms of mortality, length of stay, and cost savings, there can be no doubt that in critical care, the campaign has begun a revolution in the translation of clinical science to the bedside.

REFERENCES

1. Available at: http://www.survivingsepsis.org/back ground/barcelona_declaration. Accessed May 13, 2008.
2. Berwick DM, Calkins DR, McCannon CJ, et al. The 100,000 lives campaign: setting a goal and a deadline for improving health care quality. JAMA 2006; 295(3):324–7.
3. Dellinger RP, Carlet JM, Masur H, et al. Surviving sepsis campaign guidelines for management of severe sepsis and septic shock. Crit Care Med 2004; 32:858–73.
4. Dellinger RP, Carlet JM, Masur H, et al. Surviving sepsis campaign guidelines for management of severe sepsis and septic shock. Intensive Care Med 2004;30:536–55.
5. Dellinger RP, Levy MM, Carlet JM, et al. Surviving sepsis campaign: international guidelines for management of severe sepsis and septic shock: 2008. Crit Care Med 2008;36(1):296–327 [erratum in: Crit Care Med. 2008 Apr; 36(4):1394–6].
6. Dellinger RP, Levy MM, Carlet JM, et al. Surviving sepsis campaign: international guidelines for management of severe sepsis and septic shock. Intensive Care Med 2008;34:17–60.
7. Eichacker PQ, Natanson C, Danner RL. Surviving sepsis—practice guidelines, marketing campaigns, and Eli Lilly. N Engl J Med 2006;355(16):1640–2.
8. GRADE working group. Grading quality of evidence and strength of recommendations. BMJ 2004;328: 1490–8.
9. Guyatt G, Gutterman D, Baumann MH, et al. Grading strength of recommendations and quality of evidence in clinical guidelines: report from an American College of Chest Physicians task force. Chest 2006; 129:174–81.
10. Schünemann HJ, Jaeschke R, Cook DJ, et al. On behalf of the ATS Documents Development and Implementation Committee: an official ATS statement. Grading the quality of evidence and strength of recommendations in ATS guidelines and recommendations. Am J Respir Crit Care Med 2006;174:605–14.
11. Kumar A, Roberts D, Wood KE, et al. Duration of hypotension prior to initiation of effective antimicrobial therapy is the critical determinant of survival in human septic shock. Crit Care Med 2006;34:1589–96.
12. Rivers E, Nguyen B, Havstad S, et al. Early goal-directed therapy in the treatment of severe sepsis and septic shock. N Engl J Med 2001;345:1368–77.
13. Varpula M, Tallgren M, Saukkonen K, et al. Hemodynamic variables related to outcome in septic shock. Intensive Care Med 2005;31:1066–71.
14. Annane D, Sebille V, Charpentier C, et al. Effect of treatment with low doses of hydrocortisone and fludrocortisone on mortality in patients with septic shock. JAMA 2002;288:862–71.
15. Sprung CL, Annane D, Keh D, et al. Hydrocortisone therapy for patients with septic shock. N Engl J Med 2008;358:111–24.
16. Van den Berghe G, Wouters P, Weekers F, et al. Intensive insulin therapy in critically ill patients. N Engl J Med 2001;345:1359–67.
17. Van den Berghe G, Wilmer A, Hermans G, et al. Intensive insulin therapy in the medical ICU. N Engl J Med 2006;354:449–61.
18. Brunkhorst FM, Engel C, Bloos F, et al. Intensive insulin therapy and pentastarch resuscitation in severe sepsis. N Engl J Med 2008;358:125–39.
19. Acute Respiratory Distress Syndrome Network. Available at: http://www.ardsnet.org. Accessed June 15, 2008.
20. Gao F, Melody T, Daniels D, et al. The impact of compliance with 6-hour and 24-hour sepsis bundles on hospital mortality in patients with severe sepsis: a prospective observational study. Crit Care 2005; 9(6):R764–70.
21. Douglas IS, Marchlowska P, Rains R, et al. A statewide implementation of surviving sepsis campaign bundles by the Colorado Critical Care Collaborative. Crit Care Med 2006;34(12):A99 [abstract supplement].
22. Kortgen A, Niederprüm P, Bauer M. Implementation of an evidence-based standard operating procedure and outcome in septic shock. Crit Care Med 2006;34(4):943–9.

23. Trzeciak S, Dellinger RP, Abate NL, et al. Translating research to clinical practice: a 1-year experience with implementing early goal-directed therapy for septic shock in the emergency department. Chest 2006;129(2):225–32.

24. Micek ST, Roubinian N, Heuring T, et al. Before–after study of a standardized hospital order set for the management of septic shock. Crit Care Med 2006; 34(11):2707–13.

25. Shapiro N, Howell MD, Bates DW, et al. The association of sepsis syndrome and organ dysfunction with mortality in emergency department patients with suspected infection. Ann Emerg Med 2006; 48(5):583–90, 590.e1.

26. Nguyen HB, Corbett SW, Steele R, et al. Implementation of a bundle of quality indicators for the early management of severe sepsis and septic shock is associated with decreased mortality. Crit Care Med 2007;35(4):1105–12.

27. Ferrer R, Artigas A, Levy MM, et al. Improvement in process of care and outcome after a multicenter severe sepsis educational program in Spain. JAMA 2008;299(19):2294–303.

28. Jones AE, Focht A, Horton JM, et al. Prospective external validation of the clinical effectiveness of an emergency department-based early goal-directed therapy protocol for severe sepsis and septic shock. Chest 2007;132(2):425–32.

29. Shorr AF, Micek ST, Jackson WL, et al. Economic implications of an evidence-based sepsis protocol: can we improve outcomes and lower costs? Crit Care Med 2007;35(5):1257–62.

30. Wade N. Thomas S. Kuhn. Revolutionary theorist of science. Science 1977;197(4299):143–5.

Sepsis Strategies in Development

Steven P. LaRosa, MD[a,b],*, Steven M. Opal, MD[a,c]

KEYWORDS

- Sepsis • Therapeutics • Endotoxin • Cytokines
- Anticoagulants • Complement

Severe sepsis, defined as inflammation and organ failure due to infection, continues to result in a mortality of approximately 30% despite advances in critical care. Current therapy includes timely administration of antibiotics, source control of infection, aggressive fluid resuscitation, support of failing organs, and use of activated protein C where clinically indicated. Bacterial mediators, including endotoxin and superantigens, as well endogenous proinflammatory cytokines are considered important to the pathogenesis of sepsis-induced organ failure and are being targeted with numerous molecules and removal devices. Additional therapeutic strategies are aimed at restoring the natural anticoagulant levels, blocking deleterious effects of the complement cascade, reversing cytopathic hypoxia, and inhibiting excessive lymphocyte apoptosis. Molecules with pluripotent activity, such as interalpha inhibitor proteins and estrogen-receptor ligands, are also being investigated.

THERAPIES TARGETING ENDOTOXIN
Eritoran

Eritoran is a synthetic lipid A antagonist modeled from an unusual lipopolysaccharide (LPS) structure of *Rhodobacter spp* that functions as a competitive inhibitor of LPS at the cell membrane receptor level (the MD-2 Toll-like receptor 4 [TLR-4]).[1] Eritoran binds to the hydrophobic pocket of MD-2 and sterically inhibits the ability of active forms of lipid A from binding to this critical region of the receptor-signaling complex. Eritoran has unusually long fatty acids (with 18 carbons) adjacent to unusually short fatty acids (with 10 carbons) rather than the standard 12- to 14-carbon fatty acids found in highly active forms of lipid A. Eritoran avidly binds to MD-2 and engages TLR-4. However, eritoran blocks dimerization of TLR-4–intracellular domains essential for signal transduction.[2] If sufficient quantities are available, eritoran will completely terminate LPS signaling. This lipid A antagonist has been shown to be highly active in a variety of animal models[3] and in several phase I human endotoxin volunteer studies.[4] After demonstrating safety in cardiac surgery patients[5] and a 293-patient, multicenter, phase II sepsis trial, eritoran is now being investigated in a phase III, international, clinical trial in severe sepsis. The results of this study should be available within the next 2 to 3 years.

Recombinant Human Bactericidal/ Permeability-Increasing Protein

Bactericidal/permeability-increasing protein (BPI) is an endogenous endotoxin-binding protein found in azurophilic granules of human neutrophils. BPI is a highly cationic protein that has a hydrophobic lipid A binding domain within its amino terminus. In addition to possessing antibacterial activity, BPI is a very potent LPS inhibitor.[6] BPI possesses high affinity binding capacity to LPS and blocks access

---

Steven P. Opal and Steven M. LaRosa received investigator grants from Eisai Medical Research (maker of eritoran) and Novartis (maker of tifacogin) as members of the Ocean State Clinical Coordinating Center.

[a] Warren Alpert School of Medicine, Brown University, Providence, RI, USA
[b] Division of Infectious Diseases, Rhode Island Hospital, POB Suite #330, 593 Eddy Street, Providence, RI 02903, USA
[c] Division of Infectious Diseases, Memorial Hospital, 111 Brewster Street, Pawtucket, RI 02860, USA
* Corresponding author. Division of Infectious Diseases, Rhode Island Hospital, POB Suite #330, 593 Eddy Street, Providence, RI 02903.
E-mail address: slarosa@lifespan.org (S.P. LaRosa).

Clin Chest Med 29 (2008) 735–747
doi:10.1016/j.ccm.2008.06.007

of LPS to LPS-binding protein, an important carrier protein for LPS signaling. A variety of animal models[7] and human endotoxin volunteer studies[8] have shown that BPI can neutralize LPS-mediated toxicity if sufficient quantities are available. The protein has a very short half-life in the systemic circulation (5–10 minutes), necessitating a continuous infusion of BPI to maintain endotoxin inhibition. The N-terminal domain of BPI ($rBPI_{21}$) has been studied in a variety of clinical trials and has proven to be safe. Antineutrophil cytoplasmic antigen antibodies recognize BPI, but the epitope for this autoantibody is expressed on the carboxyl terminus of the BPI holo-protein.[9] A large international phase III trial with $rBPI_{21}$ has been completed in children with severe meningococcal sepsis.[10] BPI-treated children had statistically significant reductions in the total number of amputations and significantly improved long-term neurologic injury. Regrettably, the mortality end point and composite end point for this trial was not met and thus BPI has not been approved yet for clinical use in endotoxin-mediated diseases.[11]

Recombinant Human Lactoferrin

Lactoferrin is a neutrophil granular protein and an extracellular product produced by epithelial cells.[12] This iron chelating protein contains cationic and hydrophobic regions, making it an effective endotoxin binding and neutralizing human protein.[13] Lactoferrin also has direct antimicrobial properties, including its ability to limit the availability of iron to bacteria, to enhance phagocytic function, and to cause damage to the outer membrane of gram-negative bacteria. Lactoferrin also blunts LPS-induced tumor necrosis factor (TNF) release in macrophages.[14] Administration of lactoferrin in a variety of endotoxin challenge models, with gram-negative bacteria, and in experimental sepsis models has proven to be efficacious.[15] Talactoferrin, a recombinant lactoferrin produced from *Aspergillus niger*, has been administered orally to over 200 patients without the development of drug-related adverse events.[16] A phase II trial of talactoferrin in patients with severe sepsis will soon commence.

Recombinant Human Alkaline Phosphatase

Alkaline phosphatase is best known as a marker for intrahepatic and extrahepatic biliary obstruction. Elevated alkaline phosphatase levels are frequently observed in the cholestasis of sepsis and yet the physiologic role of alkaline phosphatase has never been clearly defined. Alkaline phosphatase has the capacity to cleave phosphate groups off the lipid A portion of bacterial endotoxin.[17] Lipid A is biphosphorylated and removal of one or both of the phosphate moieties greatly diminishes or ablates the toxicity of lipid A structures.[18] Administration of human recombinant alkaline phosphatase has proven to be efficacious as an antiendotoxin strategy in a number of animal models.[19,20] Clinical studies with this recombinant enzyme are being contemplated. The kinetics and rate of dephosphorylation of bacterial endotoxin in septic patients may be a limitation to this antiendotoxin strategy.

TAK-242

TAK-242 is a small-molecule inhibitor of intracellular signaling pathways following engagement of LPS with its cell surface receptor, the MD-2-TLR-4 complex. Intracellular signaling is blocked at the MyD88-dependent pathway and effectively inhibits cytokine generation following LPS stimulation in experimental in vitro and in vivo systems.[21,22] In the human endotoxin challenge model, TAK-242 has also proven to be efficacious in the prevention of acute phase proteins and proinflammatory cytokines and human phase I trials with endotoxin challenge.[22] The short half-life of the drug has indicated that continuous infusion is needed to be efficacious in clinical sepsis trials. A phase II trial has recently been completed with this molecule and the drug proved to be safe with favorable trends in reduction of mortality rate.[23] However, the primary end point of the study, reduction in proinflammatory cytokines, was not achieved in this phase II trial. A second phase II/III is planned in the near future with TAK-242 as an antiendotoxin therapeutic strategy.

Polymyxin B Immobilized Hemofiltration Columns

Polymyxin B is an antibacterial agent that possesses potent LPS-binding capacity via its cationic amino acids and alternating hydrophobic amino acids.[24] Polymyxin B is active against many gram-negative bacteria but has dose-limiting neurotoxicity and potential nephrotoxicity. To avoid these side effects, polymyxin B has been immobilized onto hemofiltration cartridges for extracorporal use as an endotoxin removal device.[25] There is extensive clinical experience with this endotoxin adsorption strategy in Japan. These polymyxin B–immobilized columns may remove other potentially injurious components of septic plasma, such as the high mobility group box–1 (HMGB1) protein and other negatively charged, bioactive lipid molecules.[26,27] Numerous clinical trials with these columns suggest therapeutic benefit in severely septic patients.[25,26,28] A recent review and meta-analysis of polymyxin columns support their clinical value,[29] yet no convincing, randomized, placebo-controlled, phase III trial data are available to confirm its clinical efficacy.[28,29]

Heparin-Induced Extracorporeal Lipoprotein Fibrinogen Apheresis

The heparin-induced extracorporeal lipoprotein fibrinogen or HELP system has had extensive use in the treatment of patients with treatment-resistant hypercholesterolemia. During this apheresis, blood is removed from the patient, the plasma is separated from cells, low-density lipoprotein and other lipid components are removed by heparin precipitation and filtration, and then the reconstituted blood is put back in the patient.[30] This system was also found to remove TNF-α and LPS. A modification of this system with the use of a diethylaminoethyl-cellulose (DEAE-cellulose) filter was able to effectively remove endotoxin.[31] The anion-exchange groups and hydrophobic properties of the filter are thought to be responsible for its LPS-binding ability. A pilot study was conducted with the DEAE-cellulose filter in 15 patients with severe sepsis and a plasma LPS concentration of more than 0.30 endotoxin units per milliliter. Extracorporeal treatment with this device was associated with a 35% reduction in LPS levels ($P < .001$). Statistically significant decreases in IL-6, C-reactive protein, and fibrinogen levels were also observed in the treatment arm.[32] Larger human studies of this technology are currently being considered.

Antiendotoxin Vaccines

Bacterial endotoxin, or LPS, is the principal microbial mediator capable of inducing a septic shock–like state in humans. A vaccine that could attenuate or prevent the injurious systemic consequences of LPS release could be a valuable adjunct in the treatment of severe sepsis.[33] Current vaccine strategies focus primarily on the highly conserved core glycolipid region of bacterial LPS. High-titer, polyclonal antibodies directed against this region of LPS are protective in a variety of animal models.[33,34] A detoxified LPS vaccine administered as a complex with the outer membrane protein of *Neisseria meningitidis* and immunoadjuvants has undergone phase I trials in human volunteers.[34] The vaccine was well tolerated and generated persistent antibody responses, but the vaccine-induced antibody titers were relatively low and will need to be boosted to be highly protective. Efforts to improve upon this vaccine and to make it available for a phase II clinical trials are underway.[35]

SUPERANTIGEN ANTAGONISTS

The superantigens are a related group of staphylococcal and streptococcal bacterial exotoxins that possess the capacity to induce profound activation of the immune system without the need for conventional antigen processing and presentation.[36] Superantigens bind to the class II molecules on antigen-presenting cells and link together the beta loop of the variable component of the T cell receptor (Vβ) expressed by a large number of CD4+T cells. By this mechanism, superantigens activate both T cells and monocyte/macrophage populations, resulting in the outpouring of large quantities of proinflammatory cytokines and chemokines. These superantigens are central to the pathogenesis of streptococcal and staphylococcal toxic shock syndromes.[37] Inhibition of superantigens can be accomplished through adsorption, antibody clearance, or the use of specific peptide inhibitors of superantigen activity.[37-39] Passive immunotherapy with human immunoglobulin is one of the standard adjuvant treatments for toxic shock syndromes, despite its uncertain efficacy. Improved superantigen antagonists under development may prove to be of clinical value for toxic shock syndrome states and perhaps more general use in a variety of other bacterial infections.[37] Some of these superantigens have biodefense implications and effective inhibitors have become an urgent research priority.

THERAPIES TARGETING EXCESSIVE INFLAMMATION
High-Volume Hemofiltration Systems

High-volume hemofiltration (HVHF) is postulated as a blood purification technique for septic patients by employing membranes with high porosity characteristics and high flow to efficiently clear large inflammatory proteins, such as proinflammatory cytokines, vasoactive peptides, and chemokines.[40] Removal of excess quantities of these injurious elements from the plasma of septic patients would seem to provide a survival benefit. The advantage of this system is its ability to remove a myriad of inflammatory molecules at the same time, thereby attenuating the systemic inflammatory response. Theoretically, local inflammatory reactions and paracellular cell signaling reactions remain largely unchanged by this technique.[40,41]

In addition to concerns about technical issues involved with HVHF in hypotensive patients with sepsis, there is a concern over the concomitant loss of coagulation regulators, anti-inflammatory cytokines, and other valuable plasma proteins.

Patients often require an albumin infusion to maintain oncotic pressure using this technique. Pulse dosing of HVHF and various techniques of heme absorption to remove specific inflammatory cytokines are also under study.[40,42]

The efficacy of this HVHF technique in actual clinical septic shock remains controversial. Initial evidence by Ronco and colleagues[43] indicated that HVHF with continuous veno-veno hemofiltration may be a survival benefit in severe sepsis if filtration rates were maintained at greater than 45 mL/kg/h. Several other clinical studies with HVHF have shown inconsistent results. Therefore, large prospective clinical trials currently underway will determine the practicality, safety, and efficacy of this strategy for severe sepsis.[40,44]

Renal Assist Devices

The renal assist device is an innovative strategy using hemofiltration columns lined with viable human renal tubular epithelial cells existing as a living biomembrane compartment. Renal assist devices have been developed as a treatment for acute kidney injury and severe sepsis. These renal tubule epithelial cells are biologically active and provide many metabolic, endocrine, and detoxifying processes subsumed by normal kidney function, including regulation of vasoactive substances and inflammatory cytokines in the systemic circulation in sepsis.[45] This strategy, while technically difficult and challenging to maintain, offers a novel renal support platform during continuous veno-venous hemofiltration (CVVHF). This technique has advanced to human clinical trials. A phase I safety trial confirms the safety of the technique in critically ill patients. The renal assist device showed significant declines in granulocyte colony stimulating factor, IL-6, and IL-10 in this phase I trial.[46] A phase II trial with 58 patients has been undertaken in critically ill patients with dialysis-dependent acute kidney injury. Patients were randomized to CVVHF alone versus CVVHF with the renal assist device for 72 hours. A reduction in 28-day all-cause mortality rate was observed in those patients randomized to the renal assist device (34% versus 56%).[47,48] Further studies of this technique or similar strategies are worthy of consideration in the future.

Ovine Anti–Tumor Necrosis Factor α Polyclonal Fab Fragment

TNF-α is a proinflammatory cytokine released from monocytes in response to outer membrane components of bacteria, including endotoxin, lipoteichoic acid, and peptidoglycan. This cytokine can directly cause tissue injury as well as damage to the endothelium, causing activation of the clotting cascade. CytoFab is an ovine anti–TNF-α polyclonal Fab fragment produced by immunizing sheep with human TNF-α. The theoretic benefits of such a strategy are many and include the ability to bind to multiple epitopes, a reduced risk of immunotoxicity due to absence of an antibody tail, a larger volume of distribution due to the smaller size, and more rapid clearance. CytoFab has been studied in a phase IIb randomized, double-blinded placebo-controlled trial in 81 septic patients with shock or two or more organ dysfunctions. CytoFab increased mean ventilator-free days (15.0 versus 9.8; $P = .040$) and intensive care unit–free days (12.6 versus 7.6; $P = .030$) compared with placebo. All-cause 28-day mortality rates were 26% in the CytoFab group versus 37% in placebo patients.[49] The molecule has undergone a manufacturing change to allow it to be commercially viable. A phase II safety and tolerability study began in January 2008.

Vagal Nerve Stimulation

Recently, a fascinating interaction of the nervous system and the immune response has been described. Tracey and colleagues[50] noted that stimulation of the vagus nerve led to decreased production of proinflammatory cytokines from monocytes. This action occurred via the action of the vagus' principal neurotransmitter, acetylcholine, on the alpha 7 acetylcholine receptor on monocytes. Electrical stimulation of the vagus nerve in a lethal rat model of endotoxemia decreased hepatic TNF production and prevented the development of shock. Animals that underwent a vagotomy had increased production of TNF and a shorter time to the development of shock.[50] In a second rat endotoxemia study, animals that received vagal nerve stimulation had less activation of the clotting cascade, less inhibition of the fibrinolytic system, and smaller decreases in natural anticoagulant levels.[51] The possibility exists for implantation of a vagal nerve stimulator in the setting of severe sepsis to control the inflammatory and coagulopathic response.

Alpha 7 Nicotinic Acetylcholine Receptor Agonists

Pharmacologic means could also be used to stimulate the cholinergic anti-inflammatory pathway. Pretreatment of mice with nicotine before an intraperitoneal challenge with *Escherichia coli* was associated with decreased inflammatory cell infiltrates in the peritoneal fluid and decreased cytokine levels.[52] In the cecal ligation and perforation model in mice, nicotine treatment improved survival even when delivered 24 hours after the infectious insult. Treatment with nicotine was also associated with decreased release of HMGB1, a late mediator of sepsis that functions as a proinflammatory cytokine.[53] A selective alpha 7 nicotinic acetylcholine receptor agonist, GTS-21, is currently under development. GTS-21 is devoid of nicotinic activity and should be associated with less toxicity. This molecule was associated with increased survival in both a lethal murine endotoxin challenge model and in the cecal ligation and perforation model.[54]

High Mobility Group Box–1 Protein Inhibition

HMGB1 is a nuclear and cytoplasmic protein that binds DNA and regulates transcription. Necrotic cells release HMGB1 into the extracellular fluid in response to an infectious challenge. The molecule in small amounts helps control infection by stimulating chemotaxis, by facilitating binding of neutrophils to the endothelium, and by causing the release of cytokines TNF and IL-1 from monocytes. In high concentrations, HMGB1 disrupts the endothelial barrier as well as enterocyte stability and can cause acute lung injury.[55] HMGB1 is an attractive target compared with other proinflammatory cytokines because it is a late mediator of lethality. Release of HMGB1 occurs approximately 20 hours after monocytes are challenged with endotoxin.[56] In patients with severe sepsis, high levels of HMGB1 are detected as late as 1 week into the illness, a time when other proinflammatory cytokines are undetectable.[57] Anti–HMGB1 antibodies given to mice as late as 24 hours after an endotoxin challenge or cecal ligation and puncture-induced peritonitis are protective.[58] Investigation of the HMGB1 protein revealed that it contains two DNA binding regions: the A box and the B box. Further studies have revealed that it is the B box that stimulates TNF release from monocytes and mediates lethality while the A box can competitively inhibit the HMGB1 molecule. Passive treatment with the A box 24 hours postendotoxin challenge and cecal ligation and perforation is also protective in mice.[59] Nicotine and other selective agonists of the 7 alpha acetylcholine receptor, transcutaneous vagus nerve stimulation, green tea, an lysophosphatidylcholine all are able to decrease production of HMGB1 from LPS-challenged monocytes.[53,60–62] Human trials of molecules targeting HMGB1 have not been performed to date.

Anti–Receptor for Advanced Glycation End-Product Therapies

The receptor for advanced glycation end-products (RAGE) is ubiquitously expressed on multiple cell types on both immune effector cells and epithelial and mesenchymal cells of the human body.[63] The RAGE is of special interest as it is up-regulated in acute and chronic inflammatory states while most other cytokine receptors are down-regulated in acute inflammation. The RAGE recognizes a wide array of endogenous ligands of potential significance in septic shock, such as HMGB1, S-100, and other calgranulins. The RAGE is also a counter receptor for the neutrophil adhesion molecules beta-2 integrins.[64] Inhibitors of the RAGE by soluble decoy receptors or anti-RAGE antibodies have beneficial effects in clinically relevant, experimental models of sepsis.[65,66] Clinical trials with RAGE inhibitors are currently under consideration as a treatment strategy for severe sepsis.

Suppressors of Cytokine Signaling

Suppressors of cytokine signaling (SOCS) are a family of eight endogenous, intracellular, signaling proteins that regulate cytokine, interferon, and growth factor signaling pathways. They primarily act upon the Janus kinase-signal transducer and activator of transcription (JAK-STAT) pathways.[67] SOCS-3 is prominently expressed in myeloid cells and its presence limits excess cytokine generation.[68] SOCS-1 is primarily found in T cells and prevents excess apoptosis of activated T cells during acute inflammatory states.[67] It has been hypothesized that molecules that could promote the expression of SOCS proteins could provide survival advantage in humans, as has been demonstrated in experimental animals.[69] Work on this strategy continues, although there are no clinical trials with SOCS molecules in sepsis at present.

Adenosine A2A Receptor Agonists

Adenosine can bind to adenosine A2A receptors on the surface of neutrophils and monocytes and exert potent anti-inflammatory actions. Binding of the A2A receptor on neutrophils has multiple effects, including the decreased production of oxygen free radicals, decreased chemotaxis, and decreased adhesion to endothelial cells.[70] Binding of the A2A receptor in macrophage and monocytes decreases the production of proinflammatory cytokines.[71] Platelet aggregation can also be inhibited by binding of this adenosine receptor.[72] One A2A receptor agonist, ATL146e, was protective in an LPS and live E coli challenge murine model.[73] A newer agonist, ATL 313, was associated with decreased ileal edema, hemorrhage, inflammatory cell infiltration, TNF production, and mucosal disruption in a murine model of Clostridium difficile toxin A–induced ileal enteritis.[74] None of these molecules has been taken forward into human clinical trials of patients with sepsis.

Peroxisome Proliferator–Activated Receptor-Gamma Agonists

A member of the nuclear receptor family peroxisome proliferator–activated receptor-gamma (PPAR-gamma) has been found to mediate inflammation. When PPAR-gamma is engaged by ligands, it forms a heterodimer with retinoic acid receptor and competes for coactivators of proinflammatory genes.[75] PPAR-gamma activation has been shown in animals to attenuate the hemodynamic response to sepsis, to reduce neutrophil infiltration of organs, and to decrease proinflammatory cytokine response.[76] Thiazolidinediones, including the commonly prescribed glucose-lowering agent rosiglitazone, are ligands for PPAR-gamma as are cyclopentenone prostaglandins and nonsteroidal anti-inflammatory drugs.[75] In a murine model of multiple organ dysfunction induced by intraperitoneal instillation of zymosan, rosiglitazone was associated with decreased inflammation and organ injury.[77] Curcumin, a commonly used spice, was associated with up-regulation of PPAR-gamma in the liver, decreased tissue injury and TNF levels, and improved survival in a murine cecal ligation and perforation model.[78] Human trials of ligands for PPAR-gamma are not currently underway.

Chemically Modified Tetracyclines

The tetracycline class of antibiotics has known anti-inflammatory properties in addition to their antimicrobial properties. These anti-inflammatory properties include the reduction in TNF release following endotoxin challenge, inhibition of matrix metalloproteinases, and inhibition of nitric oxide synthesis.[79,80] Modified tetracyclines have been produced devoid of antimicrobial properties. Chemically modified tetracycline CMT-3, a molecule produced by removing the dimethyl amino group at position 4, was protective as a prophylactic in the rat cecal ligation and perforation model of sepsis. This molecule was associated with decreased TNF-α levels, decreased mitogen-activated protein kinase activation, and improved mortality compared with placebo.[81] Another chemically modified tetracycline, COT-3, was studied in a porcine two-hit molecule involving superior mesenteric artery clamping followed by fecal blood clot implantation. The oral administration of COL-3 12 hours before the challenge was associated with the prevention of acute respiratory distress syndrome and septic shock compared with the control animals. Decreased lung edema

was seen in the treated animals as well as decreased bronchoalveolar lavage levels of IL-6, IL-8, IL-10, and neutrophil elastase compared with controls.[82] COL-3 was protective in the cecal ligation and perforation model when its administration was delayed as long as 12 hours after the infectious challenge.[83] Human sepsis trials with COT-3 have not been conducted to date.

3-Hydroxymethyl-3-Methylglutaryl Coenzyme A Reductase Inhibitors

3-Hydroxymethyl-3-methylglutaryl coenzyme A reductase inhibitors (statins) are effective in lowering cholesterol through their involvement in the mevalonate pathway. These agents also have potent anti-inflammatory properties mediated through the same pathway.[84] Large observational studies have shown a decreased mortality rate in patients with bacteremia who are on statins as well as decreased rate of the development of sepsis in cardiovascular patients and in patients with acute bacterial infections.[85,86] Statins have decreased mortality in the murine cecal ligation and perforation model of sepsis through maintenance of blood pressure and decreased proinflammatory cytokine production.[87] Healthy humans challenged with endotoxin had preserved blood pressure responses, decreased monocyte tissue-factor expression, decreased inflammatory markers, and decreased TLR-4 expression on monocytes when given statins.[88,89] Different statin agents are currently being studied in clinical trials of abdominal sepsis, early sepsis, and septic shock.

TARGETING THE COAGULATION CASCADE
Recombinant Tissue Factor Pathway Inhibitor

Tissue factor pathway inhibitor (TFPI) is a three–Kunitz-domain protease inhibitor that functions as endogenous anticoagulant. TFPI inhibits factor Xa by binding it at the second Kunitz domain. It is also able to limit further production of Xa by binding factor VIIa/tissue factor complex at the first Kunitz domain.[90] Factor Xa and factor VIIa/tissue factor complex can signal protease-activated receptors (PARs) 1 and 2 on the cell membrane leading to the production of proinflammatory cytokines, display of adhesion molecules, and endothelial vasorelaxation. TFPI can inhibit PAR activation by inhibition of factor Xa and factor VIIa/tissue factor.[91–93] Finally, TFPI can bind LPS and prevent its transfer to CD14 molecules.[94] Tifacogin, a recombinant tissue factor pathway inhibitor (rTFPI), was unsuccessful in a large phase III study of patients with severe sepsis. Subgroup analyses revealed a very clear drug-drug interaction between this rTFPI and heparin. In the primary efficacy population who did not receive heparin, the mortality in the rTFPI arm was 34.6% versus 42.7% in the placebo arm (P = .05).[95] An additional subgroup analysis revealed a large efficacy signal in patients with sepsis due to community-acquired pneumonia with an rTFPI mortality of 31.3% and a placebo mortality of 39.8% (P = .05).[96] A large placebo-controlled trial (Captivate trial) of rTFPI in patients with severe community-acquired pneumonia will soon be completed.

Recombinant Antithrombin

Antithrombin is a plasma protein that functions as a serine protease inhibitor and is a major regulator of the coagulation system. Antithrombin levels fall rapidly in sepsis and antithrombin replacement has been extensively tested in animal and clinical trials in septic patients for many years.[97] The largest clinical phase III trial was the KyberSept study published in 2001.[98] In this multinational trial of 2314 patients, plasma-derived antithrombin, given at 30,000 IU over 4 days, was compared against placebo in severely septic patients. The results showed no significant benefit overall, and an excess risk of bleeding in patients who received antithrombin (particularly when administered with concomitant heparin). However, in a prespecified subgroup of patients who received antithrombin but no heparin, there was a modest improvement in survival that reached statistical significance after 90 days (52% versus 44.9%; P < .05).[98,99]

A recombinant form of human antithrombin expressed in transgenic goats is now in phase II testing in sepsis-induced disseminated intravascular coagulation.[100] The results of this study should be available in the next 12 to 18 months.

Recombinant Human Soluble Thrombomodulin

Thrombomodulin is an endothelial cell surface protein that participates in the endogenous anticoagulant pathway. Thrombomodulin forms a tight complex with thrombin, inhibiting its prolongation. The complex once formed assists in the conversion of the zymogen protein C to activated protein C.[101] Activated protein C inhibits further thrombin generation via its effects on factor V and factor VIII. Thrombomodulin has anti-inflammatory effects via the activation of protein C.[102] Thrombomodulin also has direct anti-inflammatory effects, including its ability to bind to HMGB1 and interfere with complement activation.[103,104] ART-123 is a recombinant human soluble thrombomodulin that is expressed in Chinese hamster ovary cells and

consists of D1, D2, and D3 but lacks the cytoplasmic and transmembrane domains.[105] Recombinant soluble thrombomodulin has been shown to prevent the onset of disseminated intravascular coagulation in crab-eating monkeys.[106] A placebo-controlled, double- dummy design comparing ART-123 and heparin in patients with disseminated intravascular coagulation (DIC) due to either infection or malignancy was conducted in Japan. The DIC resolution rate was higher in the ART-123 compared with heparin, but the result was not statistically significant. Mortality in the subgroup with DIC due to infection was 6.6% lower (95% CI −24.6–11.3) in the ART-123 arm compared with placebo, while no difference in mortality was seen in the population with malignancy-induced DIC arm.[107] A phase II trial of ART-123 in sepsis-induced DIC is underway.

TARGETING THE COMPLEMENT CASCADE

The complement cascade is a series of proteins that serve as an arm of defense against invading organisms. The cascade can be triggered via three different pathways, all of which converge at C3 and ultimately C5a, C5b, and the C5b-C9 terminal attack complex.[108] C5a in excess during sepsis can initiate many injurious activities for the host. Excessive C5a production leads to defective neutrophil function and oxidative burst, excessive release of the proinflammatory cytokines TNF and IL-1, the expression of tissue factor on endothelial surfaces and monocytes, and lymphocyte apoptosis.[109] Beneficial effects with C5a blockade have been observed in many animal models of sepsis. In a rat cecal ligation and perforation model, polyclonal anti-C5a antibody administration was associated with improved survival, improved hydrogen peroxide production by neutrophils, and decreased bacterial counts compared with rats treated with preimmune IgG. Improved survival occurred when therapy was initiated up to 12 hours following the insult.[110] In this same model, blockade of C5a was associated with less activation of coagulation cascade and inhibition of fibrinolysis compared with preimmune IgG–treated rats.[111] A number of companies have anti-C5a molecules in preclinical development, but none have been tested in human sepsis to date.

INHIBITION OF APOPTOSIS

The vast majority of the therapeutic agents tested in sepsis have been based on the assumption that an overly exuberant proinflammatory response results in organ failure and death. Results of autopsy studies in humans who have succumbed to sepsis and in animal models of sepsis have challenged this assumption. Autopsy studies have demonstrated excessive lymphocyte cell death in the spleen and bowel as well as lymphopenia in humans who have died from sepsis compared with patients who have died from a nonseptic critical illness.[112] The mechanism of the lymphopenia occurring in sepsis has been investigated and appears to be due to excessive apoptosis or programmed cell death of lymphocytes.[113] The excessive apoptosis can be triggered by two pathways. The extrinsic pathway is triggered by cytokines released by sepsis, including TNF-α and Fas ligand. Both of these molecules can activate a death domain that ultimately activates caspase 8. The intrinsic pathway is triggered by molecules that include reactive oxygen species and corticosteroids, and results in the activation of caspase 9. Both caspase 8 and caspase 9 can activate caspase 3, which is the final effector molecule that leads to cell death via DNA fragmentation.[114]

Multiple animal studies of sepsis attempting to prevent excessive apoptosis have suggested this strategy as being of potential value. Transgenic animals that overexpress the antiapoptotic protein BCL-2 have an improved outcome in sepsis.[115] Broad spectrum caspase inhibitors have also shown improved survival in animal models of sepsis.[116] Small interfering RNA against Fas and caspases has also been developed. A Fas receptor fusion protein improved the outcome in the cecal ligation and perforation model of sepsis even when treatment was delayed 12 hours after the infection insult.[117] Antiretroviral agents, previously known to prevent apoptosis in CD4 cells, tested in the cecal ligation and perforation model were associated with decreased lymphocyte apoptosis, improved survival, increased TNF levels, decreased levels of the anti-inflammatory cytokines IL-6 and IL-10, and improved bacterial clearance compared with placebo.[118] The authors are not aware of an antiapoptotic agent currently being studied in humans with severe sepsis.

TARGETING CYTOPATHIC HYPOXIA

A state of defective cellular respiration, called *cytopathic hypoxia,* has been implicated in the organ failure seen with severe sepsis. Cytopathic hypoxia is thought to be due to depletion in the cellular stores of nicotinamide adenine dinucleotide (NAD+/NADH). The process by which this occurs begins with formation of peroxynitrite from oxygen free radicals and nitric oxide. Peroxynitrite causes DNA breaks, which activate poly–ADP-ribose polymerase (PARP) in cells. PARP causes the cleavage of NAD, an essential cofactor in glycolysis and the Krebs cycle, leading to a depletion of ATP and cell death.[119] PARP-1 also plays a role in the proinflammatory cytokine response by serving as a costimulator of NF-kappa B.[120] PARP inhibitors have also been studied in a variety of animal models. In a pig model of septic peritonitis, the PARP inhibitor PJ34 was associated with less cardiac dysfunction, attenuation of TNF-α release, and improved survival compared with animals given a placebo.[121] Animals treated with the PARP inhibitor INO-1001 had decreased lung edema, less histologic evidence of inflammation, and less deterioration in oxygenation than control animals following smoke exposure and tracheal instillation of *Pseudomonas aeruginosa.*[122] Despite the signal seen in animal models of sepsis, PARP-inhibitors have not been studied in septic humans to date.

MISCELLANEOUS AGENTS
Inter-Alpha Inhibitor Protein

The inter-alpha inhibitor protein complex consists of a family of plasma proteins covalently linked to bikunin, the active enzymatic moiety of this protein complex. Bikunin acts as a broad-spectrum protease inhibitor affecting the enzymatic activity of serine proteases in the coagulation system, complement system, fibrinolytic system, elastase, and a variety of other serine proteases. Levels of inter-alpha inhibitor proteins rapidly fall in severe sepsis[123] and replacement therapy has proven to be protective in preclinical sepsis models.[124] For many years in Japan, urinary trypsin inhibitor (a component of the I-alpha-I family) has been in clinical use for systemic inflammatory states following pancreatitis.[123] Clinical trials with inter-alpha inhibitor components in severe sepsis have been completed in China.[125,126] In a phase II trial of 342 patients, the 28-day mortality rate was significantly reduced by urinary trypsin inhibitor (38.3 versus 25.1; $P < .01$).[126] Further clinical trials with this treatment strategy are contemplated in the near future.

Estrogen-Receptor Ligands

Estradiol has two functional receptors in human physiology: the estrogen-receptor alpha (ER-α) and estrogen-receptor beta (ER-β).[127] ER-β agonists are of particular interest as a variety of other physiologic effects are mediated by ER-β signaling, such as reduced apoptotic activity, membrane sparing, endogenous nitric-oxide synthase activity, and reduced inflammatory mediator synthesis.[128,129] Because women have a decided advantage with a significantly lower incidence of septic shock compared with their male counterparts, ER-β agonists are speculated to provide a survival benefit for the prevention and treatment of sepsis. Experimental studies with specific ER-β agonists support the potential utility of this approach in treatment of septic shock.[130,131] Clinical trials with these agents are being planned for sepsis studies in the near future.

REFERENCES

1. Visintin A, Halmen KA, Latz E, et al. Pharmacological inhibition of endotoxin responses is achieved by targeting the TLR4 coreceptor, MD-2. J Immunol 2005;175(10):6465–72.
2. Kim HM, Park BS, Kim J-I, et al. Crystal structure of the TLR4-MD-2 complex with bound endotoxin antagonist eritoran. Cell 2007;130:906–17.
3. Solomon SB, Cui X, Gerstenberger E, et al. Effective dosing of lipid A analogue E5564 in rats depends on the timing of treatment and the route of Escherichia coli infection. J Infect Dis 2006;193(5):634–44.
4. Lynn M, Rossignol DP, Wheeler JL, et al. Blocking of responses to endotoxin by E5564 in healthy volunteers with experimental endotoxemia. J Infect Dis 2003;187(4):631–9.
5. Bennett-Guerrero E, Grocott HP, Levy JH, et al. A phase II, double-blind, placebo-controlled, ascending-dose study of eritoran (E5564), a lipid A antagonist, in patients undergoing cardiac surgery with cardiopulmonary bypass. Anesth Analg 2007;104(2):378–83.
6. Elsbach P. The bactericidal/permeability-increasing protein (BPI) in antibacterial host defense. J Leukoc Biol 1998;64(1):14–8.
7. Heyderman RS, Ison CA, Peakman M, et al. Neutrophil response to Neisseria meningitidis: inhibition of adhesion molecule expression and phagocytosis by recombinant bactericidal/permeability-increasing protein (rBPI21). J Infect Dis 1999;179(5):1288–92.
8. Jellema WT, Veerman DP, DeWinter RJ, et al. In vivo interaction of endotoxin and recombinant bactericidal/permeability-increasing protein (rBPI23): hemodynamic effects in a human endotoxemia model. J Lab Clin Med 2002;140(4):228–35.
9. Schultz H, Weiss J, Carroll SF, et al. The endotoxin-binding bactericidal/permeability-increasing protein (BPI): a target antigen of autoantibodies. J Leukoc Biol 2001;69(4):505–12.
10. Levin M, Quint PA, Goldstein B, et al. Recombinant bactericidal/permeability-increasing protein (rBPI21) as adjunctive treatment for children with severe meningococcal sepsis: a randomized trial. rBPI21 Meningococcal Sepsis Study Group. Lancet 2000;356(9234):961–7.
11. Giroir BP, Scannon PJ, Levin M. Bactericidal/permeability-increasing protein—lessons learned from the phase III, randomized, clinical trial of rBPI21 for adjunctive treatment of children with severe meningococcemia. Crit Care Med 2001;29(7Suppl):S130–5.
12. Japelj B, Pristovsek P, Majerle A, et al. Structural origin of endotoxin neutralization and antimicrobial activity of a lactoferrin-based peptide. J Biol Chem 2005;280(17):16955–61.
13. Andrä J, Gutsmann T, Garidel P, et al. Mechanisms of endotoxin neutralization by synthetic cationic compounds. J Endotoxin Res 2006;12(5):261–77.
14. Ellison RT III. The effects of lactoferrin on gram-negative bacteria. In: Hutchens TW, Rumball SV, Lönnerdal B, editors. Lactoferrin: structure and function. New York: Plenum Press; 1994. p. 71–90.
15. Zimecki M, Artym J, Chodaczek G, et al. Protective effects of lactoferrin in Escherichia coli-induced bacteremia in mice: relationship to reduced serum TNF alpha level and increased turnover of neutrophils. Inflamm Res 2004;53(7):292–6.
16. Andersen JH. Technology evaluation: rh lactoferrin, Agennix. Curr Opin Mol Ther 2004;6:344–9.
17. Bentala H, Verweij WR, Huizinga-Van der Vlag A, et al. Removal of phosphate from lipid A as a strategy to detoxify lipopolysaccharide. Shock 2002;18(6):561–6.
18. Verweij WR, Bentala H, Guizinga-Van der Vlag A, et al. Protection against an Escherichia coli-induced sepsis by alkaline phosphatase in mice. Shock 2004;22(2):174–9.
19. van Veen SQ, van Vliet AK, Wulferink M, et al. Bovine intestinal alkaline phosphatase attenuates the inflammatory response in secondary peritonitis in mice. Infect Immun 2005;73(7):4309–14.
20. Su F, Brands R, Wang Z, et al. Beneficial effects of alkaline phosphatase in septic shock. Crit Care Med 2006;34(8):2182–7.
21. Yamada M, Ichikawa T, Li M, et al. Discovery of novel and potent small-molecule inhibitors of NO and cytokine production as antisepsis agents: synthesis and biological activity of alkyl 6-(N-substituted sulfamoyl)cyclohex-1-ene-1-carboxylate. J Med Chem 2005;48(23):7457–67.
22. Land WG. Innate immunity-mediated allograft rejection and strategies to prevent it. Transplant Proc 2007;39(3):667–72.
23. Bernard GR, Wheeler AP, Rice TW, et al. TAK-242 treatment for severe sepsis: a randomized controlled trial [abstract 264]. In: editors. Programs and Abstracts for the Society for Critical Care Medicine Meeting. Honolulu (HI): 2008. p. 946.
24. Kushi H, Miki T, Nakahara J, et al. Hemoperfusion with an immobilized Polymyxin B fiber column improves tissue oxygen metabolism. Ther Apher Dial 2006;10(5):430–5.

25. Uriu K, Osajima A, Hiroshige K, et al. Endotoxin removal by direct hemoperfusion with an adsorbent column using Polymyxin B–immobilized fiber ameliorates systemic circulatory disturbance in patients with septic shock. Am J Kidney Dis 2002;39(5):937–47.

26. Kushi H, Miki T, Okamaoto K, et al. Early hemoperfusion with an immobilized Polymyxin B fiber column eliminates humoral mediators and improves pulmonary oxygenation. Crit Care 2005;9(6):R653–61.

27. Sakamoto Y, Mashiko K, Matsumoto H, et al. Relationship between effect of Polymyxin B–immobilized fiber and high-mobility group box-1 protein in septic shock patients. ASAIO J 2007;53(3):324–8.

28. Cruz DN, Bellomo R, Ronco C. Clinical effects of Polymyxin B-immobilized fiber column in septic patients. Contrib Nephrol 2007;156:444–51.

29. Ronco C. The place of early haemoperfusion with Polymyxin B fibre column in the treatment of sepsis. Crit Care 2005;9(6):631–3.

30. Eisenhauer T, Armstrong VW, Wieland H, et al. Selective removal of low density lipoproteins (LDL) by precipitation at low pH: first clinical application of the HELP system. Klin Wochenschr 1987;65:161–8.

31. Samtleben W, Bengsch S, Boos KS, et al. HELP apheresis in the treatment of sepsis. Artif Organs 1998;22:43–6.

32. Bengsch S, Boos KS, Nagel D, et al. Extracorporeal plasma treatment for the removal of endotoxin in patients with sepsis: clinical results of a pilot study. Shock 2005;23:494–500.

33. Opal SM, Palardy JE, Chen W, et al. Active immunization with a detoxified endotoxin vaccine protects against lethal polymicrobial sepsis: its use with CpG adjuvant and potential mechanisms. J Infect Dis 2005;192:2074–80.

34. Cross AS, Opal SM, Palardy JE, et al. Phase I study of detoxified Escherichia coli J5 lipopolysaccharide (J5dLPS)/ group B meningococcal outer membrane protein (OMP) complex vaccine in human subjects. Vaccine 2003;21:4576–87.

35. Opal SM. The host response to endotoxin, anti-LPS strategies and the management of severe sepsis. Int J Med Microbiol 2007;297:365–77.

36. Visvanathan K, Charles A, Bannan J, et al. Inhibition of bacterial superantigens by peptides and antibodies. Infect Immun 2001;69(2):875–84.

37. Hong-Geller E, Gupta G. Therapeutic approaches to superantigen-based diseases: a review. J Mol Recognit 2003;16(2):91–101.

38. Miwa K, Fukuyama M, Matsuno N, et al. Physiological response to superantigen-adsorbing hemoperfusion in toxin-concentration-controlled septic swine. Blood Purif 2006;24(3):319–26.

39. Hong-Geller E, Möllhoff M, Shiflett PR, et al. Design of chimeric receptor mimics with different TcR Vbeta isoforms. Type-specific inhibition of superantigen pathogenesis. J Biol Chem 2004;279(7):5676–84.

40. Honoré PM, Joannes-Boyau O, Gressens B. Blood and plasma treatments: the rationale of high-volume hemofiltration. Contrib Nephrol 2007;156:387–95.

41. Honoré PM, Joannes-Boyau O. High volume hemofiltration (HVHF) in sepsis: a comprehensive review of rationale, clinical applicability, potential indications and recommendations for future research. Int J Artif Organs 2004;27(12):1077–82.

42. Joannes-Boyau O, Rapaport S, Bazin R, et al. Impact of high volume hemofiltration on hemodynamic disturbance and outcome during septic shock. ASAIO J 2004;50(1):102–9.

43. Ronco C, Bellomo R, Homel P, et al. Effects of different doses of continuous veno-venous haemofiltration. Lancet 2000;356:26–30.

44. Cornejo R, Downey P, Castro R, et al. High-volume hemofiltration as salvage therapy in severe hyperdynamic septic shock. Intensive Care Med 2006;32(5):713–22.

45. Humes HD, MacKay SM, Funke AJ, et al. Tissue engineering of a bioartificial renal tubule assist device: in vitro transport and metabolic characteristics. Kidney Int 1999;55(6):2502–14.

46. Issa N, Messer J, Paganini EP. Renal assist device and treatment of sepsis-induced acute kidney injury in intensive care units. Contrib Nephrol 2007;156:419–27.

47. Tumlin J, Wali R, Brennan K, et al. Effect of the renal assist device (RAD) on mortality of dialysis-dependent acute renal failure: a randomized, open-labeled, multicenter, phase II trial [abstract]. Presented at the American Society of Nephrology (ASN) 38th Annual Meeting. Philadelphia, February 2–6, 2008.

48. Humes HD, Weitzel WF, Bartlett RH, et al. Initial clinical results of the bioartificial kidney containing human cells in ICU patients with acute renal failure. Kidney Int 2004;66:1578–88.

49. Rice TW, Wheeler AP, Morris PE, et al. Safety and efficacy of affinity-purified, anti–tumor necrosis factor-alpha, ovine Fab for injection (CytoFab) in severe sepsis. Crit Care Med 2006;34:2271–81.

50. Borovikova LV, Ivanova S, Zhang M, et al. Vagus nerve stimulation attenuates the systemic inflammatory response to endotoxin. Nature 2000;405:458–62.

51. van Westerloo DJ, Giebelen IA, Meijers JC, et al. Vagus nerve stimulation inhibits activation of coagulation and fibrinolysis during endotoxemia in rats. J Thromb Haemost 2006;4:1997–2002.

52. van Westerloo DJ, Giebelen IA, Florquin S, et al. The cholinergic anti-inflammatory pathway

regulates the host response during septic peritonitis. J Infect Dis 2005;191:2138–48.

53. Wang H, Liao H, Ochani M, et al. Cholinergic agonists inhibit HMGB1 release and improve survival in experimental sepsis. Nat Med 2004;10:1216–21.

54. Pavlov VA, Ochani M, Yang LH, et al. Selective alpha7-nicotinic acetylcholine receptor agonist GTS-21 improves survival in murine endotoxemia and severe sepsis. Crit Care Med 2007;35:1139–44.

55. Mantell LL, Parrish WR, Ulloa L. HMGB-1 as a therapeutic target for infectious and inflammatory disorders. Shock 2006;25:4–11.

56. Wang H, Bloom O, Zhang M, et al. HMG-1 as a late mediator of endotoxin lethality in mice. Science 1999;285:248–52.

57. Sunden-Cullberg J, Norrby-Teglund A, Rouhiainen A, et al. Persistent elevation of high mobility group box-1 protein (HMGB1) in patients with severe sepsis and septic shock. Crit Care Med 2005;33:564–73.

58. Yang H, Ochani M, Li J, et al. Reversing established sepsis with antagonists of endogenous high-mobility group box 1. Proc Natl Acad Sci U S A 2004;101:296–301.

59. Li J, Kokkola R, Tabibzadeh S, et al. Structural basis for the proinflammatory cytokine activity of high mobility group box 1. Mol Med 2003;9:37–45.

60. Huston JM, Gallowitsch-Puerta M, Ochani M, et al. Transcutaneous vagus nerve stimulation reduces serum high mobility group box 1 levels and improves survival in murine sepsis. Crit Care Med 2007;35:2762–8.

61. Chen X, Li W, Wang H. More tea for septic patients?—Green tea may reduce endotoxin-induced release of high mobility group box 1 and other pro-inflammatory cytokines. Med Hypotheses 2006;66:660–3.

62. Chen G, Li J, Qiang X, et al. Suppression of HMGB1 release by stearoyl lysophosphatidylcholine: an additional mechanism for its therapeutic effects in experimental sepsis. J Lipid Res 2005;46:623–7.

63. Schmidt AM, Yan SD, Yan SF, et al. The multiligand receptor RAGE as a progression factor amplifying immune and inflammatory responses. J Clin Invest 2001;108:949–55.

64. Chavakis T, Bierhas A, Al-Fakhri N, et al. The pattern recognition receptor (RAGE) is a counterreceptor for leukocyte integrins: a novel pathway for inflammatory cell recruitment. J Exp Med 2003;198:1507–15.

65. Liliensiek B, Weigand MA, Beirhaus A, et al. Receptor for advanced glycation end products (RAGE) regulates sepsis but not the adaptive immune response. J Clin Invest 2004;113:1641–50.

66. Lutterloh E, Opal SM, Pittman D, et al. Inhibition of receptor for advanced glycation endproducts as a novel treatment strategy in severe sepsis. Crit Care 2007;11(6):122–30.

67. Grutkoski PS, Chen Y, Chung CS, et al. Sepsis-induced SOCS-3 expression is immunologically restricted to phagocytes. J Leukoc Biol 2003;74(5):916–22.

68. Chung CS, Chen Y, Grutkoski PS, et al. SOCS-1 is a central mediator of steroid-increased thymocyte apoptosis and decreased survival following sepsis. Apoptosis 2007;12(7):1143–53.

69. Watanabe H, Kubo M, Numata K, et al. Overexpression of suppressor of cytokine signaling-5 in T cells augments innate immunity during septic peritonitis. J Immunol 2006;177(112):8650–7.

70. Sullivan GW, Rieger JM, Scheld WM, et al. Cyclic AMP –dependent inhibition of human neutrophil oxidative activity by substituted 2-propynlcyclohexyl adenosine A (2A) receptor agonists. Br J Pharmacol 2001;132:1017–26.

71. Eigler A, Greten TF, Sinha B, et al. Endogenous adenosine curtails lipopolysaccharide-stimulated tumor necrosis factor synthesis. Scand J Immunol 1997;45:132–9.

72. Hourani SM. Purinoreceptors and platelet aggregation. J Auton Pharmacol 1996;16:349–52.

73. Sullivan GW, Fang G, Linden J, et al. A2A adenosine receptor activation improves survival in mouse models of endotoxemia and sepsis. J Infect Dis 2004;189:1897–904.

74. Cavalcante IC, Castro MV, Barreto ARF, et al. Effect of novel A2A adenosine receptor agonist ATL313 on Clostridium difficile toxin A–induced murine ileal enteritis. Infect Immun 2006;74(5):2602–12.

75. Zingarelli B, Cook JA. Peroxisome proliferator-activated receptor-gamma is a new therapeutic target in sepsis and inflammation. Shock 2005;23:393–9.

76. Collin M, Murch O, Thiemermann C. Peroxisome proliferator-activated receptor-gamma antagonists GW9662 and T0070907 reduce the protective effects of lipopolysaccharide preconditioning against organ failure caused by endotoxemia. Crit Care Med 2006;34:1131–8.

77. Cuzzocrea S, Pisano B, Dugo L, et al. Rosiglitazone, a ligand of the peroxisome proliferator-activated receptor-gamma, reduces the development of nonseptic shock induced by zymosan in mice. Crit Care Med 2004;32:457–66.

78. Siddiqui AM, Cui X, Wu R, et al. The anti-inflammatory effect of curcumin in an experimental model of sepsis is mediated by up-regulation of peroxisome proliferator-activated receptor-gamma. Crit Care Med 2006;34:1874–82.

79. Solorzano CC, Ksontini R, Pruitt JH, et al. A matrix metalloproteinase inhibitor prevents processing of tumor necrosis factor alpha (TNF alpha) and

abrogates endotoxin-induced lethality. Shock 1997; 7:427–31.

80. D'Agostino P, Ferlazzo V, Milano S, et al. Anti-inflammatory effects of chemically modified tetra-cyclines by the inhibition of nitric oxide and interleukin-12 synthesis in J774 cell line. Int Immunopharmacol 2001;1:1765–76.

81. Maitra SR, Bhaduri S, Chen E, et al. Role of chemically modified tetracycline on TNF-alpha and mitogen-activated protein kinases in sepsis. Shock 2004;22:478–81.

82. Steinberg J, Halter J, Schiller H, et al. Chemically modified tetracycline prevents the development of septic shock and acute respiratory distress syndrome in a clinically applicable porcine model. Shock 2005;24:348–56.

83. Halter JM, Pavone LA, Steinberg JM, et al. Chemically modified tetracycline (COL-3) improves survival if given 12 but not 24 hours after cecal ligation and puncture. Shock 2006;26:587–91.

84. Diomede L, Albani D, Sottocorno M, et al. In vivo anti-inflammatory effect of statins is mediated by nonsterol mevalonate products. Arterioscler Thromb Vasc Biol 2001;21:1327–32.

85. Liappis AP, Kan VL, Rochester CG, et al. The effect of statins on mortality in patients with bacteremia. Clin Infect Dis 2001;33:1352–7.

86. Almog Y, Shefer A, Novack V, et al. Prior statin therapy is associated with a decreased rate of severe sepsis. Circulation 2004;110:880–5.

87. Merx MW, Liehn EA, Graf J, et al. Statin treatment after onset of sepsis in a murine model improves survival. Circulation 2005;112:117–24.

88. Steiner S, Speidl WS, Pleiner J, et al. Simvastatin blunts endotoxin-induced tissue factor in vivo. Circulation 2005;111:1841–6.

89. Niessner A, Steiner S, Speidl WS, et al. Simvastatin suppresses endotoxin-induced upregulation of toll-like receptors 4 and 2 in vivo. Atherosclerosis 2006; 189:408–13.

90. Creasey A. New potential therapeutic modalities: tissue factor pathway inhibitor. Sepsis 1999;3: 173–82.

91. Rhewald M, Ruf W. Mechanistic coupling of protease signaling and initiation of coagulation by tissue factor. Proc Natl Acad Sci U S A 2001;98(14): 7742–7.

92. Senden NHM, Jeunhomme TMAA, Heemserk JWM, et al. Factor Xa induces cytokine production and expression of adhesion molecules by human umbilical vein endothelial cells. J Immunol 1998;161: 4318–24.

93. Schaeffer P, Mares AM, Dol F, et al. Coagulation factor Xa induces endothelium-dependent relaxation in rat aorta. Circ Res 1997;81:824–8.

94. Park CT, Creasey AA, Wright SD. Tissue factor pathway inhibitor blocks cellular effects of endotoxin by binding to endotoxin and interfering with transfer to CD14. Blood 1997;89(2):4268–74.

95. Abraham E, Reinhart K, Opal S, et al. Efficacy and safety of tifacogin (recombinant tissue factor pathway inhibitor) in severe sepsis. JAMA 2003;290: 238–47.

96. Opal S, Wunderink R, Laterre PF, et al. Therapeutic rationale for tissue factor pathway inhibitor for severe community-acquired pneumonia (CAP) [abstract 234]. In: editors. Final program and abstracts of the 42nd annual meeting Infectious Disease Society of America. Boston: 2004. p. 76.

97. LaRosa SP, Opal SM, Utterback B, et al. Decreased protein C, protein S, and antithrombin III levels are predictive of poor outcome in gram-negative sepsis caused by Burkholderia pseudomallei. Int J Infect Dis 2006;10(1):25–31.

98. Warren BL, Eid A, Singer P, et al. High-dose antithrombin III in severe sepsis (the KyberSept trial). JAMA 2001;286:1869–87.

99. Weidermann CJ, Hoffman JN, Juers M, et al. High dose antithrombin III in the treatment of severe sepsis with high risk of death. Crit Care Med 2006; 34(2):285–92.

100. Levy JH, Despotis GJ, Szlam F, et al. Recombinant human transgenic antithrombin in cardiac surgery: a dose-finding study. Anesthesiology 2002;96(5): 1095–102.

101. Mohri M, Sugimoto E, Sata M, et al. The inhibitory effect of recombinant human soluble thrombomodulin on initiation and extension of coagulation—a comparison with other anticoagulants. Thromb Haemost 1999;82:1687–93.

102. Uchiba M, Okajima K, Murakami K, et al. Recombinant human soluble thrombomodulin reduces endotoxin-induced pulmonary vascular injury via protein C activation in rats. Thromb Haemost 1995;74:1265–70.

103. Abeyama K, Stern DM, Ito Y, et al. The N-terminal domain of thrombomodulin sequesters high-mobility group-B1 protein, a novel antiinflammatory mechanism. J Clin Invest 2005;115:1267–74.

104. Van de WM, Plaisance S, De VA, et al. The lectin-like domain of thrombomodulin interferes with complement activation and protects against arthritis. J Thromb Haemost 2006;4:1813–24.

105. Nakashima M, Kanamura M, Umemura K, et al. Pharmacokinetics and safety of a novel recombinant soluble human thrombomodulin, ART-123, in healthy male volunteers. J Clin Pharmacol 1998; 38:40–4.

106. Mohri M, Gonda Y, Oka M, et al. The antithrombotic effects of recombinant human soluble thrombomodulin (rhsTM) on tissue factor-induced disseminated intravascular coagulation in crab-eating monkeys (Macaca fascicularis). Blood Coagul Fibrinolysis 1997;8:274–83.

107. Saito H, Maruyama I, Shimazaki S, et al. Efficacy and safety of recombinant human soluble thrombomodulin (ART-123) in disseminated intravascular coagulation: results of a phase III, randomized, double-blind clinical trial. J Thromb Haemost 2007;5:31–41.

108. Haeney MR. The role of the complement cascade in sepsis. J Antimicrob Chemother 1998;41(Suppl A): 41–6.

109. Guo RF, Riedemann NC, Ward PA. Role of C5a-C5aR interaction in sepsis. Shock 2004;21(1):1–7.

110. Czermak BJ, Sarma V, Pierson CL, et al. Protective effects of C5a blockade in sepsis. Nat Med 1999;5: 788–92.

111. Laudes IJ, Chu JC, Sikranth S, et al. Anti-c5a ameliorates coagulation/fibrinolytic protein changes in a rat model of sepsis. Am J Pathol 2002;160:1867–75.

112. Hotchkiss RS, Swanson PE, Freeman BD, et al. Apoptotic cell death in patients with sepsis, shock, and multiple organ dysfunction. Crit Care Med 1999;27:1230–51.

113. Hotchkiss RS, Tinsley KW, Swanson PE, et al. Sepsis-induced apoptosis causes progressive profound depletion of B and CD4+ T lymphocytes in humans. J Immunol 2001;166:6952–63.

114. Oberholzer C, Oberholzer A, Clare-Salzler M, et al. Apoptosis in sepsis: a new target for therapeutic exploration. FASEB J 2001;15:879–92.

115. Hotchkiss RS, Chang KC, Swanson PE, et al. Caspase inhibitors improve survival in sepsis: a critical role of the lymphocyte. Nat Immunol 2000;1: 496–501.

116. Hotchkiss RS, Tinsley KW, Swanson PE, et al. Prevention of lymphocyte cell death in sepsis improves survival in mice. Proc Natl Acad Sci U S A 1999;96:14541–6.

117. Chung CS, Song GY, Lomas J, et al. Inhibition of Fas/Fas ligand signaling improves septic survival: differential effects on macrophage apoptotic and functional capacity. J Leukoc Biol 2003;74:344–51.

118. Weaver JG, Rouse MS, Steckelberg JM, et al. Improved survival in experimental sepsis with an orally administered inhibitor of apoptosis. FASEB J 2004;18:1185–91.

119. Fink MP. Bench-to-bedside review: cytopathic hypoxia. Crit Care 2002;6:491–9.

120. Oliver FJ, Menissier-De Murcia J, Nacci C, et al. Resistance to endotoxic shock as a consequence of defective NF-kappaB activation in poly (ADP-ribose)

polymerase-1 deficient mice. EMBO J 1999;18: 4446–54.

121. Goldfarb RD, Marton A, Szabo E, et al. Protective effect of a novel, potent inhibitor of poly(adenosine 5'-diphosphate-ribose) synthetase in a porcine model of severe bacterial sepsis. Crit Care Med 2002;30:974–80.

122. Murakami K, Enkhbaatar P, Shimoda K, et al. Inhibition of poly (ADP-ribose) polymerase attenuates acute lung injury in an ovine model of sepsis. Shock 2004;21:126–33.

123. Opal SM, Lim Y-P, E Siryaporn E, et al. Longitudinal studies of inter-alpha inhibitor proteins in severely septic patients: a potential clinical marker and mediator of severe sepsis. Crit Care Med 2007; 35:387–92.

124. Garantziotis S, Hillingworth JW, Ghanayem RB, et al. Inter-α-trypsin inhibitor attenuates complement activation and complement-induced lung injury. J Immunol 2007;179:4187–92.

125. Zhongguo WE, Zhong Bing J, Jue Y, et al. Clinical study on effects of ulinastatin on patients with systemic inflammatory response syndrome. Chinese Crit Care Med 2005;17(4):228–30.

126. Lin HY. Clinical trial with a new immunomodulatory strategy: treatment of severe sepsis with Ulinastatin and Maipuxin. Zhonghua Yi Xue Za Zhi 2007;87(7): 451–7.

127. Harris HA, Katzenellenbogen JA, Katzenellenbogen BS. Characterization of the biological roles of the estrogen receptors, ER alpha and ER beta, in estrogen target tissues in vivo through the use of an ER alpha-selective ligand. Endocrinology 2002;143:4172–7.

128. Deshpande R, Khalili H, Pergolizzi RG, et al. Estradiol down-regulates LPS-induced cytokine production and NFkB activation in murine macrophages. Am J Reprod Immunol 1997;38:46–54.

129. Kuebler JF, Jarrar D, Toth B, et al. Estradiol administration improves splanchnic perfusion following trauma-hemorrhage and sepsis. Arch Surg 2002; 137:74–9.

130. Opal SM, Keith J, Cristofaro P, et al. The activity of estrogen receptor pathway selective ligands in experimental models of sepsis and inflammation. Shock 2005;24(6):535–40.

131. Cristofaro P, Opal SM, Keith J, et al. WAY202196, a selective estrogen receptor beta agonist, protects against death in experimental septic shock. Crit Care Med 2006;34(6):2188–93.

Index

Note: Page numbers of article titles are in **boldface** type.

Clin Chest Med 29 (2008) 749–754
doi:10.1016/S0272-5231(08)00101-9

Moving?

Make sure your subscription moves with you!

To notify us of your new address, find your **Clinics Account Number** (located on your mailing label above your name), and contact customer service at:

E-mail: elspcs@elsevier.com

800-654-2452 (subscribers in the U.S. & Canada)
1-407-563-6020 (subscribers outside of the U.S. & Canada)

Fax number: 407-363-9661

Elsevier Periodicals Customer Service
6277 Sea Harbor Drive
Orlando, FL 32887-4800

*To ensure uninterrupted delivery of your subscription, please notify us at least 4 weeks in advance of move.

United States Postal Service

Statement of Ownership, Management, and Circulation
(All Periodicals Publications Except Requestor Publications)

1. Publication Title
Clinics in Chest Medicine

2. Publication Number
0 0 0 - 7 0 6

3. Filing Date
9/15/08

4. Issue Frequency
Mar, Jun, Sep, Dec

5. Number of Issues Published Annually
4

6. Annual Subscription Price
$232.00

7. Complete Mailing Address of Known Office of Publication (Not printer) (Street, city, county, state, and ZIP+4)

Elsevier Inc.
360 Park Avenue South
New York, NY 10010-1710

Contact Person
Stephen Bushing

Telephone (Include area code)
215-239-3688

8. Complete Mailing Address of Headquarters or General Business Office of Publisher (Not printer)

Elsevier Inc., 360 Park Avenue South, New York, NY 10010-1710

9. Full Names and Complete Mailing Addresses of Publisher, Editor, and Managing Editor (Do not leave blank)

Publisher (Name and complete mailing address)

John Schrefer, Elsevier, Inc., 1600 John F. Kennedy Blvd. Suite 1800, Philadelphia, PA 19103-2899

Editor (Name and complete mailing address)

Sarah Barth, Elsevier, Inc., 1600 John F. Kennedy Blvd. Suite 1800, Philadelphia, PA 19103-2899

Managing Editor (Name and complete mailing address)

Catherine Bewick, Elsevier, Inc., 1600 John F. Kennedy Blvd. Suite 1800, Philadelphia, PA 19103-2899

10. Owner (Do not leave blank. If the publication is owned by a corporation, give the name and address of the corporation immediately followed by the names and addresses of all stockholders owning or holding 1 percent or more of the total amount of stock. If not owned by a corporation, give the names and addresses of the individual owners. If owned by a partnership or other unincorporated firm, give its name and address as well as those of each individual owner. If the publication is published by a nonprofit organization, give its name and address.)

Full Name	Complete Mailing Address
Wholly owned subsidiary of	4520 East-West Highway
Reed/Elsevier, US holdings	Bethesda, MD 20814

11. Known Bondholders, Mortgagees, and Other Security Holders Owning or Holding 1 Percent or More of Total Amount of Bonds, Mortgages, or Other Securities. If none, check box. ☐ None

Full Name	Complete Mailing Address
N/A	

12. Tax Status (For completion by nonprofit organizations authorized to mail at nonprofit rates) (Check one)
The purpose, function, and nonprofit status of this organization and the exempt status for federal income tax purposes:
☐ Has Not Changed During Preceding 12 Months
☐ Has Changed During Preceding 12 Months (Publisher must submit explanation of change with this statement)

PS Form 3526, September 2006 (Page 1 of 3 (Instructions Page 3)) PSN 7530-01-000-9931 PRIVACY NOTICE: See our Privacy policy in www.usps.com

---

13. Publication Title
Clinics in Chest Medicine

14. Issue Date for Circulation Data Below
September 2008

15. Extent and Nature of Circulation

		Average No. Copies Each Issue During Preceding 12 Months	No. Copies of Single Issue Published Nearest to Filing Date
a. Total Number of Copies (Net press run)		3400	3300
b. Paid Circulation (By Mail and Outside the Mail)	(1) Mailed Outside-County Paid Subscriptions Stated on PS Form 3541. (Include paid distribution above nominal rate, advertiser's proof copies, and exchange copies)	1667	1528
	(2) Mailed In-County Paid Subscriptions Stated on PS Form 3541 (Include paid distribution above nominal rate, advertiser's proof copies, and exchange copies)		
	(3) Paid Distribution Outside the Mails Including Sales Through Dealers and Carriers, Street Vendors, Counter Sales, and Other Paid Distribution Outside USPS®	821	797
	(4) Paid Distribution by Other Classes Mailed Through the USPS (e.g. First-Class Mail®)		
c. Total Paid Distribution (Sum of 15b (1), (2), (3), and (4)) ▲		2488	2325
d. Free or Nominal Rate Distribution (By Mail and Outside the Mail)	(1) Free or Nominal Rate Outside-County Copies Included on PS Form 3541	75	96
	(2) Free or Nominal Rate In-County Copies Included on PS Form 3541		
	(3) Free or Nominal Rate Copies Mailed at Other Classes Mailed Through the USPS (e.g. First-Class Mail)		
	(4) Free or Nominal Rate Distribution Outside the Mail (Carriers or other means)		
e. Total Free or Nominal Rate Distribution (Sum of 15d (1), (2), (3) and (4)) ▲		75	96
f. Total Distribution (Sum of 15c and 15e) ▲		2563	2421
g. Copies not Distributed (See instructions to publishers #4 (page #3)) ▲		837	879
h. Total (Sum of 15f and g) ▲		3400	3300
i. Percent Paid (15c divided by 15f times 100)		97.07%	96.03%

16. Publication of Statement of Ownership
If the publication is a general publication, publication of this statement is required. Will be printed in the **December 2008** issue of this publication. ☐ Publication not required

17. Signature and Title of Editor, Publisher, Business Manager, or Owner

[signature]
Stephen Bushing/Tanucci – Executive Director of Subscription Services

Date
September 15, 2008

I certify that all information furnished on this form is true and complete. I understand that anyone who furnishes false or misleading information on this form or who omits material or information requested on the form may be subject to criminal sanctions (including fines and imprisonment) and/or civil sanctions (including civil penalties).

PS Form 3526, September 2006 (Page 2 of 3)